For Mr. Mack:

Healers in World War II

Happy Birthday, "Mr. Mack"!
We love you,
Bob, Joy, and Sarah

See pp. 139-142

This book is dedicated to my parents, Campbell and Bethel,
who lived and loved through the war years,

and

to "Mum" and her daughters
who befriended an American GI, my dad,
a kindness he never forgot.

Healers in World War II

Oral Histories of Medical Corps Personnel

Edited by
Patricia W. Sewell

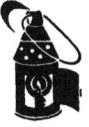

McFarland & Company, Inc., Publishers
Jefferson, North Carolina, and London

Library of Congress Cataloguing-in-Publication Data

Healers in World War II : oral histories of Medical Corps personnel / edited by Patricia W. Sewell
    p.   cm.
   Includes index.
   ISBN 0-7864-0933-9 (softcover : 50# alkaline paper) ∞
   1. World War, 1939–1945—Personal narratives. 2. Medicine, Military—Biography. 3. World War, 1939–1945—Medical care. I. Title: Healers in World War Two. II. Title: Healers in World War 2. III. Sewell, Patricia W., 1951–
D811.5.H387   2001
940.54'75'0922—dc21   2001041068

British Library cataloguing data are available

©2001 Patricia W. Sewell. All rights reserved

No part of this book may be reproduced or transmitted in any form or by any means, electronic or mechanical, including photocopying or recording, or by any information storage and retrieval system, without permission in writing from the publisher.

Manufactured in the United States of America

Cover photograph ©2001 Corbis Images

McFarland & Company, Inc., Publishers
   Box 611, Jefferson, North Carolina 28640
   www.mcfarlandpub.com

Table of Contents

Acknowledgments   viii
Preface   1

1. A Medic Tells His Story   3
   Les Habegger
2. Recollections of an Infantry Battalion Doctor   10
   Frank R. Ellis, M.D.
3. Dr. Kurt Lekisch   13
   Sol Schwartz
4. "How Long You Been Here, Boy?"   16
   Alan King, M.D.
5. The Neapolitan Typhus Epidemic   21
   Vincent Stephen Conti, M.D.
6. One Hundred Pounds and Five Feet Tall   24
   Mary A. Breeding
7. Beanie, Ernie, and More   27
   James Marion Kirtley, M.D.
8. From Med School to France   41
   Shelley M. Strain, M.D.
9. Nearsighted and Flatfooted   44
   Stanley A. Kornblum, M.D.
10. A World War II Remembrance of Luis Castillo   57
    Al Castillo

11. Picking Up the Dead *Grady Forsyth*	60
12. The Miracle Day *Desmond T. Doss*	63
13. Stateside *George S. Barnes, M.D.*	67
14. From the States to Down Under *Samuel E. Warshauer, M.D.*	69
15. Into Enemy Fire *Arthur V. O'Connell*	77
16. ASTRP and an "Opportunity" *Daniel Seftel, M.D.*	79
17. A Physician Scientist in the Army *Richard J. Bing, M.D.*	81
18. Corregidor *Logan W. Hovis, M.D.*	85
19. Medical Supply *Glen A. Fookes*	94
20. An Unbroken Chain *Jeremiah Henry Holleman, M.D.*	100
21. Minefield *Gregory S. Kirchner*	111
22. "Young and Foolish as We Were" *Daniel E. DiIaconi, M.D.*	117
23. Ambulance Driver in the Italian Campaign *Des Ball*	122
24. "I Was Doing Something Good" *Daniel Goolsbee*	139
25. "You Did What You Had to Do" *Julia Parrish Sadler*	143
26. The Balkan Nurses *Judith A. Bellafaire* and *Diane Burke Fessler*	147
27. POW of the Germans *Richard John Feltham, M.D.*	150

28. The CBI Theater . . . 181
    Thomas J. McKenna, M.D.
29. H.M.N.Z.H.S. *Maunganui* . . . 187
    Herbert Matthew Robson and *Grace Robson*
30. The U.S. Army Nurse Corps . . . 213
    Lee Threlkeld Jansak
31. Physical Therapy in the South Pacific . . . 218
    Forrest Walker
32. British Red Cross Nurse . . . 239
    Mona Stanton
33. Treating the Wounded in the Battle of the Bulge . . . 245
    Henry M. Hills, Jr., M.D.
34. Memories of Naval Medicine in World War II . . . 260
    Norton L. Francis, M.D.
35. More on the War . . . 262
    Various Authors

Afterword . . . 273
Index . . . 275

Acknowledgments

I would like to express my appreciation to all those who assisted me in some way. There have been so many that I could not try to list them all for I risk forgetting someone.

To all those who contributed their personal accounts: You have my deepest gratitude. I know that some of these were composed under difficult personal circumstances. I am grateful to the spouses, children, grandchildren, and others who helped make this possible.

To all those in the various veterans' associations, medical organizations, and those who just took the time to contact me with a possible lead, I am indebted. I will always remember the many people in the United States, Australia, and New Zealand who assisted me so professionally and with such kindness.

I wish to express my gratitude to the authors who wrote to me graciously offering their autobiographies. It was very kind of Dr. Holleman and Dr. Kirtley to accord me this privilege. Diane Burke Fessler generously allowed me to use excerpts about the Balkan Nurses from her book *No Time for Fear*. Mona Stanton granted me the privilege of using excerpts from her book *Four Glorious Years*. I would like to thank Mona for her encouragement.

Jenny Setchell offered me her father's detailed account of his imprisonment, which gives the reader an intimate view of the lives of those whose freedom was taken while trying to win freedom for others. Jenny has proven herself a faithful friend.

I owe a debt of gratitude to Al Castillo for the many photographs he allowed me to use in my book, as well as for inviting me to a military show to view the many items he had collected from World War II. I will always remember his patience as I rummaged through the medic's kit.

Les Habegger's account was the first one I received for this book. I am indebted to him for his encouragement, for answering my endless questions, and for all the times he has made me laugh.

I would like to thank my son, Jordan, for his patience and assistance during the writing of this book.

Preface

I am not an historian. I am a storyteller—or in this instance, one who relates the stories of the men and women who served in the Medical Corps during World War II, whether in the front line, the rear, or on the home front. For the last, Dr. George S. Barnes stated, "Some of us never heard a shot fired in anger, but we did what we were ordered to do."

My goal was to represent the many personnel who comprised the medical corps, not only the doctors and nurses but also those who assisted in caring for the ill and wounded, from the ambulance drivers and frontline medics and navy corpsmen to those in air evacuation teams and hospital ships. I have also included some volunteers, such as the women who served in the Voluntary Aid Detachment (voluntary nursing aids) from New Zealand.

Most of the accounts are in the first person, composed by the individuals themselves. Some I have taken from donated autobiographies, interviews, and cassette tapes. Some were interviews that were sent to me.

As much as possible I have attempted to keep first person accounts just as they were when submitted. It is my hope that I have retained the personality and character of each contributor. In some instances I have changed British spelling to American unless I felt this detracted from original documents. At times I have adjusted punctuation, added or removed capitalization, and corrected obvious typographical or grammatical errors. If there was more than one way to spell a word that was repeated, I chose one spelling and used it throughout the manuscript. Some overly long paragraphs were broken down into several shorter ones. Sometimes it was necessary to use the third person narrative so as to condense accounts and allow space for more pertinent information in the first person.

Many of the contributors to this work were decorated for their valor and devotion to duty. All, I am certain, have the gratitude and respect of those for whom they cared so compassionately.

During the time I collected these accounts I was struck by the humility of these men and women. None of them seemed to think that they had done anything out of the ordinary personally. They went where they were sent because their skills were needed. It was as simple as that. Some volunteered, many were drafted, but they all served.

Chapter One

A Medic Tells His Story
LES HABEGGER

Less Habegger, 1st Battalion, 274th Infantry Regiment, recounts his experiences as a medic. Les came from an Amish background.

Habbeger's regiment was part of the 70th Infantry Division, which provided the following division history:

> The Medical Detachment, 275th Infantry, was activated June 15, 1943, at Camp Adair, Oregon, as a unit of the 70th Infantry Division with cadre mainly from the 91st Infantry Division, then at Camp White, Oregon. Basic training was given with the aid of infantry officers, and unit technical training by assigned Medical Corps officers. Men showing aptitude as technicians were sent to Medical and Surgical Technicians Schools at Fitzsimmons General Hospital, O'Reilly General Hospital and Beaumont General Hospital.
>
> The 70th Division moved from Camp Adair to Ft. Leonard Wood, Missouri, in July 1944 and continued training. The 275th Infantry moved by train starting November 16th to Camp Miles Standish, Massachusetts.
>
> The 275th, together with the 274th and 276th Infantries composed Task Force Herren. Final supply and qualifications essentials were completed and all personnel were given the required inoculations at Miles Standish. On December 6th the organization sailed from Boston for permanent change of station outside the continental United States.
>
> On December 15th the organization arrived and debarked at Marseilles, France, moving by motor to Staging Area CP-2, a short distance north of the city. Administrative bivouac was established in the cold and muddy fields. On December 22nd the organization departed the staging area by train and motor. On December 31st Task Force Herren was attached to the 45th Infantry Division, and received orders for immediate movement. A night motor march brought the 275th Infantry into Niederbronn,

France, during the early hours of January 1st, and troops were quartered in a large abandoned wire factory for the remainder of the night.

On the morning of January 1, 1945, the Regimental Medical Detachment moved into Niederbronn and established all aid stations in the forward, northwestern end of town. The regimental command post (CP) was in the center of Niederbronn, approximately ten blocks away.

The Medical Battalion of the 45th Division made contact and attached a liaison sergeant and six ambulances to the detachment. These were assigned one to each aid station, two in reserve.

The regimental mission was the defense of the north flank of the 45th Division salient pointed at German-held Bitche. The lines ran across mountainous, heavily wooded terrain, creased by narrow, north-south running valleys, and facing German forward positions at Baerenthal and Dambach.

The Second Battalion was on the left flank of the regiment in the hills facing Baerenthal, where a small group of houses comprising the village of Muhlthal was used as the Battalion CP. The Second Battalion Medical Section established an aid station in one of the houses, chosen for a direct litter entrance, convenient location, and sturdy construction.

The Third Battalion had the ground to the right, over rugged terrain leading to the next valley; the town of Phillipsburg was just ahead of their first positions. The 62nd Battalion of the 14th Armored Division had just stopped a German advance immediately to the front of Phillipsbourg and were preparing to withdraw.

On the morning of January 2, 1945, the First Battalion moved up from Niederbronn into Phillipsbourg on the right of the Third. Its mission was the defense of the town and the hilly area to its right front, with the highway that formed the main street of the town being the boundary between the First and the Third Battalions. The Third Battalion aid station set up in a beer hall at the north end of town where all forward roads leading to their lines converged. When the First Battalion moved into Phillipsbourg they chose the vestry of a church as their aid station, as it had two entrances without stairs, and the church courtyard offered parking space for the vehicles.

My parents didn't enter me in the first grade until I was seven years of age; consequently I was 18 years old in my senior year in high school. I turned 18 in November 1942 and received my notice to report for my physical in March '43. Because I had not graduated yet my local draft board gave me a deferment. As soon as I walked out the door of the school on the last day "my friends and neighbors" gave me an invitation to report.

I had never been out of the state of Indiana, where I was born and raised, and had hardly ever been out of the little town of 1,800 people in northeastern Indiana named Berne. So when I was inducted I was one homesick puppy. I had been at the reception center at Fort Benjamin Harrison

1. A Medic Tells His Story

near Indianapolis for a while awaiting assignment when one day the shipment bulletin board had several pages of names which said "Shipment to Oregon" on them. I had heard of Oregon only because of some class we had to take in high school, but as far as I knew it was like any other "foreign country," and I knew that they certainly didn't play basketball out there, which for a "Hoosier" was important.

Of course my name was one of those on the list. Why was I being shipped overseas directly from the reception center was my question. I could not imagine how I was going to survive that far from home. My fears and anxiety were heightened when in the wee hours of an August morning I stepped off a troop train and stared straight at a cross rifle insignia. Infantry? Me? What in the world was I doing in the infantry? At the reception center I had signed a paper stating that I wanted to be in the air corps, so why was I at Camp Adair? I was one frightened, young, Indiana farm boy. Little did I know then what real fear I would encounter in December 1944.

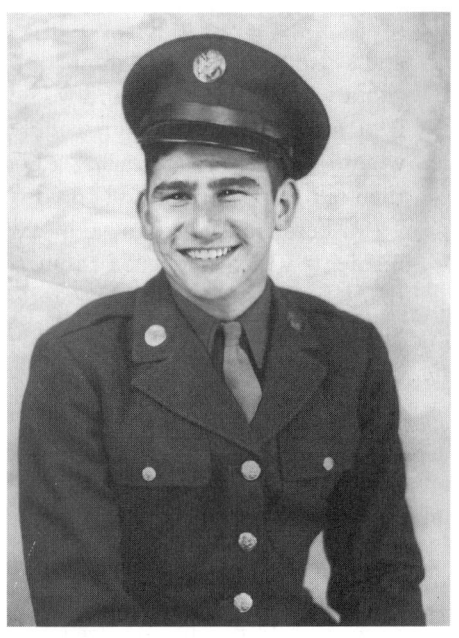

Les Habegger. *Courtesy of Les Habegger.*

I have often thought that as 18 year olds they asked us to become men in a split second. And in so doing we lost our youth, never really having had the chance to enjoy what every 18, 19, 20 year old enjoys doing. We left right out of high school and came back 21, 22 year olds. When I returned home in April 1946, I realized immediately that I was different from the rest of my family. There were five of us sons in the service, but I was the only one who saw combat.

All of us who gather together at our reunions, I am sure, had many experiences which caused us to wonder and ask, "How did I ever survive that?" Those horrors that we endured for days, weeks, and months had an affect on all of our lives that will stay with us forever.

I was a medic with First Battalion, 274th. I alternated between litter bearer and company aid man. What do I remember from those days? Incessant barrages of 88s, mortars, machine gun fire, rifle fire, snow up to my armpits, severe, unbelievable cold weather, living in foxholes like rats, and at times being so frightened that I had a discussion with my partner about whether giving a hand would be worth it to get out of combat, and if we did stick our hand out, would that be classified as SIW [self-inflicted wound]. I remember wearing a hood to keep my ears from freezing but then taking it off because I couldn't hear the incoming 88s. Freezing ears was a better option than taking a direct hit. But there are two specific incidents which happened to me that are deeply imbedded in my mind that I want to relate. These, to me, are in the category of, "How did I survive that?" There is no explanation short of the miraculous to explain my survival.

The first incident happened when we were in Phillipsbourg. We were in a factory outside of Niederbronn being briefed by our CO, Capt. Frank Ellis. As he sent us down the road toward Phillipsbourg, following behind A Company, he said, "Good luck, be careful; we have reports that the Germans are shooting at medics."

I was with a litter squad walking down the road thinking this is just like going out on a problem in Oregon and Missouri—nothing tough about this. In the distance we heard artillery, but no big deal; we had also heard that at Adair and Leonard Wood. Gradually the artillery got louder and closer. All of a sudden shells landed in the middle of the road, and as I dove for the ditch I thought, "Holy cow, what are they doing? Why is our artillery sending rounds on top of us?" It was then that I heard the cry, "Medic, medic," and realized this was the real thing.

We had been in Phillipsbourg for several days when one evening my litter squad was ordered to go up into the hill to the west of town to get some wounded who had been lying up there for a few days because the Germans had the company surrounded. I don't recall which company it was. The message from the company said these men needed to be evacuated now but because there were still Krauts in the area, a rifle squad should accompany us. It was midnight, pitch black, snow up to our necks, bitter cold as we climbed up to rescue the wounded. We finally reached the area where they were without encountering any Krauts. We placed the severely wounded on the litters. There was one rifleman who had a shrapnel wound in his left shoulder but was able to slowly walk along. It became my duty to place one arm around his waist, let him lean on me, and help him get back to the aid station.

We headed back to Phillipsbourg without incident and eventually reached the main road back in town. Our aid station was located in a house at the southern tip of Phillipsbourg. When we entered town we were a considerable distance from the aid station. The rifle squad, assuming we

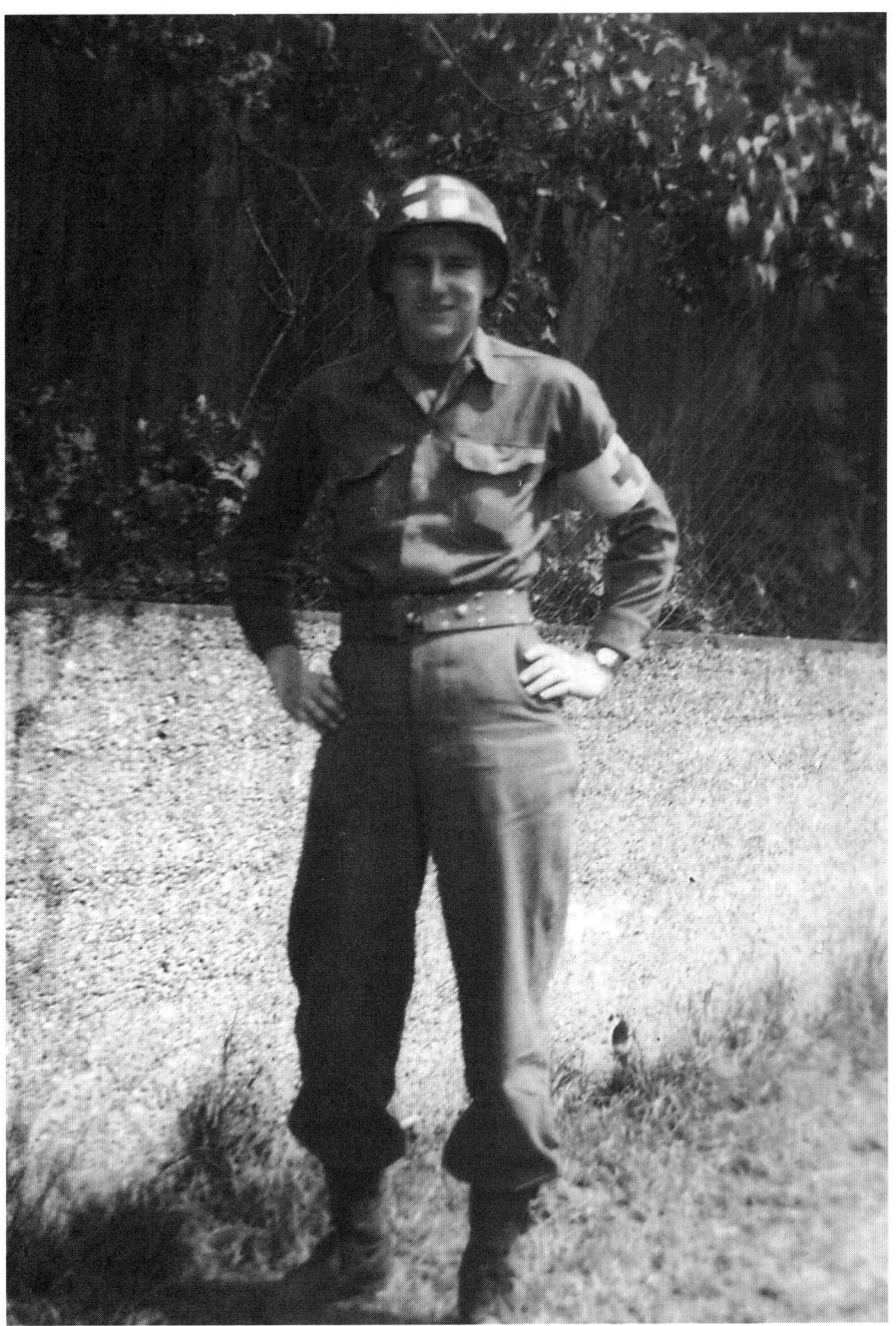

Les Habegger in ETO. *Courtesy of Les Habegger.*

were out of danger, took off down the road followed by the litter bearers, leaving me alone with the walking wounded. It was slow going for me because of his injury, so in a short while he and I were all alone, a considerable distance behind the riflemen and litter bearers. We were shuffling along when all of a sudden out of the corner of my eye I saw a figure jump out from behind one of the buildings on the west side of the road. We had been warned that there were Germans wearing our uniforms who had infiltrated our lines. The distinguishing feature between them and us was that they did not wear our helmet liner or helmet, although they did wear our wool skullcap. As this figure ran up to me I saw a man wearing our uniform, a skull cap, but no helmet. He stuck a pistol into my side and in English asked, "Where are you from?"

I looked at him, and my mind and heart were racing a mile a minute. What should I do? If I yelled for the rifle squad who were long gone by now, it would do no good. He could pull the trigger and take off. "What is my duty," I thought. There was no doubt in my mind that he was a Kraut and even if it was a GI who had gone nuts, what could I do? Helping an injured soldier walk and carrying only medical supplies, I hardly was a match for the man with pistol in my side. I answered back, "What do you mean, where am I from?"

He shoved the pistol harder into my side and said, "You know what I mean. What state are you from?"

I have often had a few laughs recalling how my thinking went. I can't tell him the truth (name, rank and serial number only—right?). So I gave him the name of a state other than Indiana where I was from. Then he asked, "What city are you from? What is the name of the city?"

Again my mind said, "Tell him a city that is not in the state that I told him I was from." Then I thought, "Jeez, what if he knows American geography well enough to know that city isn't in that state?" Anyway, he continued walking with me for a few more steps, which seemed like miles, and disappeared behind the buildings that he had jumped out from, as fast as he had appeared.

When I got to the aid station I reported what had happened to Captain Ellis. A rifle squad was sent on patrol but the Kraut was long gone. Why didn't he take me prisoner? There were probably several good reasons why. But not pulling the trigger is something else.

The second incident happened when our aid station was located in Etzlingen. I was at that time assigned to A Company as an aid man. We had taken a woods, and for some unknown reason, four riflemen and I stood in a group talking and only one of the group had started digging a fox hole, and his was hardly deep enough to take care of his body. As we stood there talking we heard the unmistakable sound of an incoming 88. All five of us dove for the one hole. I, being the farthest away, landed on top of the other four so that I was a considerable distance above the ground and obviously totally exposed. The shell landed close by and covered me with dirt and rocks but no shrapnel. The only one of the group that got hit was the first rifleman in the hole, lying on the bottom covered by four of us. He was severely wounded, severely enough that we heard from him later that he had been sent back to the States.

How could that possibly happen? All of us, no doubt, can relate similar experiences, and all of us have asked, "How did I survive that?" There are no scientific explanations to what happened to us "up there." I, being a believer in God and a Christian, choose to believe, "Only by the grace of God can it be explained."

Chapter Two

Recollections of an Infantry Battalion Doctor

FRANK R. ELLIS, M.D.

Dr. Ellis served as a captain in the medical corps of the United States Army. He was First Battalion Surgeon with the 274th Infantry Regiment, 70th Infantry Division.

Even after more than a half-century, some experiences of youth continue to be indelibly etched in my memory: growing up during a monumental economic depression; being exposed to first-hand discipline and the work ethic while in the Civilian Conservation Corps; and carefree years attending the University of Michigan. Altogether, these provide an everlasting background upon which the horrors of war intruded on an impressionable young physician.

Although a sense of high adventure was tempered by worry of danger during weeks of training after entering the army, the stark reality of war quickly emerged. Less than a half year after qualifying to practice medicine I was in northeastern France with a new infantry division facing an aggressive German offensive dubbed *Nordwind*. The process of becoming accustomed to seeing dead Americans had begun before we headed for the front line. A soldier's head was crushed by a box when a truck carrying supplies overturned. And during our initial approach march to the line of contact with the enemy we passed the bodies of several yanks killed minutes before as our troops moved forward. Unsettling of course, such incidents created deep anxiety among all personnel. It has not been forgotten to this day.

But once the unit became engaged in fighting, we were so busy caring for wounded there was little time to worry about personal injury or, for that matter, personal discomfort. And as day followed day seeing the physical destruction of buildings, dead animals and humans—the utter devastation of our surroundings—it should hardly be surprising that one became cynical. This loss of the sense of perhaps becoming "the next one" may have been the result of an emotionally protective shield against losing one's mind completely.

Emotional stress coupled with abject physical exhaustion often became so severe as to defy description. While riflemen were consistently more likely to become casualties in this way, front-line medical personnel and members of other branches whose duties kept them in the same environment were also at risk of such incapacity. I do not know the official figures of so-called "battle fatigue," but its incidence among our personnel was amazingly infrequent. Having said that, however, it remains a personal belief that everyone has a level of tolerance that, once exceeded, will result in collapse and the total loss of composure.

There were myriad encounters with wounded troops that surface still. Many result from tales related by old comrades in arms during periodic reunions of the 70th Infantry Division Association still going on. Almost everyone I know who has been in combat acknowledges having endured an unusual sense of fear of personal injury or death. They also largely share the view that war solves little in spite of its cost in property and lives. I suspect they may also agree that any politician promoting the use of military force should be required to spend at least 30 days during the winter as a PFC [Private First Class] in a foxhole under hostile fire before being entitled to cast his vote.

Phillipsbourg, France, January 1945

During the German offensive *Nordwind*, launched on New Year's Eve 1944, the three rifle regiments of the 70th Infantry Division operating as Task Force Herren were committed to combat barely two weeks after landing in France. The 274th Infantry was sent into Phillipsbourg on January 3rd to relieve its sister 275th Infantry which had been severely mauled by a German counterattack during the preceding 24 hours.

Our First Battalion aid station operated in a building for several days which also housed the D Company Command Post. The house was under sporadic mortar fire most of those days—usually three or four rounds at a time—occasionally bracketing the building. Shelling regularly followed any vehicular activity at the site during daylight hours.

During one early-morning site inspection from the front steps of the house, overnight change in impact pattern and size was noted. Two or three craters with twice or more the diameter and depth of before, and much wider margins of dirt strewn about the periphery of these holes provided convincing evidence that larger weapons were now firing on this target. After notifying the units we were supporting, we withdrew the aid station a few hundred meters to the barn of a house we had occupied earlier, clearing the site by midmorning.

Shortly after noon the same day the building we had just vacated took a pickle-barrel hit with a delay-fused artillery shell which exploded in the room in the basement being used for D Company's CP [Command Post]. Nearly all of the officers and troops in the room being briefed on battle plans for later in the day were either injured or killed. Lt. Joseph Dito, one of the few survivors who had started out the door to answer a field telephone, was blown out of the building by the explosion. He jeeped to the aid station to notify us of the disaster. I shall never forget the bewildered expression of horror on Dito's dust-covered face and clothing as he described the scene.

Lt. John Passanisi returned with him to assist in and oversee evacuation of several ambulance loads of wounded from that site. The shell had fallen through the first floor room we had been using to care for casualties.

Chapter Three

Dr. Kurt Lekisch

Sol Schwartz

I saw him treat the wounded with such care and compassion that tears still well up in my eyes to this day at his concern.
—Sol Schwartz remembers Dr. Kurt Lekisch

I was the radio repairman and a radio operator in the First Battalion, HQ [Headquarters] Company of the 275th Regiment, 70th Infantry Division. Early in our combat action several wounded men were brought to our battalion command post. I helped man a stretcher to carry a severely wounded GI to the battalion aid station a couple of hundred yards down a road, it was fairly out of sight of infiltrators and the mortar and artillery fire they directed at the CP.

At the aid station I saw the medics and Dr. Lekisch working on wounded men (nothing at all like the scenes in *M*A*S*H* which I could never warm to). He immediately came over to the GI we had just brought in and started to reassure him, and gave him an injection of morphine to ease his pain. He was gentle, compassionate, and he worked swiftly removing shreds of shattered bone and torn flesh and preparing him for evacuation. It was not a sight that I could bear, so I went back to the CP.

I saw him on several other missions of mercy. I said to myself and to my buddies, "He's the kind of doctor I want to take care of me in war or peace."

I never saw him again after those dreary days in early January 1945, 54 years ago. He was one of the world's good guys.

From The Trailblazer, *the magazine of the 70th Infantry Division:*

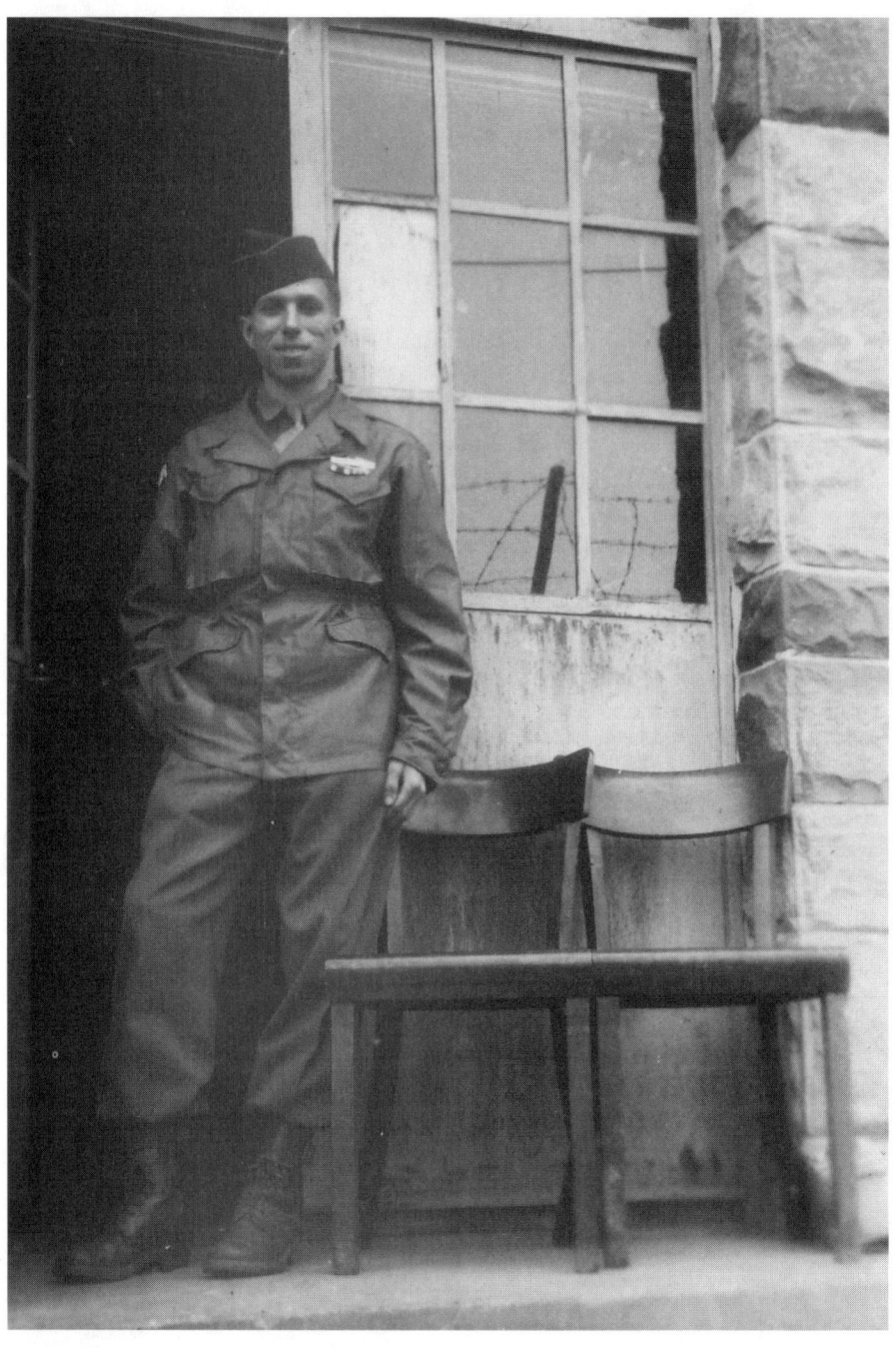

Sol Schwartz in Arolsen, Germany. *Courtesy of Sol Schwartz.*

3. Dr. Kurt Lekisch

Surgeon Hero Hears Taps

Death has claimed one of the Patriarchs of the Platoons: Dr. Kurt Lokeisch[*sic*]. He was battalion surgeon for 2nd B/275. He died May 27, 1994, at the age of 83.

He was born in Germany to a Jewish family that had at least one surgeon in every generation since 1634. In 1939 his family fled the Nazi persecutions and came to the United States. Grateful to his new country, the doctor volunteered for army duty and came to the 70th.

When the Trailblazers came through Mainz, Germany, he found that all that remained of his previous home was the front steps. He also found a cousin who had been hidden and saved by a Catholic priest when Hitler wreaked his "final solution."

His death was reported by George Barten who was battalion commander and a close personal friend. George recalls stories of the great deprivations in Germany in the years following World War I. Kurt told how his family wore suits and dresses for 10 years, then took them apart, turned the cloth inside out and resewed the garments to wear 10 more years.

The surgeon worked heroically treating not only GIs, but also civilians and German POWs. Barten recalls when our troops took Grossbliederstroff during the Saar campaign, they found villagers huddled in a limestone mine. Many were sick, and Dr. Lokeisch [*sic*] cared for them whenever he had a moment free from treating wounded Trailblazers.

Chapter Four

"How Long You Been Here, Boy?"
ALAN KING, M.D.

Compiled in gratitude for my release as a POW in Germany by American troops.
—Dr. Alan King, South Perth, Australia

Dr. King sailed from Fremantle, West Australia, on September 22, 1940, to the Middle East, arriving at the Suez Canal October 12. He then went by train to Beit Jirja, Palestine, where he trained. He served in campaigns in Egypt, close to the action in the battles of Bardia and Tobruk. He eventually ended up in Greece, where his unit was involved in the bloody Greek campaign of 20 days from April 6 to April 26. They ran advanced and main dressing stations north and south of the Brallos Pass. Dr. King said he will never forget a poignant moment at the foot of the pass when they buried a number of those killed, and their bugler blew the last post. Their losses in Greece were heavy: 310 killed in action, some 494 wounded, and 2,030 taken prisoner by the Germans. His unit was evacuated from Megara Beach to Crete on April 25, ANZAC (Australian and New Zealand Army Corps) Day. It was on Crete that he was captured, by German alpine troops at an aid post at the schoolhouse in Neon Korion.

They were quite pleasant to us, so I was in the bag with nothing much to do but look after those in my care, some 30 wounded. We were there for three to four days, when our victors transported the wounded to what had been the British Seventh General Hospital near Maleme.

I then found myself with 16 captured medical officers at Imros, but as usual was picked to do some work and became the MO [Medical Officer] for some 1,100 captured Australian and New Zealand troops in a barbed wire camp near Maleme, with limited facilities.

I acted as a lookout while three of my friends (they eventually got to Egypt and Australia) went "under the wire," and somehow Jerry knew I was involved, and I was thrown into solitary confinement for a day or so till the padre in the camp got me released to continue my medical duties. I would have liked to join the escapees, but I had to remain as MO to the thousand-plus troops. I managed to get any very sick transferred to the main POW hospital. Eventually, in groups, the whole camp was transferred via Greece to Germany.

Our losses in Crete were again heavy with 274 killed in action, 504 wounded and 3,109 POWs. (The total number of Allied POWs in these two campaigns in Greece and Crete was some 16,000.) However, the German losses were so much larger among paratroopers and personnel in the seaborne invasion (who were lost at sea): 3,986 killed or missing and 2,594 wounded, and 220 aircraft including gliders destroyed. It is said that Hitler never used his paratroopers again because of the losses at Maleme; these also delayed his advance on Russia for some six weeks, which was important at the time.

Then in groups we were transferred to Greece to the old Turkish Barracks at Salonica. A little story: I had some ten walking wounded in my care; we were paraded on the wharf. I took my courage in both hands, left the ranks, marched up to the German major in command, saluted and with my limited German said, "Ich habe verwundeted." He beckoned me to one side—I got transport to the Salonica POW Barracks and my poor self-appointed batman Private Dodds had to lug our two "swags" to the camp some two or three miles away.

Salonica was a hell camp. The first morning I woke with my eyes closed due to the bites from bed bugs; the food was terrible; and during the five weeks I was there, I believe two trying to escape at night through the wire were shot.

Then finally off to Germany, 40 to a "cattle truck," with occasional stops to stretch our legs. The high spot was a stop at Belgrade station for ablutions. The Yugoslav Red Cross ladies helped with tins of jam to revive us. Eventually we arrived at Lamsdorf Stalag VIIIB, lower Silesia, a POW camp of many thousands, mostly British from Dunkirk. It was pretty well organized, and the food rations were augmented with British Red Cross parcels.

We were detoured through a special delousing station, our clothes heat sterilized because of typhus. The Germans had driven many thousands

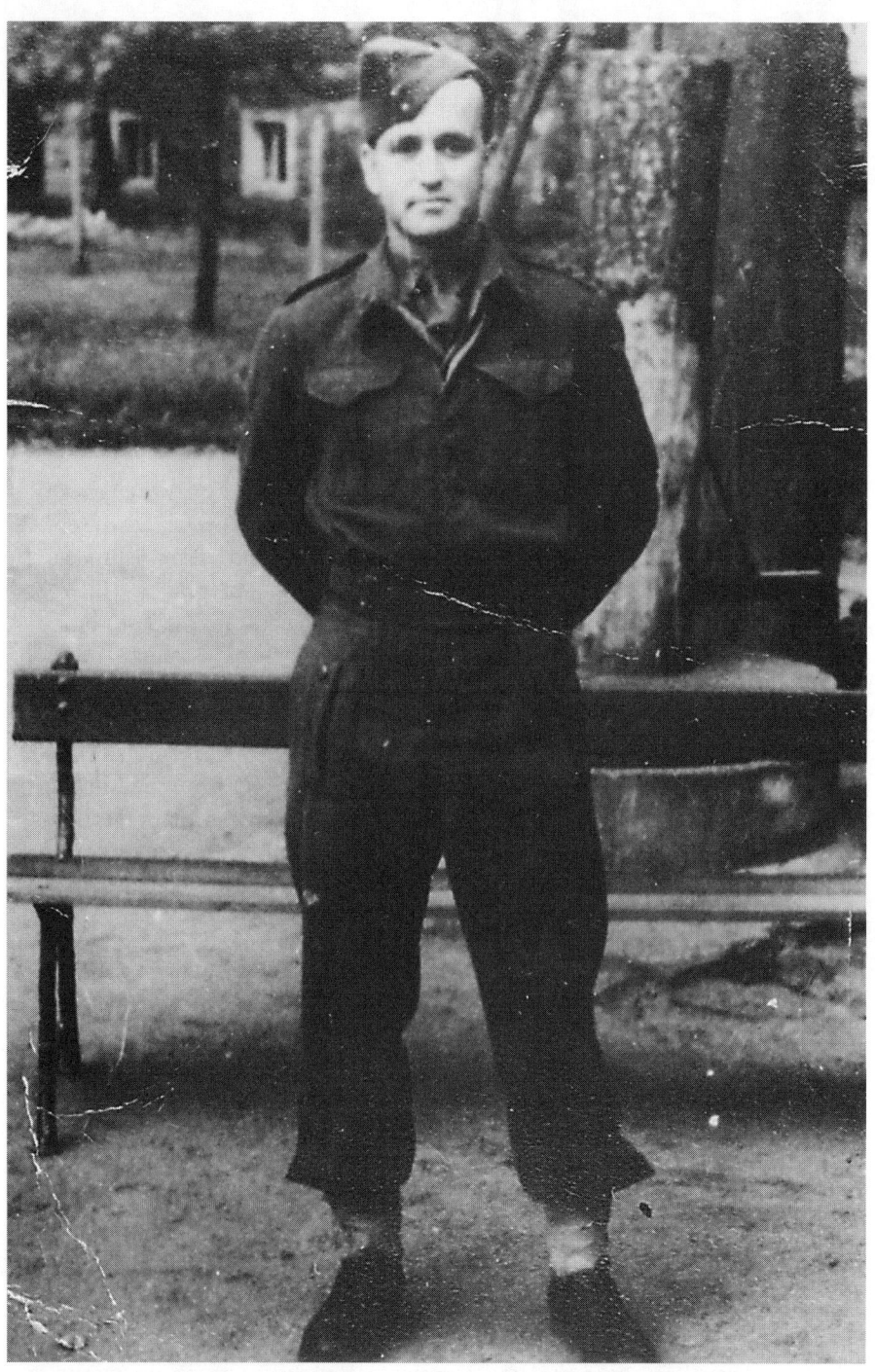

Dr. Alan King. *Courtesy of Dr. Alan King.*

of Russians out of their homes. They were camped in the open, outside our camp; many died. Two of our MOs who went to help in a makeshift hospital eventually died of typhus. I had been friendly with one of them and had to write to his wife (we were allowed a small postcard to write home every couple of months); I still have several that arrived with my relatives.

I was at Lamsdorf for some four months; there being so many surplus MOs I seized the opportunity when offered to "volunteer" to go and help treat Allied POWs suffering from pulmonary tuberculosis. This resulted in the highlight of my stay in Germany, a trip with a German officer "Dollmecher" (interpreter). We stayed with his relatives in Dresden (a butcher who seemed to have only German sausage). We had a good feed and an escorted trip through Dresden Museum the next day! Eventually we arrived at Konigswartha, an old converted "Blind Home," with extra barracks with two-tier bunks for the sick, some hundreds altogether, French, Polish, Yugoslavs, and British, and even two Australians.

There I was for 15 months, February '42 to May '43, being taught how to treat TB [tuberculosis] by some six French doctors, and particularly a TB specialist, Maurice Blondeau, who taught me how to perform "artificial pneumothoraces," and to operate on the adhesions, if any (pneumolysis). No drugs for TB in those days, only isolation and bed rest, plus "artificial pneumothoraces," to rest the lungs.

By coincidence, after 12 months some five other Australian doctors arrived to help me, three from my own unit, including my field ambulance commanding officer, which lightened my load.

French patients were being repatriated; British numbers were growing, and we were transferred to a six-ward, standard German army hutted hospital at Elsterhorst, Stalag IVA. Here I had charge of one 90-bed ward, but did many operations (pneumolyses), as we had a special operating-room block and pharmacy. Here we were for 20 months, May 1943 to February 1945. Two groups of patients were repatriated in October '43 and January '45; two of our Australian doctors went with them.

The Russians were moving towards us from the east; we could hear their guns. We were regarded as hostages and transported to the west; patients and all on the floors of cattletrucks, we were a week meandering through Czechoslovakia and Germany with one night in the Dresden railyards. Finally we arrived at a small town, Hohenstein-Ernstahl, and went to a previous charity home with extra huts. Our numbers built up to over 1,000 including sick and wounded. I personally looked after a number of American troops suffering from severe frostbite; they had been captured at Bastogne and marched ten days through the snow without succor.

We were there for two months, February 24 to April 26, 1945. The great day of liberation arrived mid-April with General Patton and his Third Armored Division. I was at the top of the main building watching aerial dogfights when I saw a vehicle slowly coming down the road.

The Jerry guards had disappeared. I was first down to greet a jeep carrying a Lieutenant Kaplan and three American soldiers. He said to me, "How long you been here, boy?" On my reply of "Four years," he said, "I guess you need this, boy" and produced a bottle of French brandy. It took about ten days for the Americans to evacuate our hospital; then we staff were trucked to Erfurt, and recuperated there from April 26 to May 12— real white bread, etc.!

To the airport there; many planes. One Australian pilot said, "Where do you want to go?" We said, "England." He just took off without formality (or clearance), and I saw the White Cliffs of Dover from the nose of a Lancaster bomber. Home on May 12, 1945.

I wished to complete my surgical studies, having been in Edinburgh when war broke out. They didn't want us during the "Phoney War" [the months immediately after the U.K. declared war on Germany on September 3, 1939, in which there were no real hostilities], but after the conflict the Australian army mission in London decided I was needed in Australia to treat the large numbers of ex-servicemen being found with TB on discharge, and it arranged a six-month postgraduate tour of England, Wales, Canada, and the United States of America for me. In the United States I caught up with some of my American patients at the Fitzgerald Hospital near Denver. Couldn't find Kaplan in Chicago (there were so many of them in the phone book).

On return to Australia I became Specialist Major in charge of TB patients in all the States after submitting two reports to the army in February 1946. I was finally discharged from the army January 16, 1947.

Chapter Five

The Neapolitan Typhus Epidemic
VINCENT STEPHEN CONTI, M.D.

Dr. Conti was awarded the Typhus Commission Medal and the Bronze Star for his work fighting typhus in Naples, Italy, in 1943 and 1944. The following information comes from his treatise on the epidemic, The Neopolitan Typhus Epidemic.

Typhus fever took its first foothold in the city of Naples, Italy, about March 1943. The first case recorded, in conjunction with this epidemic, was in an Italian soldier who had returned from the Russian front. Cases occurred sporadically, three to six a month, until the beginning of November when it started to take on epidemic proportions. The disease reached its peak in January 1944 when as many as 80 to 100 cases were admitted daily. Because of the growing danger to Allied troops in this area, the Typhus Commission was formed under the command of Brig. Gen. L.A. Fox. This group with the help of the civil authorities in the city of Naples was responsible for the control of the epidemic.

Typhus fever is an acute infectious disease. The epidemic form (European type) as found in Naples is transmitted to man by the body louse (Pediculus humanus). The onset of the disease is abrupt: the patient complains of a severe headache, frontal or occipital, accompanied by a chill and general malaise. The temperature rises with the onset of the disease and usually is elevated from 102 degrees to 103 degrees F. The headache is persistent and usually lasts throughout the period of illness, which is from 12 to 14 days. The rash is first noted on the fourth [or] fifth day. The patient first becomes stuporous, and it is quite difficult to arouse him. Later he may go into an excited stage terminating with coma and death.

From Lee D. Cady, Commanding Officer of the 21st General Hospital in his recommendation for Dr. Conti to receive the Typhus Commission Medal:

> Practically the entire civil population was infested with typhus-bearing lice, and many thousands of homeless and fearful people were living in squalor in greatly crowded caves, tunnels, *ricoveros* (air raid shelters), and dilapidated, half-destroyed buildings. Mere presence in the streets of these areas meant almost certain infestation with lice. Some of these miserable people not only had thousands of lice on them, but one to two ounces of them! There was no fuel, soap, bath water, and no insecticide, and no relief of any sort until such workers as Captain Conti were sent to take charge. After a preliminary period of widespread dusting activities, Captain Conti became a case-finder or diagnostician in one-sixth of the Naples area. He hunted down all cases of typhus and contacts to see that they were properly handled and immunized and dusted. Since the Italian people were moving about at all hours of the day and night, so did Captain Conti work such long, fatiguing hours. He permitted nothing to discourage him or prevent his disagreeable work of mercy. Thousands of civilians owe their lives to his personal services.
>
> As a worker, ordered to serve in this ... dangerous mission merely because he was a doctor who spoke Italian, Captain Conti was also serving as a human "guinea pig" test animal for the efficiency of our vaccine against typhus for it was not generally known how efficacious it was. He faced his dangers as unfalteringly as he faced other duties and with the courage of driving professional conscience.

For this service Dr. Conti was awarded the Typhus Commission Medal and the Bronze Star.

Dr. Conti was graduated from Boston University and received his M.D. in 1938. He served his internship and residency, in obstetrics and gynecology, in Metropolitan Hospital in New York from 1938 to 1942. It was at this time that he met and fell in love with his future wife, Rose, an anesthesiology resident at Metropolitan.

Rose Conti has provided the following further information: Vincent Conti was almost 31 years old when he was inducted into the army in 1942. Lt. Conti was sent on maneuvers at Camp Claiborne, Louisiana. In March 1943 when they were alerted that they were being sent overseas, he persuaded Rose to go down to Louisiana and get married. By the time he was sent overseas in April 1943, Rose was pregnant. Lt. Conti sailed on an LST and spent 26 days on the high seas on the way to Oran, Africa.

He was then sent to Naples, Italy, where he distinguished himself in the typhus epidemic. Rose delivered their son while Dr. Conti was en route to Naples. He didn't find out about the birth until weeks later (for which delay he was very bitter). It was a sad and lonely time for him, a new husband and a new father. His son was almost two years old when he first saw him.

After Naples the 21st General Hospital was sent to Nancy, France. The hospital was bombed on Christmas Day 1944, and the German pilot was shot down on the hospital grounds.

Dr. Conti had been alerted to go to Japan when the A-bomb was dropped, and the war ended. He was sent home in September 1945.

Chapter Six

One Hundred Pounds and Five Feet Tall

MARY A. BREEDING

Mary Breeding was 21 years old when she served with the U.S. Army Nurse Corps in the 17th General Hospital in France.

I graduated from the Mercy Hospital School of Nursing in Springfield, Massachusetts, in 1943. Between 1943 and 1944 I did private duty because it was my intention to join the ANC soon after my 21st birthday in 1944. I was referred to as a general duty nurse.

On August 4, 1944, I was sworn in as a second lieutenant in the United States Army Nurse Corps. Upon my induction I was sent to Fort Devens–Lovell General Hospital in Ayer, Massachusetts. There our basic training took place. Training included familiarizing us with army medical procedures, keeping of medical records and, of course, drills in marching, bivouacs, and survival tactics. We were assigned to hospital wards taking care of many D-Day veterans. Soon the time came. Our whole hospital staff and unit were ready to go. We were the 174th General Hospital.

From a port somewhere in New Jersey we embarked on the *Queen Mary*. I don't remember how long it took us to cross the ocean but we made it to a port in Scotland. There we boarded trains, under blackout precautions, that traveled all night, taking us to Southampton, England. There we boarded an English transport ship called the *Empire Lanee*. We had a view of the White Cliffs of Dover. Off we went until we reached the shores of France (Normandy). We called it Utah Beach. It was October 22, 1944.

6. One Hundred Pounds and Five Feet Tall 25

We got off the mother ship and were picked up by LSTs taking us to shore. All I could see were trucks, jeeps, and soldiers knee-deep in mud preparing to haul us to our destination in a little town called La Haye-du-Puits, south of Cherbourg. As we rode along we could see devastation. There was no fanfare, but an eerie silence as we rode along.

Finally in a cow pasture surrounded by hedgerows was our tent hospital, with the big red cross. I remember it was so cold our Chief Nurse, Major Roby, told us to sleep with our clothes on. (I failed to mention we were in our combat uniforms, helmets and all.) Two pot-bellied stoves were our source of heat. We replaced the 42nd General Hospital whose staff moved on to the front, so our patients were there already to care for. Our hospital was something like you see on the sitcom M*A*S*H, but our operation was strictly serious with a determined desire to do our duty the best we knew how.

As for native contact, there was very little. We were confined away from the town, although I did find a hairdresser to give me a perm. People pretty much kept to themselves.

Our work began the morning after we arrived. We went to our designated wards. More patients were being brought in either by plane or train.

Snow, cold, and in December the war was escalating. Many wounded GIs were coming in from the front. We were in full alert. News of the Bulge filtered down to us. Our boys were hurting. Where did they come from? Belgium, Ardennes, Metz, Luxembourg, Antwerp, and Liège—and more. There were trench foot, scabies, section eights (psycho), many with shrapnel wounds. These I can account for, but I know there were others more seriously hurt that didn't come to us. They were sent to the United Kingdom or back to the States. At that part of the war we had so many wounded we acted more

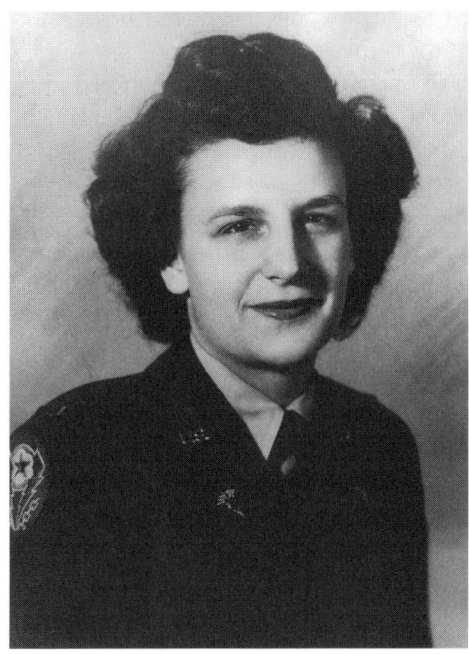

Mary A. Breeding. *Courtesy of Mary Lou James.*

like an evac hospital. We were sending men to the United Kingdom and, much to my sorrow, back to duty.

In spite of all the pain and misery around us, our gallant men never complained. There was a spirit of love of our country and the urge to get the job done. Everyone was helpful. I had one young man in particular who had a terrible leg wound who took it upon himself to make up his own bed. A little thing, but very meaningful.

Because I was only 100 pounds and five feet tall, I was called the "Little General" by my patients. Also, being short, when I tried to reach for something they would say "Lieutenant, do you want a piece of paper to stand on?" They just loved to tease me—so-o-o good to hear them laugh. So it wasn't all gloom and doom.

Soon the tide turned. We noticed as our boys were being discharged our beds were being filled with wounded German POWs. Our doctors were replaced by German doctors. The patients were a result of our finally winning the war. These patients were in terrible shape. Severed cords, paralysis, bed sores so bad you could see their tail bones (coccyx). Our boys did a number on them to be sure. We cared for them not as prisoners, but as we would take care of our own in hopes that their side was doing the same for our personnel. I didn't lose any one of our boys, but for some of the German prisoners, it was the end of the line.

There are a few things I'd like to make note of. When I entered my ward every morning, I would hear this loud command in German, "Achtung!" All patients would sit or stand rigid until I said something that sounded like "Gualemula." I was told it meant "at ease." What a shock it was to me at first not being used to this type of respect.

Another incident I wish to mention concerns a prisoner who came to my ward in a coma. A few days later as I was taking his pulse he opened his eyes and said something in German that made the entire ward laugh. No one would tell me what he said.

Finally the ward was staffed by German medics. The only remaining personnel were military police. Now it was time to leave; the war was over in Europe. We were not finished yet. We traveled by box cars, slept on floors, ate K rations until we reached Marseilles only to be redeployed for the Pacific. Then the news—V-J Day. Our orders were changed. Manila—no, United States—yes! How sweet those words—homeward bound.

Chapter Seven

Beanie, Ernie and More
JAMES MARION KIRTLEY, M.D.

From Kirtley Kronicles: The Life and Times of James Marion Kirtley, M.D. *(pp. 75–133), published by the Montgomery County Historical Society (Montgomery County, Indiana) in 1997.*

In 1940 Dr. Kirtley was ordered to Fort Knox, Kentucky, for active duty, but it was quite evident that preparations were being made for some serious military involvement by the United States. His duty there was supposedly for one year and after that he was told he could return to civilian life. By the summer of 1941, few of the physicians believed this.

I had sought and received a leave for Christmas and was fairly relaxed and looking forward to being home with the family and planning to see Lee [Dr. Kirtley's future wife], too. On Sunday afternoon, December 7, 1941, I was lying on my bunk listening to one of the name bands on the radio. The announcer said, "We interrupt this program to announce that the great naval base of Pearl Harbor in Hawaii has been bombed by an enemy and there has been much destruction. More information will be given later."

"Did you hear that?" I yelled. "Hear what?" someone else yelled. "The Japs have bombed Pearl Harbor and we're in it now," I said....

Major Kirtley, now married, shipped out for England on January 18, 1944, on the Capetown Castle, a British passenger liner which had been converted into a troopship.

Routine sick call and shot makeup took most of our time and the ship's doctor even had a few medical conferences on current ideas and procedures. He had a well-equipped "surgery" and told us that we would be in charge of any surgery that might be needed because he was not a surgeon himself. One day one of the boys became ill with vomiting and pain in his right side and it was quite obvious that we had an acute appendicitis on our hands. A hurried consultation was held and Bob Miller, of Argos, Indiana, volunteered to be the anesthetist and we got our patient prepped and ready for the procedure. We did have ether and a mask for administering it and, with the equipment furnished, the job was done. The young man recovered nicely and was carried ashore in Liverpool to recuperate in a medical installation there.

My good friend, Chaplain Bill Boice, became very ill during this time and apparently developed a bad case of influenza. He, too, had to leave us at Liverpool and wound up, after recovering from the flu, in the infamous ... Replacement Depot, run by some sort of despot who made life miserable for all personnel, officers and enlisted men alike. When Bill returned to us in Devon he was the happiest man in the regiment and regaled us with tales of life in the ... Repledepple. Later we had similar reports of bad treatment but did not learn if the place got any better....

Major Kirtley arrived in Liverpool, England on January 29, 1944. His medical detachment was taken to Denbury Camp in Devon.

Training again began in earnest and everyone was aware that a serious approach to it was essential if we were to accomplish our mission. Staff meetings at regimental headquarters were frequent and I was responsible for checking on our various small medical detachments scattered over a large part of Devon. Field Marshall Montgomery visited our camp at one time and addressed us while standing on the hood of a jeep in our motor pool area. It was a damp, squally day when he came and he had us remove our helmets, "so I can see your faces," he said. I developed a "doosey" of a head cold shortly, and Dr. Dave Raynes, one of my dentists, told me to blame Monty for it!...

At last, during the third week in May, came the orders to prepare to be taken to the area nearer to our port of embarkation where we would be held in guarded fields until the loading time came. These fields were known as marshaling yards and we found ourselves quartered in pyramidal tents that were placed inside a wire enclosure around the periphery of small fields. Once inside, there was no movement to the outside and we knew that military police were on duty to see that there was no communication with anyone but our own people. We were encouraged to write letters home but were told that they would not be processed until the invasion had actually taken place. This was so there would be no hint of what was going on in case letters fell into enemy hands....

On June 4, 1944, we were alerted to break camp and were taken to our assigned vehicles to go to our waiting seacraft. Sgt. Stanley Osowski, my faithful driver of [our jeep] "Beanie" [Dr. Kirtley, about to become a father, christened his jeep with the nickname for the baby they were expecting], was ready to roll, and we joined the convoy which moved to the "hards," which were cobblestoned areas from which the tanks, trucks, cannon, and other equipment could be loaded aboard their assigned craft. My medical headquarters group of the regiment was assigned to a LCT, and we were loaded with other vehicles of the regimental headquarters. Since I was the senior officer aboard, but in no way in command, my jeep would be the first off the craft and so it was loaded last. The front end of "Beanie" was facing the front of the boat and immediately behind the ramp, which was pulled to the upright position when we were all aboard. It was evening by the time all was in readiness and we prepared to take to the open sea. Our port was Plymouth and we were intrigued by the fact that the Pilgrims had named their first landfall in the New World after this very same place.

I had retained some of the anti-seasick pills we had been trying during the invasion training exercises in Florida and I fixed a litter on the deck in front of the jeep, arranged my blankets and took the pills. I had expected to awake to the sound of artillery fire but instead I awoke in a quiet spot in the port of Portsmouth. We had joined the seagoing convoy on schedule and had made our way into the English Channel on the night of June 4–5 but, because of the terrific storm, had been called back to the safety of Portsmouth. After a day of waiting, I again prepared myself and on the morning of June 6, 1944, I was wakened by the sounds of firing from the battleship, cruisers, and destroyers who were sending heavy shells flying toward the vaguely seen shore of Normandy, France [Utah Beach]....

Troopships could be seen in our vicinity unloading soldiers by way of cargo nets strung over their sides, the soldiers climbing down to drop into the assault craft or Higgins boats. The sea was still very rough and it was a real job to get the boys onto the small craft without injury. As the boats became loaded, they scooted away to join a great circle that was preparing to get into proper alignment for their run to the shore....

We were waiting for our orders to move toward the shore and by 1000 [10:00 A.M.]we were on our way. We were unable to see to our front because of the ramp being in place but very soon the coxswain of our craft let us know that we were at our designated spot and he dropped the ramp with a splash. There was no enemy activity in our immediate region and I prepared to leave the craft, since I was the senior aboard. I stepped off the ramp into the water and was happy to see that we had been landed close to shore and the water was about chest high. Stanley Osowski gave "Beanie" the gun and the little car and its trailer hit the water and, without hesitating, made its way to dry land. The other vehicles got off safely and we made our way to the shelter of the concrete seawall that was supporting a large sand dune. A navy Beachmaster came up shortly and told us to move out as quickly as possible to the exit-way from the beach which had been constructed by engineers who blew out a section of the wall with dynamite. The roadway through the sand had a base of perforated steel plates to keep our heavy trucks from bogging down and traffic was moving nicely.

There were very few wounded soldiers in our view and the ones we did see were being cared for by the beach-party medics, probably navy people. Looking out to sea we observed watercraft of all descriptions making their way ashore. The amphibious trucks or DKWs, known as "ducks" by our guys, were making trips seaward and back and bringing in supplies from craft offshore. As soon as our turn came, we moved up to the opening in the seawall and made our way to a small roadway inside the dune line. We stopped at a little crossing and noted German captives carrying some of their wounded in blankets to the aid station on the beach. Our stopping where we did was certainly not wise for crossroads are prime targets for enemy gunners or snipers and we did actually hear the whine of a bullet over our heads.

The Germans had flooded large areas of land back of the dunes by diverting water from a nearby river. They had constructed causeways at wide intervals so that the flooded areas could be crossed. They had zeroed in their weapons on these paths but our combat troops who had landed soon after H-Hour had been able to make their way forward and had eliminated most of the danger. So we followed the soldiers moving ever-farther inland and could see a little village to our front. St. Marie du Mont was one of the first of these and it had been badly damaged by artillery fire. The church was still standing but the belfry had been destroyed. This is always done by attacking troops because these steeples made fine observation posts for ... [enemy] spotters to bring down fire on the invaders. Since we were the invaders, it was necessary to remove as many advantages for the defenders as possible.

Near St. Martin de Varreville the regimental command post was established and our detachment settled down in foxholes for our first of many nights and days that we would face the enemy.

7. Beanie, Ernie and More

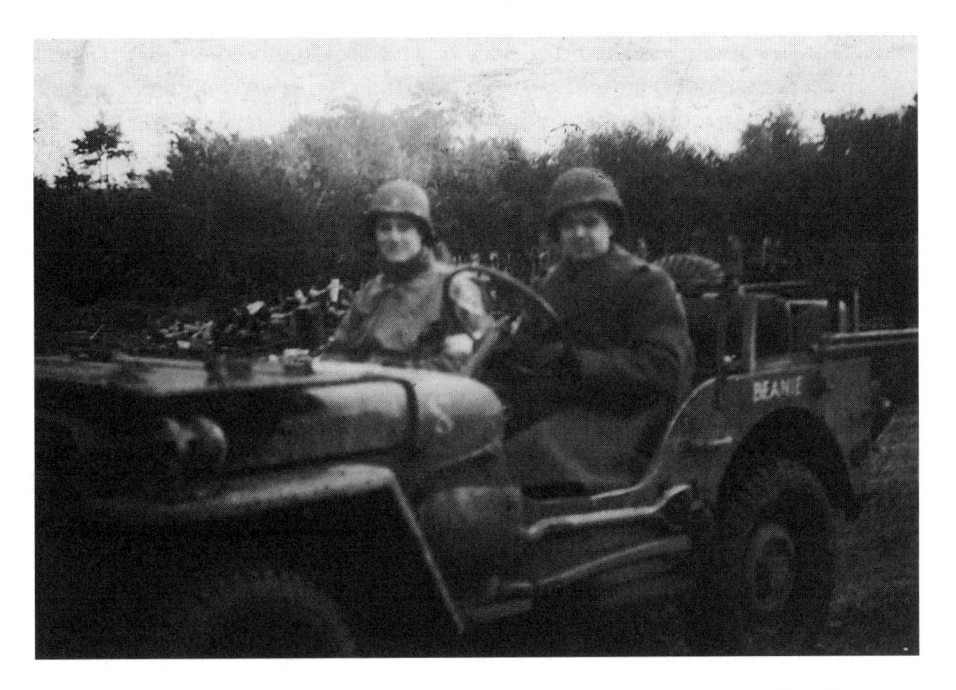

Major James M. Kirtley with his driver, T-4 Stanley Osowski in "Beanie," their Jeep, named for Dr. Kirtley's son David J. Kirtley. *Courtesy of Dr. James M. Kirtley.*

On this first night ashore, we were thankful for the relative ease of our landing and were enthralled by the fireworks display we could see from our foxholes. Anti-aircraft batteries were firing at inquisitive German aircraft and the tracer bullets of lavender, white, and red gave forewarning of what we would see in the future.

Utah Beach and on to Germany

The first night's bivouac near St. Martin de Varreville was spent with a feeling of thanksgiving that we had been able to get ashore so easily and that our regiment had had so few casualties. However, there were some heartbreaking events and the one that stands out in my mind was the accidental death of one of our fine officers. He was marching down a road just in front of one of our tanks when the gunner in the turret was thrown against his weapon, discharging it and killing the young father who left a small child for his wife to raise. This tragedy would be repeated many times in the coming months, not in the same way but in the deaths of the flower of young manhood. War is senseless!

Cherbourg was the prize that we were striving for and the German soldiers that stood in our way were determined that we would not reach it. One regimental combat team of the Ninetieth Infantry Division landed soon after our three regiments were ashore and they were assigned the task of knocking out the fortifications on our right flank. They moved very slowly and the corps commander was not pleased with their progress. One of the first tough objectives was the village of Ozeville, and we found the Germans in excellent defensive positions and with plenty of firepower to impede our progress. Sergeant Osowski and I went forward to check on the evacuation of wounded and were told by some of our front-line guys to get the heck out because there was no help that we could give them by our presence....

When I returned to my aid station one day, after an inspection trip, I heard of the complete collapse of one of my battalion surgeons who ... [was suffering] from extreme battle neurosis and had [had] to be strapped to a litter so that he could be evacuated to the rear. He was certain that his entire group was going to be killed and that the Germans were moving toward us in an unstoppable fashion. He was the only officer I lost in such a way but there might have been many more [elsewhere] because of the long times they had to serve. I think that there should have been a better way of relieving front line troops than waiting until they were killed or wounded. We had no system of rotation of medical officers that would have allowed fresh men to assume the duties of their peers and let them get away from such stressful responsibilities....

Paris Freed

On the night of August 25-26, 1944, there was some small arms fire to be heard but the artillery pieces were not being put into action. A few of us Twenty-second Headquarters medics had made the unofficial visit to the heart of Paris but had returned to our own area prior to midnight. Orders were issued that night for the motor march through Paris the next day and there was a feeling of exhilaration in all our souls.

There was some concern that German snipers might be stationed along the line of march but we heard not one explosion as we moved along. The Free French partisans (FFI) were to be seen watching the background for any evidence of hostile action. These people were truly patriots and many of them were caught and executed summarily in the months before the Allied invasion. They were the true heroes of the resistance.

By 0800 hours our turn had come to get into the convoy which was moving into the city and our jeep "Beanie" was loaded with our equipment and we joined the parade of joy. In the very outskirts of Paris there was not much activity by the locals but within a short time crowds of people began gathering on the sidewalks and were waving French and American flags and shouting their thanks to us. Flowers were tossed to the men on the trucks and wine and cognac ... [were] was offered to the guys by people running along the side of the column. There were many times when the march would stop and this gave the happy people time to give hugs and kisses to the not-embarrassed GIs....

As darkness approached we were given a general area to camp for the night, ... [which was] close [to] the headquarters of our regiment. We found a walled garden behind one of the houses and our medics climbed over and bedded down, feeling some security because of the brick and mortar that made up the wall. There was no reaction from the people inside the house but we were sure that they were aware of our presence. The next morning the boys broke out the little stove to heat our C-Rations for breakfast and the people in the house now made themselves known and told us that we were most welcome to use their facilities. Their names were Mr. and Mrs. Legrin, living in the Livry-Gargan section of Paris.

Our movement from this time on was not too rapid and on the afternoon of the 27th we were parked and instructed to stay there until the general movement got going again. Some of my medics had not been able to go on our first foray into downtown Paris and they asked permission to use my jeep and do a little sight seeing. Being the usual fall guy, I agreed and our First Sergeant ... was put in charge. Time marched on and our headquarters moved out but I was left on a curb silently burning and wondering when the nuts would return for me—if ever! They finally showed up and I vented my spleen, particularly [on the] Sergeant ... but I decided not to reduce him in rank because he knew how to run the outfit and this was no time to train a replacement....

Ernest Hemingway

The next part of my story involves the eminent author Ernest Hemingway, who was a war correspondent for several periodicals and an adventurer of the first order. He was attached to the First United States Infantry Division for the Omaha Beach landing and, for some reason, he later attached himself to the Twenty-second Infantry Regiment for several weeks....

Ernest Hemingway was his own man and sometimes bent the rules for his own advantage. For one thing, he always was armed, whether with an Army .45 or a Thompson submachine gun. Correspondents were supposed to be protected by the Geneva Convention, as were chaplains and medics, but Ernie never knew when he might meet a Kraut who didn't care a fig about the Geneva Convention. In addition, he felt that he had a special right to get into Paris as soon as he could, and he threaded his way through the streets of that city, heading for his favorite headquarters, the Ritz Hotel.

Parenthetically, let me say that I had met Mr. Hemingway at the behest of Colonel Lanham who suggested that I make a "housecall" on the writer when he complained of having a cold. This occurred before we had reached the outskirts of Paris and when we were bivouacked in a small French town. He was most gracious to me and apologized for any inconvenience he had caused. I am sorry to say that our medical supplies carried few medicines for respiratory infections so I think I checked his throat and gave him a few aspirin tablets. I believe another writer, Jimmy Cannon, was with him at the time, and he thanked me, too....

Pursuit

Although the Twenty-second Infantry was not completely motorized, as we had been at one time at home, there were enough trucks available to transport the foot soldiers on the rapid ride through northern France. By September 7, 1944, our command post had reached Graide, Belgium, and we had the satisfaction of entering the environs of another foreign country....

The Twenty-second Infantry Regiment had been given the mission of getting into Germany as quickly as possible and this was accomplished on the 11th of September when Lt. C.M. Shugart of the Double Deucers led a patrol across the border into Germany at 2130 hours (9:30 P.M.). They brought back a container of German soil that was to be sent to President Roosevelt. I wonder if he ever received it.

I don't recall just how I happened to be in the right vicinity at the right time, but Stan Osowski, "Beanie," and I were in a small column near the village of Buchet and we stopped to have our first view of the dragon's teeth impediments of the famed Siegfried Line on September 12, 1944. There was no doubt that Germans occupied the bunkers that were part of the line, but we were not fired on at that time. The dragon's teeth were tetrahedral concrete structures placed in a staggered manner and designed to impede the progress of our armored vehicles, primarily tanks. Thus they acted much in the same way that the hedgerows in Normandy [did in holding] up tank action. The enemy artillery and bazookas could then attack the slowed down tanks and destroy them.

The Twenty-second Infantry was able to mount an attack against the "Siegfried Line" on September 14, 1944, and were successful in penetrating several hundred yards against a determined German resistance and a counterattack that had one battalion surrounded for a while until it was relieved by our reserve battalion. There were several casualties among our boys and some were killed.

The unit remained in the area paralleling the Siegfried Line for several weeks and some soldiers did have a chance to return to nearby Belgium and be entertained by USO people and to have regular meals served by our field kitchens. An area near a small stream near Buchet was picked to set up a bath unit complete with showers with hot water and everybody received a change of underwear, which had not been possible for some time! The bath units were amenities furnished by the army and were much appreciated.

The small streams furnished the water, but it was purified and heated by the mobile equipment generic to such a unit. In my whole time in the combat zone I can remember but two such luxurious events. The usual "washing the body" procedure was accomplished by getting hot water from the field kitchen and using the steel helmet as a wash bowl....

Hurtgen Forest, the Bulge, Across the Rhine, and the End of the War

I cannot speak for ... combat [in the whole of] ... other than the European Theater of Operations, but I do know [about] a small conflict that ranks as one of the deadliest battles endured by the American soldiers. It is said that the Battle of the Hurtgen Forest is akin to Château-Thierry, the Meuse-Argonne, ... [and] even Antietam [or] ... the Wilderness.

The Fourth Division had spent most of September and October of 1944 refitting and training replacement troops who filled in the depleted ranks of the fighting units. The Twenty-second Infantry Regiment of the Fourth had lost many men in battle....

On November 9th the regiment moved from the fairly quiet area in Belgium to the forbidding darkness of deep woods, south and east of Aachen, Germany, to the Zweifall entrance to the Hurtgen Forest. The Fourth Division was to take over the holding mission of the Twenty-eighth

Division and the lineup was Twelfth Regiment on the left or northern flank, The Twenty-second Regiment in the middle, and the Eighth Regiment on the right flank....

Preparations were being made [from] the 10th to the 15th of the month for the coming offensive by digging foxholes and setting up mortar and machine gun sites for the initial jump-off toward the Cologne plain. It was the mission of the Fourth Division to break through the deep woods and open a path for following troops to pursue rapidly the Germans who hopefully would be retreating to their fatherland across the Rhine.

Any battle plan sounds plausible, given the expertise inherent in the planners, but it had to be remembered that while objectives were easily reached on the battle maps, a determined enemy, fighting on his own ground, could make success much more difficult.

The forest itself was a magnificent mass of mostly conifers that had grown into a woods that presented the toughest type of resistance to our penetration. There were many poorly marked trails and a series of very narrow firebreaks at irregular intervals. The Germans had prepared the trails carefully with mines, booby-traps and trip wires and had mortar and machine gun emplacements that could make any movement of an invader most unpleasant....

Contact with the enemy was immediate and severe with mortar fire and machine gun fire cutting the first soldiers to pieces as they advanced. German artillery fire was extremely bad and our boys were subjected to another terrible hazard, the tree bursts of the artillery shells that rained a deadly shower on them.

No one could accuse our men of cowardice for they moved forward in spite of the hellish fire and gained ground up to 500 yards, routing out determined Germans from their small fortifications. Because of the tree-bursts and the shrapnel that descended straight down, it was necessary, when there was no active attack, to dig into the forest floor and place heavy logs on top of a hole with several feet of earth ... [on top of them]. This arrangement made a fairly secure hidey-hole unless one was unfortunate enough to get a direct hit from a mortar shell or aerial bomb from the sometimes active German Luftwaffe.

Severe casualties were encountered during the entire battle and our aid men were real heroes in responding to the calls for medics and going to the fallen comrades without regard for their own safety. Litter bearers were doing the same type of heroic duty and carried the wounded many yards back to the battalion aid station that was always situated just behind the fighting line. Here the wounded received their first professional medical care from battalion surgeons, but the aid men had already done the

7. *Beanie, Ernie and More* 37

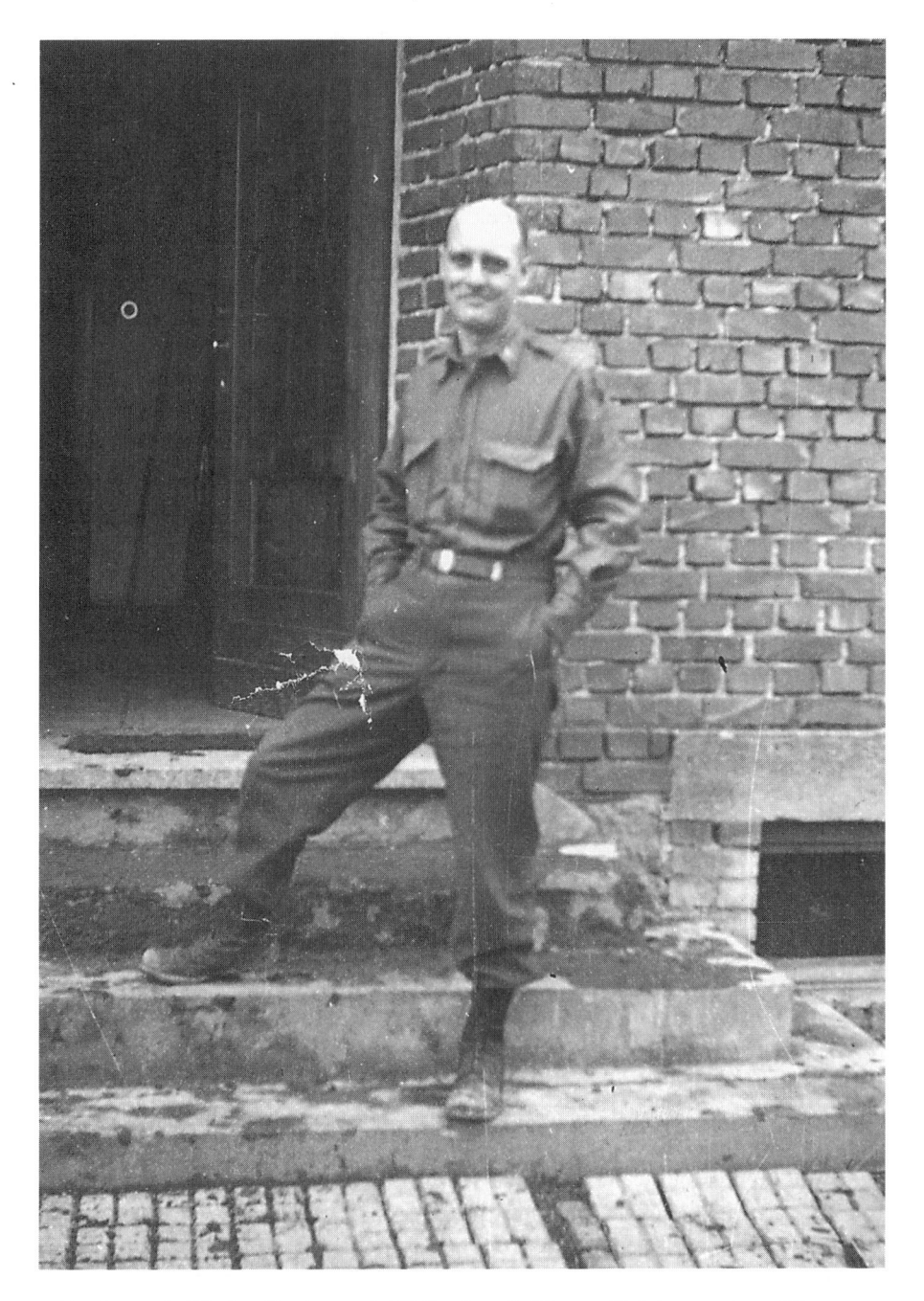

Dr. James A. Kirtley, Regimental Aid Station, Bullingen, Belgium, prior to Hurtgen Forest. *Courtesy of Dr. James M. Kirtley.*

primary job of dressing wounds and giving the boys morphine as indicated. Company C of the Fourth Medical Battalion was the supporting unit for the Twenty-second Infantry. Their ambulances moved forward to the aid stations to relieve them of their burden by evacuating the wounded to their own medical installation. Their dressings were inspected, replenished, and shock victims treated with blood plasma, if needed.

The regimental command post was a converted German trailer that had been "liberated," and [from it] Colonel Charles T. Lanham and his staff were able to keep track of the activities of the fighting battalions. The site of the command post was on top of a small hill and was accessed from the rear by one of the roads through the forest. One day a jeep came roaring up the hill and out jumped Ernest Hemingway with his Tommy-gun at the ready, for we were under German mortar fire that often meant an enemy attack in progress. Mr. Hemingway consulted with our commander, and after that he made frequent visits until we were relieved.

The immediate objective of the Twenty-second was the village of Grosshau and a nearby hamlet called Gey. Grosshau was finally captured after a terrible battle, for the Germans had fortified every house and they had to be reduced, one by one. We were in and out of Gey several times because the enemy counterattacks were difficult to meet and we were relieved by elements of the Eighty-third Division before that place was securely in our hands....

It is difficult to recount the terrible privations that the soldiers endured in the battle. The weather was very bad most of the time with rain and snow making them miserable. Most foxholes were inhabited by two men and the companionship they developed was life giving. Water in the holes could not be drained out and even the sturdy GI boots did little to give protection. Overshoes were distributed later but not in time to make much difference.

Dry socks were delivered when rations were carried forward, which wasn't too often. The men were encouraged to remove their shoes frequently, and each man massaged his companion's feet so that circulation was encouraged. Wet socks were wrung out as completely as possible and then put inside the undershirt next to the skin so as to help dry them. In spite of this many soldiers developed "trench foot," and most had to be evacuated, some to lose toes or portions of the foot because of the gangrene that developed. These were called "non-battle casualties," but they were just as devastating as wounds from shrapnel or rifle fire.

The frightful conditions of the foxholes, the never-ending enemy cannon and mortar fire, the lack of warm food, combined to produce another sort of non-battle casualty which was called "battle fatigue," or stress syndrome. These poor soldiers had to be evacuated, hopefully to receive psychiatric care and possibly to return to their units in due time. Many, however, did not make [a] good recovery and were the victims of a complex mental-physical condition that remained for many years.

The doleful statistics for the Twenty-second Infantry Regiment for the period November 16 through December 3, 1944, attest the terrible punishment suffered by our men. They are: Killed in action—enlisted men, 126, officers, 12; Wounded in action—enlisted men, 1,782, officers, 77; Missing in action (mostly POW)—enlisted men, 178, officers, 6; Non-battle casualties—enlisted men, 489, officers, 8. Total casualties: enlisted men, 2,575, officers, 103. Grand total: 2,678.

On the plus side, however, is the fact that twenty-five enemy units were met and decimated or annihilated during this period of time. The troops they met and defeated were not home guard or poorly trained soldiers, but some of the best the Germans had because they realized that if we were not stopped, the future for them was bleak indeed.

We were to fight many more battles before the Germans were finally defeated, but in none of these ... [were] the intense suffering and the number of casualties so pronounced. Hurtgen Forest has been called "The Place of Death," and for good reason.

Horrors of Hurtgen Forest Battle Not Forgotten

The horrors of the Hurtgen Forest battle were not forgotten, but it was with a sense of thankful relief that the Fourth Division began pulling out of that fearful area on December 4, 1944, having been relieved by the Eighty-third Infantry Division.

The Eighty-third had been guarding the banks of the Moselle River in Luxembourg, and the Fourth was to take their positions in this relatively quiet sector. The 130 mile road march from the Hurtgen area to Luxembourg was without incident, and I remember our column moving along the streets of Luxembourg City in silence, but no longer dread. Our destination was the village of Senningen, east of the capital city....

Headquarters of the Twenty-second moved to Mondorf on December 10th, and remained there until the 21st when it again moved to Rodenbourg and occupied the nice home of the village priest. My detachment was placed in a pleasant little house, still occupied by the owners, who seemed to be content to have us there. A friendly white cat by the name of Robert (pronounced in the French fashion by the family) got a lot of attention from my boys, and he was wise enough to know where the goodies were coming from. We all tried our French on the family and a regular routine was "Ou est Robert?" The answer, "Ah! Robert a parti, promenade avec bon ami." ["Where is Robert?" "Robert is gone. He is walking with his good friend."]

As Christmas neared our boys were not going to let the season pass unnoticed, and they produced a small tree and made some decorations for it. Headquarters also had a tree with trimmings, and it was almost pleasant except for the fact that von Rundstedt had already launched his forces against our thin line at Echternach where the Twelfth Infantry Regiment was on guard.

We had heard about some of Mr. Hemingway's escapades and that he was separated from his current wife, war correspondent Martha Gelborn. Who should show up at Headquarters but Martha herself, and she decided to share Christmas with us. I don't know just what Ernie's reaction was, but I think he was gracious enough to have Christmas dinner with her....

Post "Bulge" Activity

The Fourth Division met with sporadic resistance as we moved to the east, but on some days many miles were passed without a shot being fired. President Roosevelt's death in April sent a shiver through the armies, but President Truman's determination to carry out the policies of Roosevelt's administration became known and the war went on to victory in May of 1945....

The Twenty-second Infantry wound up its drive in the city of Ansbach, and the regimental headquarters was housed in a needle factory; yes, a sewing needle works. It was clean and comfortable, and we were glad to be anywhere in peace. A beautiful little town of Heilbronn was the last command post for my detachment, and we soon moved to an area south of Bamberg where we prepared for our return to the United States....

The division finally settled at Camp Old Gold near the French port of Le Havre, and we went aboard a clean little ship, the army transport, *General Parker*, on July 3, 1945, and were greeting the Statue of Liberty on July 11. What a wonderful sight!

Chapter Eight

From Med School to France
SHELLEY M. STRAIN, M.D.

Dr. Strain recalls his work at the front in Europe, as well as some unusual recreational time.

I graduated from Case Western Reserve University Medical School at Cleveland, Ohio, in June 1942. At the time of my graduation there were two universities, Case and Western Reserve, located across the street from each other. Several years ago they merged. Case was primarily an engineering school. Reserve featured an undergraduate college and schools of medicine, pharmacy, and dentistry. It also had a school of nursing. I interned in Pathology July 1–31, 1942, at the Institute of Pathology, CWRU, under Howard Karsner, M.D., Professor of Pathology. Then from January 1, 1943, to December 31, 1943, I interned in Internal Medicine at New York Postgraduate Hospital, New York City.

I entered the U.S. Army Medical Corps on December 31, 1943, with the rank of first lieutenant. My first six weeks were spent at Carlisle Barracks, Pennsylvania, with about 600 physicians and dentists being taught how to be army officers. It was anything but amusing, interesting, or even ridiculous. I rode the train from Harrisburg to Penn Station in New York City almost every weekend to see my wife, who was employed in engineering at Gibbs & Cox, Marine Architects.

I arrived in the ETO [European Theater of Operations] in November 1944 onboard the USS *Westpoint* (formerly the USS *America*—a passenger ship), via Camp Miles Standish and Boston, in Massachusetts, and Liverpool, England. The English were friendly to us Americans and glad we were there.

I first attended wounded in a U.S. general hospital in Rheims, France, which occupied a previous French private hospital on the edge of town. It was much like treating patients at home who had been admitted to an emergency room. At the age of 27 years, physical and mental stress did not exist for me. At the general hospital hours were essentially eight or ten each day, except when I was OD (officer of the day).

I joined the Ninth Evac as a replacement in January 1945 at Rambervillers and stayed until August 1945 when the Ninth Evac came home. The Ninth Evac's is an interesting story. The *M*A*S*H* television series with Alan Alda resembled the Ninth Evac except most of the patients arrived by ambulance, rather than helicopter. The Ninth Evac was a reserve hospital from Roosevelt Hospital in New York City. The medical staff and nurses had some connection with this hospital, and most of the enlisted personnel were from Brooklyn. The hospital had arrived in England at an early date, and when North Africa was invaded to confront Rommel, the Ninth Evac went in at Oran. They supported the conflict across North Africa to Bizerte, Tunisia, until Rommel surrendered. Next they went to Sicily, thence to Naples, Italy, where they set up in the Naples Fairgrounds and functioned as a French general hospital for nine or ten months. Most of the team became fluent in French. Next was the invasion of Southern France and a rapid sweep up the Rhone Valley.

In the Ninth Evac Hospital where I was on a surgical team, we worked 12-hour shifts in surgery and postoperative care of patients. When the front was nearby, it was busy, with 90 to 100 surgeries in 24 hours. Off-duty activities ranged from sleeping to skiing, to sailboating and faltboating.

In March 1945 the Ninth Evac was still in Rambervillers, France. The active front had moved ahead, and we were finished receiving new patients until we also moved ahead. Three of our surgeons who were from New England states and liked to ski went to nearby Grenoble (a French ski resort) for several days of skiing. I went one day, accompanying the group that took them food. Later in 1945 at the close of most military action in Germany, the Ninth Evac Hospital was in Landsburg. These same three spent several days in Innsbruck, Austria, skiing down a 6,000 foot mountain that is ascended by three cable cars from (practically downtown) and is the old Olympic ski run.

Dr. Larry Poole, the neurosurgeon, was acquainted with Munich where he had worked in the summer between his junior and senior medical school years. He looked up a German physician, Ludwig Saenger, who lived on the Ammer See. He was the author of books on sailing and owned many small sailboats some of which Larry arranged for us to sail.

Larry went to Rosenheim and arranged the factory purchase of about 30 faltboats (folding boats) by the physicians. Larry had a father and two brothers who were prominent New York City surgeons. They were members of the New York Boat Club, and Larry had been on two around-the-world sailings in his youth.

We used the faltboats on nearby streams when we were in Landsburg, the summer of 1945. The boat folds into two packs, one for each man to carry. There are also single-person boats. The trip (which I did not do) was a two-day trip down the Inn River from Innsbruck to Rosenheim. From Rosenheim to Munich was a short electric train ride back.

I returned home in late November 1945.

Chapter Nine

Nearsighted and Flat Footed

STANLEY A. KORNBLUM, M.D.

With poor vision, Dr. Kornblum was turned down by the navy, air force, and marines before finally serving with the U.S. Army.

My father was a physician; he graduated from the Long Island College of Medicine in 1909. I graduated from the same school in 1940. I started to intern on July 1, 1940, at King's County Hospital in Brooklyn, New York. On Pearl Harbor Day, December 7, 1941, I was on duty at the hospital.

I returned to my home in Monticello, New York, for a Christmas visit to my folks. Monticello is a small village, the county seat of Sullivan County, about 100 miles northwest of New York City. We decided at that time that I would apply for active duty as we felt, the family felt, that it was our job to take care of the Nazis. Even though I was deferred from the draft because I had a residency coming up on July 1, 1942, in Chicago, the feeling was still the same. Accordingly, upon my return to New York City during January 1942, I applied to the navy, air force, and to the marines, only to be turned down because of my poor vision. I was markedly nearsighted at that time. I finally applied to the Army Medical Corps, and was ordered to Fort Hamilton in Brooklyn, New York, for my physical in March 1942. It was a very interesting phenomenon. When they took my blood pressure my systolic (the upper number) was below 100, and the corporal informed me that I could not pass the physical. I informed him that if I jumped up and down 50 times that I was sure I could raise my blood pressure to the required level, which I accordingly did. My blood pressure was then acceptable.

Next came my eyes. Since I could not even see the letters on the board, the captain came in and told me to tell him how many fingers he was holding up. I said, "Five fingers." He said, "Take one pace nearer. How many fingers?" I said, "Four." He said, "One pace nearer. How many fingers?" I said, "Three." He said, "Fingers, eighteen feet." Accordingly, I was then acceptable to the Army Medical Corps after I had signed my name to many forms, waivers, as it were, because of my poor eyesight and my flatfeet. On this basis I was allowed to enter the Army Medical Corps as a physician on limited service—limited service meant I wasn't allowed to go into any combat or be with any combat troops.

I continued with my duties as an intern until finally, towards the end of April 1942, I received a telegram from the War Department in Washington ordering me to Fort Sam Houston. I did not know where Fort Sam Houston was. I then arranged to take the train in the beginning of May of 1942 and traveled to San Antonio, Texas.

Now the telegram said to report to the commanding general, so I walked into the headquarters and asked to see the general. The colonel looked at me and said, "Lieutenant, you can see me. I'm the adjutant here; the General is busy."

So I reported to this colonel, and all I had to do along with several dozen other reserve army officers of the Medical Corps, recently inducted, was to report every morning to him to see if any orders had been cut. I was assigned to the Eighth Service Command, and finally, after ten days, ordered to Fort Sill in Lawton, Oklahoma.

When I got to Fort Sill I pulled up to the BOQ, the bachelor officers' quarters, and reported to the colonel in charge of the station hospital. I was assigned two wards, and when I went to see what my assignment was, the sergeant in charge of the two wards gave me some forms to sign, which I did. I asked what I was signing for. He told me all the equipment from the linens right on down to the bedpans and urinals, all of which I was responsible for. If anything was missing when I gave up this post, I would have to pay for it out of my army pay.

I was the only Yankee in the BOQ, and the rest of the officers were West Pointers, or National Guard, or Reservists from that area of the country. I was unique. Here I was, a Yankee, a New Yorker, and Jewish. Some fun! However, I got along very well with my peers; they had never seen a Jewish chap before, and they realized I didn't have horns, or cloven feet, or a tail. As a matter of fact, Fort Sill is an artillery post, and they took me out into the field and taught me how to run a battery of four 75 millimeter guns. In those days we did not know much about hearing and loud noises, and we didn't cover our ears or anything. I want to tell you, when I bracketed the target and had the battery of 75 go off, my head rang for over a day.

Now there I was at Fort Sill. I rolled out of bed at 5:30 in the morning, had breakfast, and had to get to the station hospital by seven o'clock for sick call. I'll never forget the time I was standing on the corner waiting for a bus, and a dumpy old man in a uniform came by in this miserable weather with a whole bunch of chaps behind him and he yelled out, "Where's that salute, Lieutenant?" I looked around. "Who the hell is he talking to?" Then it dawned on me that I was the lieutenant he had referred to, and he was a colonel, a lieutenant colonel, leading his brigade, or platoon, or whatever it was, on some sort of march. As an aside, you must realize that I spent four years in the service, and no one ever told me who I was to salute, or who I was not to salute.

Today Killeen, Texas, about 40 miles west of Waco, is a city of over 50,000 or 60,000. Back in 1942 it was a village of maybe 500 people. I was very much impressed with Camp Hood because when I asked the soldier, the guard, at the entrance gate where the station hospital was, he knew where it was. I reported to the adjutant of the hospital whose name was Joe Bassett, who was an old army sergeant who because of the war situation had been promoted to the temporary rank of major.

First thing he asked me was, "What do you need, Lieutenant?"

And I said, "I need some hot water. Of course, I want to take a shower and get my clothes cleaned up."

No way! They were still building the hospital station.

I was assigned to the outpatient department at Camp Hood, and I wrote to my father telling him how things were going, what things were like. I explained to him that I rode to Killeen and Waco, changed my clothes, took a shower, took my dirty laundry to a Chinese laundry, and then drove back to Camp Hood. The next week I would repeat this. In other words, I was riding roughly 140 miles once a week in order to have a clean shirt.

My wife was a nurse who trained at Bryn Mawr Hospital, Bryn Mawr, Pennsylvania. I met her in September or October 1942 at Camp Hood. It was a very interesting romance. It started about November 1942, and a couple of years later we got married before we went overseas to the European theater. We had to keep the marriage secret while at Camp Hood because husbands and wives couldn't be stationed together. It was okay to be boyfriend and girlfriend, but not married.

One of the things that did happen in Texas as a part of my job was that I had to review all officers that were ordered overseas to make sure they were physically fit. And I did some other jobs. My colonel liked me very much in that I always produced.

My father got very lonely; he was a widower, and he thought he would come down to see his only son. And I'll never forget how embarrassed I was when he finally came down to Killeen, Texas. I told him the closest hotel with any sort of accommodations was in Waco, roughly 40 miles away, or Temple, Texas, which was 35. Ultimately, he put up in the visitors' barracks, which he wasn't too happy with either, so I asked my colonel if he could possibly stay with me in my quarters in the BOQ, and he said "Yes," and that's what my dad did for about the week he spent with me. I'll never forget I introduced him to my colonel, and guess what my father said? Here I am a physician, an army officer, and he said to the colonel, "How's my boy doing?" like I was in the third grade. For some reason the colonel liked my father, and he really seemed to like him very much, and he always asked me for years afterward whenever I met him at various places around the country how my father was.

As part of my duties, I was a member of a group of three officers which had to pass everyone that went overseas. I was the junior member but knew all the rules and regulations. One day I had an army colonel come in for duty overseas who was asthmatic, and I told him he couldn't go overseas, and he really got furious with me. Slapped down his orders which were bordered in red, labeled top secret, and told me the following story. We had discovered we could use light tanks in the CBI (China, Burma, India Theater). He was a tank expert just back from Iceland, he was going out to the CBI to be Joe Stilwell's deputy chief of staff, and the army knew all about it. He was a West Pointer, and if he took a little adrenaline his asthma would not flare up. I asked him why he didn't take a little bit of adrenaline before he came in to see me, seeing he was wheezing like a calliope, and even my staff sergeant could hear him.

My experiences at Camp Hood were great, except that I almost got shot several times going out into the field with the ambulance whenever they went on maneuvers. One time when I fell asleep, some damn fool set up a machine gun right above me. Thank God, I rolled to one side when they started shooting live ammo. Another time the air corps came in strafing, and they were a little bit short, and the bullets went right through the ambulance. Thank God, I was not in the ambulance. I was lying off to one side watching all this training.

We were killing about five or six men a week in training. They were shot going through the "Nazi Village" and the infiltration course, and in accidents on maneuvers.

I spent several months treating German POWs in a camp at Mexia, Texas. I had one of their men assigned to me who spoke English. He was my sergeant. I had some very interesting experiences doing this. I spent several months in the POW camp before I came back to Camp Hood. One of the things that most impressed me was that there were two distinct age groups: 18 to 20 and 25 and up. I didn't understand what had happened to the men 20 to 25. I discovered that most of them were tied up at the Russian Front.

I also had the experience of asking about a medal, an Iron Cross. I had my sergeant snap to attention and tell me about it. "Sir! He got that at the Eastern Front."

Another chap had what I thought was a Polish-sounding name, and I made the mistake of asking if he came from Poland. Whoa! boy, did he really jump on me! Thank God, I was in uniform, and I had my MPs around.

I went home on leave in '43. When I came back I discovered that a lot of the medical officers and most of the personnel in my station hospital, who were on limited service like me, were using their eyesight as an excuse to get out of going overseas. They had been ordered to the ETO [European Theater of Operations], actually England, to man hospitals there in preparation for D-Day.

I told the colonel (I felt very strongly about it) that if my eyes were as bad as they were, and I believed I could go overseas, then these other characters could. So I decided to pass everybody and, of course, I became very unpopular. Before I knew it I was about the only one of the old gang still at Camp Hood.

The colonel one day called me in and said, "…I've kept you here for 18 months because you've done a great job, and now I've got to ship you out. Where do you want to go?"

"Well, I don't want to go to the CBI or to the South Pacific. I know nothing about tropical diseases and don't like what I did see from the men coming back. I'll take my chances in the ETO."

So the old man fixed me up, and I went off to the ETO. I was assigned to the 123rd General Hospital, and most of the staff that joined that hospital knew their way around. Came from the Midwest, Ohio, Indiana, some of us from New York, some from Pennsylvania.

We went overseas on the *Queen Mary*. We had 15,000 troops onboard. We had a very nice cabin. We had about sixteen in my cabin and bunk beds, four-tiered bunks, one above the other.

Someone in one of the combat outfits came into our area and wanted to know if we played poker. I played nickel-and-dime poker back in Texas. I said, "Yeah."

We sat down, and they told me it was table stakes. I had never played table stakes before, and I was horrified at the amounts of money coming

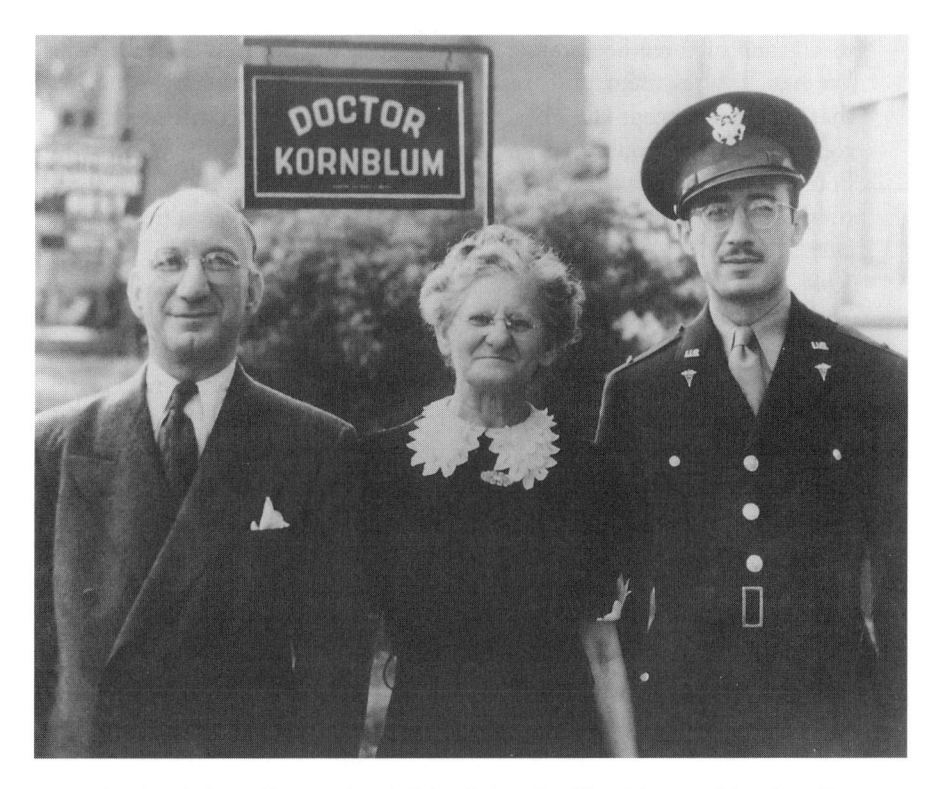

Dr. Stanley A. Kornblum, right, with his father, Dr. Kornblum, and his Aunt Rae in May 1942. *Courtesy of Dr. Stanley A. Kornblum.*

out, not only American money, but also foreign money; where they got it in the States, I don't know. I say foreign money, I mean English money. However, when I got off the vessel in Glasgow, Scotland, I ended up with $1,200, which was a large sum of money in 1944. This money was of no use to me because I couldn't buy anything in England; everything was rationed. So I sent the money home to my dad to hold for me when I got out of the service so my wife and I would have something to start with.

It took us approximately a week, six days to cross the Atlantic, zigzagging across, and we ended up at Glasgow in the middle of the night. We were put on trains and went south to a place outside Hereford, England. We got dumped out in the middle of nowhere about two o'clock in the morning and still pitch black, even at that time. This was June 1944, and I turned on my flashlight to look for my duffel bag, and some limey said, "Put that light out, or I shoot!" And I heard the bolt going back, so I put out my light mighty fast!

We were put up at a place called Foxly Manor. Then we were assigned to a group of three hospitals, including one American and one British. We had lectures there, and treated war wounds, so forth and so on. At that time the concept of early ambulation was just coming in and also the concept that you could debride wounds that were packed open over in France and do what they call secondary closures. Now, as a part of my training just two years before back in '40, '41, '42, that was a no-no, but over here we were able to do it. We also got our first penicillin in August 1944.

We were told not to go into London because of the buzz bombs coming in. However, we—this colonel at the 123rd General Hospital and I—decided to go in. We went in and stayed at the Princess Margaret Hostel which was set up for troops that were coming into London and run by the Red Cross. There were two types of buzz bombs. The V-1s: you could hear the "putt, putt, putt, putt…", then they cut out and went into their dive, and there was a big explosion when they hit the ground. The V-2s were rockets and you never heard them until they hit with a massive explosion. As long as you heard the explosion, you knew you were alive.

That first night in town we had tickets for the theater. There's a lot of beautiful theater all through England, legitimate theater, and during intermission this colonel and I went into the bar attached to the theater for a highball, and while we were there (we were the only Americans in the bar) the glasses on the bar started to jump up and down. There was a loud noise, and this limey, this English officer, turned around to us after I had made a remark that they must have built the subway very close to the bar. He said to me, "You bloody Yanks! That was a buzz bomb that went off!"

Well, that night, all night long, the buzz bombs were going off. So the next morning, I said to the colonel, "You know, we should get better quarters. We're going to get killed if we stay around here." So we went over to one of the largest hotels, I can't think of its name now, and I went up to the desk clerk, and I asked for a room. The desk clerk said there was nothing available. When I insisted that they must have a room in a hotel this size, he replied, "You know, Captain, we have half of SHAEF [Supreme Headquarters Allied Expeditionary Force] here; the other half is in France. We have the Free Dutch, the Free French, the Free Danish governments also housed here, plus others. We just don't have any room."

While he was telling me this I saw someone checking out, so I asked if we could not have his room. The desk clerk looked at us and told us that his room was not a room, it was a suite of rooms, and that the cost would be 16 pounds, which was the equivalent of $64—a lot of money for a night's sleep, a lot of money back in 1944.

9. Nearsighted and Flatfooted

Well, now that we had a suite of rooms, I had to push all the buttons. It was the first time I had seen a bidet; I didn't know what it was. I sure was a naïve young man. I called the colonel and said, "Look! Look at this thing. It must be a water fountain built for midgets." Neither one of us apparently knew. Shows how unsophisticated we were.

That night we went out for a meal on the black market, cause even though the food we could get at the hotel was nice, we wanted to sample some real food outside of the quarters. So we found a "black market" restaurant and paid an atrocious price for a meal, something like $25 or $30, which was a lot of money in those days, as I mentioned, but we had a very grand meal. On the black market you could get anything, even in England during the war.

I was sightseeing in a castle where King John put out the Magna Carta. Met two RAF officers doing the same thing. I had then been in the service over three years. I had two ribbons—one for the American theater and one for the ETO. Mind you there were 50 million people in Britain with no ribbons! The RAF men had a ribbon apiece with a small cluster on it. I asked them what the ribbon was for. Answer: 200 missions. The cluster a second 200. They were permanently grounded! We were sending our flyboys back after 50 missions. Asked how long they had been in the service. Answer: since 1939! I had to shut up and could not complain about my time in the service.

We would get convoys of wounded coming in at least once a week. I remember the *Stars and Stripes* in either October or November 1944 stating that there was light action in the Hurtgen Forest, and my God, we were getting back wounded like I could not believe. We operated for three or four days, day and night, and at the end of that period there would be a lull. There wouldn't be any more convoys coming in for a couple of days or a week, then a new convoy would come in. Those were the men we were able to get into fairly decent shape; we sent them to our rehab center. In the rehab center we took blood from them; we had them all typed. So we had a working bank for any blood we needed.

Among these convoys, invariably there would be someone asking for me by name. It was obvious that my wife's outfit was following Patton's army. The 189th General was acting as an evacuation hospital. This was the system. The front-line battalion aid stations were allowed to keep casualties for 96 hours; that's four days. They operated on them, emergency stabilized them, then shipped them back to us in the United Kingdom, in England. This was all done via the airstrips. There'd be someone asking for Captain Kornblum, and I would find out and speak to the soldier, and he'd say, "I saw your wife at airstrip A-15, or A-17, or

A-18." In view of this, I figured, boy, maybe I can get over and visit my wife.

I had done a skin graft on a sergeant from the Troop Carrier Command that was stationed in Oxford, England. And I spoke to him, and he said, "Yeah, our boys are always flying over there supplying Patton's army. And we fly to these various airstrips." A-18, or something like that was the last one my wife mentioned. I said, "How about that one?" He said, "Yeah, Doc, we can get you there."

I felt so good about that that I gave him a three-day pass. This was in December '44, and I got a three-day pass for myself and another physician who had a girlfriend over there in the same area as my wife's outfit. First Lieutenant Jack Voskamp came; he got a pass, also. We went down to the Troop Carrier Command. Now I can tell you during World War II, even though I was at a general hospital, the food was lousy. We had more dried milk, and dried eggs, and oh, stuff like that. K rations stuff, as far as I was concerned. But the air corps and the navy, they had real milk, real food, real eggs. There was ice cream; it was tremendous. Real meat! It was great! Accordingly, we took off in December '44, the three of us. Got to Oxford and arrangements were made for us to get aboard the airplanes which were Flying Boxcars, so-called, the C-130s. We were on the line around four o'clock in the morning when suddenly the field was closed down, and we were told to get off. They unpacked whatever they had on board and started packing the plane with jeeps and ammo and parapacks and other medical supplies as well as war supplies. We had no idea what was going on, and we spent the day lolling around playing with a Link trainer. The second day we could not find out anything, so that night I went to the colonel in charge of the airfield and told him that we would all be AWOL [absent without leave], including his mess sergeant, if we didn't get back to our outfit. So he gave us special dispensation to get off the post and get back to our outfits so we would not be AWOL. What had happened? The famous Battle of the Bulge where von Rundstedt, the German commander, broke through with troops and then blasted the hell out of the Ardennes Forest. We had a very thin line of troops there. We got back to the 123rd General, and sure enough, they started pulling all our ward boys, all our personnel that could handle a gun, and shipping them off to the front. As a matter of fact, as I read history, if von Rundstedt had broken through, he would have stopped the Allied front, driven a wedge between us, between our northern and southern portions. Then he may well have extended the war, or we may even have possibly lost.

It was the only time we got back mixed wounded; that is, normally the American hospital would get back American troops, the British hospital British troops, French hospital French troops, so forth and so on. Here we got back all kinds: Free French, Free Dutch, American troops, New Zealanders, Australians, South Africans; you name it, we got 'em. Now, of course, after we took care of these convoys of wounded, they went up to rehab, the bulk of them. There might be one that had to be sent back to the States, bad burns, other surgery that we could not accomplish very well in our setup; or they were so wounded or deformed that they had to be sent back to the States for rehab.

Anyhow, about April '45, a month before the end of the war, I suddenly got a phone call that my wife was at the railroad station in Hereford. I was really shocked! I was in a hot poker game; I had four aces in that hand, a big pot of money in the middle. My executive officer was a lieutenant colonel.... He said, "Yeah, take my jeep; you'd better pick her up. Throw in your hand." He took the whole pot.

I picked up my wife, and she was very indignant when she discovered, here she was living in a tent with the earth as a floor, having a helmet of water for washing purposes, drinking purposes, and here I was living in a Quonset hut, with hot water, hot showers, so forth and so on. I thought I was really roughing it, but I wasn't. She was the one who really roughed it.

In May '45, following the end of the war, V-E Day, our outfit broke up and I was transferred to southern England to Bournemouth, and I was amazed to see there were palm trees there along with all the barbed wire along the beaches. And I wondered, "Why palm trees?" After all, Bournemouth was at the same level as Hudson Bay in Canada. The reason for it, as I discovered, was the Gulf Stream which keeps the area warm and almost subtropical.

From Bournemouth I was transferred over to Europe to the continent itself. Before I left the 123rd I was taking a shower and one of the men taking a shower at the same time pointed out to me that I had a bulge in my groin. Sure enough, I had a hernia which had to be repaired, and I was not too happy with the thought. I flew from Bournemouth into Orly Field in Paris. They put me up overnight at the damnedest quarters I've ever seen, mirrored room. I didn't know what it was at all, but I found out later on, as I will remark very shortly.

When I got to this outfit, I presented myself for a physical to get ready to go over to the CBI, to Japan, to the South Pacific front, and I pointed out I had a hernia which had to be repaired, and it was done. As I mentioned earlier this was the time early ambulation was first coming in. I was trained just a few years before, and then hernia patients were kept in bed for at least two weeks. They could not do anything for several months. The army had a rule that you could not be on active duty for at least six weeks following a hernia repair. Well, I decided to stay in bed after my hernia was done, and I managed to do it for 11 days before the colonel who operated on me, a chap from the Chicago Medical School, blasted me loose, got me out of bed, and made sure I walked around. My wife was visiting me because we were located near Mourmelon-le-Petit, where her outfit was, which was about 40 kilometers south of Reims, France. She managed to get me transferred into her outfit, the 189th General. I was put in charge of the officers' ward, as I was a patient and couldn't do anything for six weeks. My wife and I had a lot of fun traveling around. We went up to Reims, looked at the cathedral, went to Paris, to the palace at Versailles, and did all the sightseeing there was to be done. As a matter of fact, we stayed at the George V Hotel in Paris. We saw the Duke and Duchess of Windsor pull up in a car, get out; I wanted to take their pictures, but my wife stopped me, but I wish I had insisted on taking them. My wife had liberated a German camera and got me started in photography. Anyhow, the stay in Paris was a good one.

Because my wife had the required number of points (she had more points than I did; in fact she had several battle stars for the same length of time in the service that I had), she was eligible to go home. I had to stay behind. When she left France, my wife was already pregnant. We apparently had planted our daughter in the George V Hotel in Paris.

Anyhow, in the 189th there was another officer from the States, a friend of mine by the name of Sam.... Sam was also assigned temporarily to the 189th as I was, and we were roommates. It was very interesting. Sam, one day, asked me if I'd play chess, and I said, yes, I'd be happy to play chess with him. And we did. As Sam was shaving, I'd call out my moves, and he didn't even bother to look at the board. He'd call out his moves, and I was checkmated in no time at all. After three games in a row like this at a dollar a throw or so, I refused to play any more and asked him how come he could do this. Then he confessed to me that he and I could play 15 games, come back a year later, and he'd be able to recite every move he and I had made in all those games.

Anyhow, Sam and I went into town one time, several times as a matter of fact, but this one time we went into town the European phase was well over. It was in the fall of 1945, and there were a lot of displaced persons wandering all over Europe. Many of these people who could speak a little bit of English were picked up and employed as guards around army installations. So we went into Mourmelon-le-Petit; I never knew what Mourmelon-le-Grand was, but le-Petit was a little hamlet with cows wandering around the streets, and chickens and so on. We had a few beers, and were coming back to camp, and this DP [displaced person] guard yelled, "Who goes there?" My friend Sam, who was a real wise guy, said in German..., "We are two American officers." I heard the guard pull the bolt back on his gun, and shouted, "Americans; don't shoot!" I hit Sam, we both hit the ground, and, thank God, the guard didn't shoot.

So that shows you all the enemy action I saw in four years in the service; V-1s and V-2s in London, in July or August of '44, and this DP guard who might have shot Sam and me if I hadn't cut my wise-guy friend off in time. That was it.

I did end up in a poker game and lost all my money the day before I was to go to Cannes, in southern France, on R&R [rest and relaxation].

I remarked earlier that I was in these very bizarre officers' quarters in Orly Field. Everyone laughed at me.

"You know where you were, Doctor?" one of them asked.

I said, "No."

Well, let me tell you what he told me. When they took over Orly Field, they took over all the "houses of ill repute," too, the red light district around the field. The room I was in was nothing more than one of the rooms in one of the "houses of ill repute." I spent the night in a French whorehouse and never knew it!

Now, I got down to Paris. Of course, in those days cigarettes were money, and I sold a carton of cigarettes for the equivalent of $20. The train ride to southern France was a long one because of frequent stops, and we had to spend the night on board the train till we got to the Rhone Valley. In southern France, they put us up in a beautiful hotel. The meals were excellent.

I was most curious about the medical situation there. I went to the local hospital, and through the Red Cross, was introduced, to the head of the hospital, the chief surgeon. He explained to me how the Germans had wiped out everything. What they could not take with them, they had destroyed. There was very little equipment in the hospital. He had a bottle of sulfa pills he had gotten from the American Embassy in Paris, which was a great thing, as he could take care of some of the infections that he was seeing.

I offered to take him to dinner. I was allowed to have one guest each night at dinner, so I was going to invite him, his wife, the children, and his mother-in-law on subsequent nights. He refused, saying that the only people who accepted such invitations were collaborators, the "riff-raff," hookers, and he wouldn't be linked with those types of people. He did invite me to his house for dinner one night, and it was a sad thing. There was very little to eat; it was all tinned meat from "Care" packages. When I got back to the States, my wife and I used to send his family "Care" packages every month for about a year.

Now my financial situation on this R&R was precarious. It was the only time I broke the law. What I did was, I would take all my old clothes, my army uniform and whatnot, down to the black market, and sell them high. Then I would go into the PX locally and buy a full new army uniform at low prices. I would wear that the next day, then take it down to the black market and sell it. And so on.

Finally my orders came through to return home. We shipped out of Antwerp, Belgium, on Christmas Eve, December 24, 1945. We had a layover in the estuary in the river because of the storms and mines in the Channel. We were onboard a Victory ship of about 10,000 or 11,000 tons, I would guess. This was the North Atlantic, and man alive, I never saw waves so big in all my life! It was a precarious voyage from my point of view. Everyone was seasick, including me, and I had the best deal. There I was lying in the ship in sick bay, passing out so-called seasick pills to the troops. All of them did very well, including myself. Within 48 hours we were under control, except for one man I had to fit with an I.V. so he would not get dehydrated from vomiting.

Now it seemed to me that the ship would go three knots forward and two knots backward with the weather that we had. On the way over we got a signal that someone had been injured on another vessel, and we were close by. We would go ahead and try to help this individual. The captain called me up and told me he would ship me over to the other ship on some sort of coxswain's something-or-other, and I didn't like the thought. The ship, my God, was rolling roughly 45°, it seemed to me, on each side of the center. The captain assured me that this wasn't bad weather for the North Atlantic during the middle of the winter. Fortunately, another ship got there first, and my services were not called upon.

We finally arrived three weeks later, about January 12, 1946, in New York City. Two weeks later I was still "rolling" as if I was aboard ship. I was discharged in April 1946 through Camp Dix. Our daughter, our first child, was born on June 16, 1946....

My final rank was major, Army Medical Corps, AUS [Army of the United States]. My wife's name was Caroline E. Holts Kornblum.... She is deceased. She died on May 30, 1993.

I should like to point out that war is a pile of ... nonsense. It doesn't accomplish anything. I've seen its death and destruction. War is made by old men and fought by young men. It is really wrong. Actually, it is fought by young men and women. And it's *really* wrong.

Chapter Ten

A World War II Remembrance of Luis Castillo

My father always said that the medics had a very hard job. Risking their lives in many cases for what were dead men.
—Al Castillo

Cpl. Luis Castillo, Company I, 9th Infantry Regiment, 2d Infantry Division, was 24 years old when he was drafted. This account was contributed by his son, Al Castillo, who taped an interview with his father before his father's death.

During the battle for Leipzig, Germany, in April 1945, I was an assistant squad leader. Our squad was attacking down a sunk road when we captured a German soldier hiding in a foxhole. He told us his company was ahead waiting in ambush. We sent him back in a jeep and continued to walk forward. We came to a crossroad, so Sgt. William McDonald ran across to the other side and hid among the bushes. Joe the Indian then ran across with Sergeant McDonald, who was signaling us to come over one at a time.

The lieutenant started to run across when a machine gun opened up on him. He dropped to the ground in the middle of the road to take cover. A bullet struck him in the top of the head. Our medic ran out to help. When he kneeled down, a string of machine gun bullets cut across his chest, killing him instantly. He slumped over, holding the lieutenant. When I saw this I got real mad. I never hated Germans as much. Some of the men were firing back by then. Sergeant McDonald kept giving me signals from across the road to call in artillery.

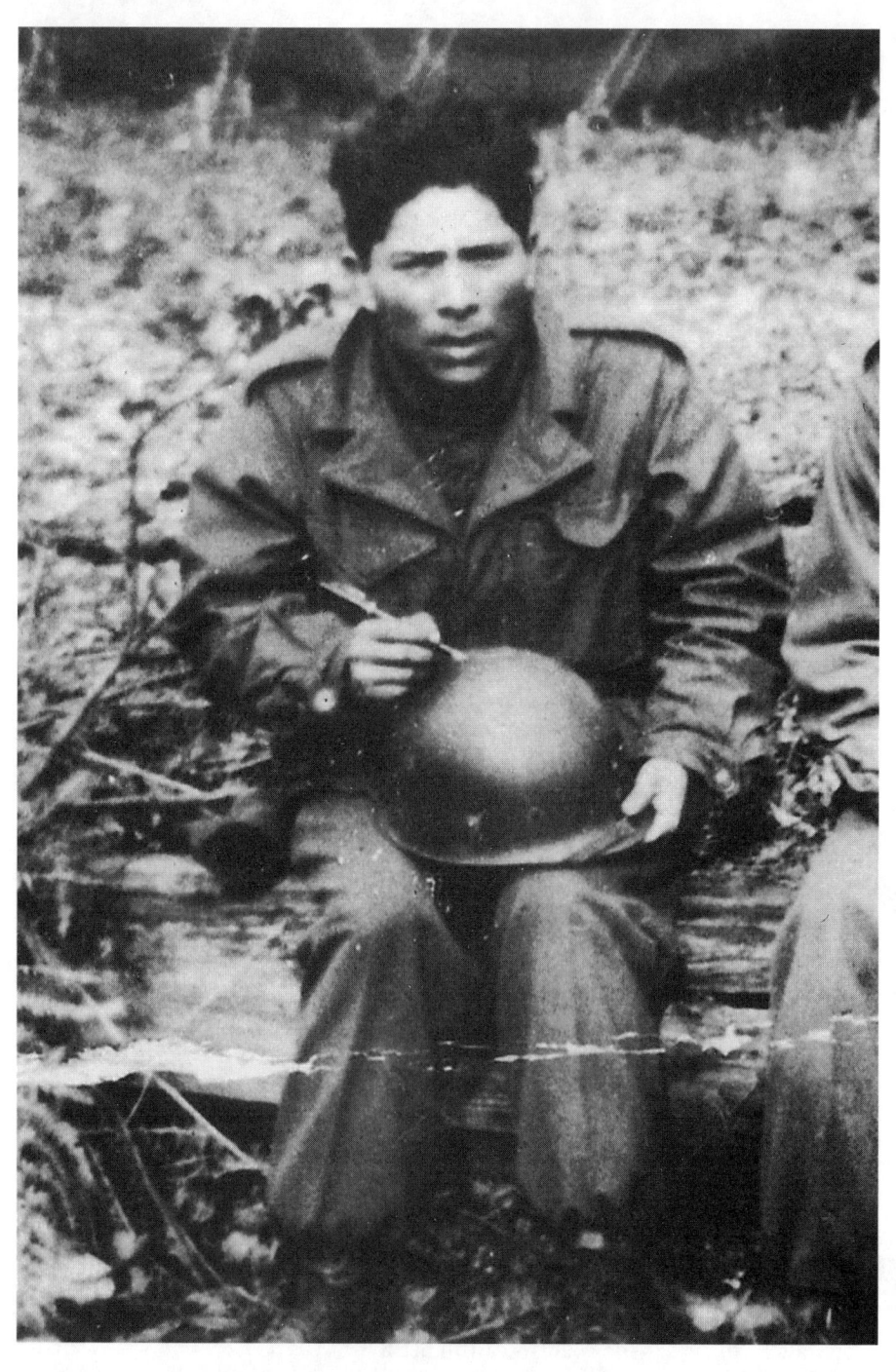

Corporal Luis Castillo. This picture was taken in April 1945 shortly after the incident involving the death of the lieutenant and medic. *Courtesy of Al Castillo.*

As the radioman came forward with the pack radio, a bullet struck him in the heel of his right boot. His leg just trembled as it squirted blood. We pulled the boot off and tied up his foot as he called artillery in on the Germans. The 105mm shells came streaking overhead, and it didn't take too many shells to convince the Germans to surrender. We took 160 prisoners that day. Yes, we roughed them up a bit, and they were lucky we didn't shoot some of them because of what had happened earlier.

Chapter Eleven

Picking Up the Dead

GRADY FORSYTH

Al Castillo conducted a taped interview with Grady Forsyth in 1990 at his home in Rome, Georgia. The following account is from that interview and Mr. Forsyth's written response to questions submitted by Mr. Castillo. Grady Forsyth died May 11, 1996.

I was sworn in at Fort Benning, Georgia. I was 33 years old and married. I was then stationed at Camp Grant, Illinois, and I took training in Camp Ellis, Illinois. I was a first aid man. I took care of the wounded.

I went overseas after about six months of basic training. I left Camp Ellis, boarded a train, and got on the boat. I went to France, to Germany, to close to Paris, then finally back to San Francisco. I boarded a ship there named *General Pope*, and my next stop was Japan. My journey to Japan was 30 days.

I was stationed while I was overseas with the Third Army Engineers, General Patton, as a first-aid man. I was not transferred to another unit. I worked with a platoon squad. I was not eager to see action, but when I did, I was proud to help my fellow man and to make him feel better. It is a pitiful sight to see your buddy wounded and more pitiful to see him dead.

My first combat experience was sad and made me feel scared. Combat is a sad thing; seeing your own buddies being killed it makes you think your time will be next. I was in the Battle of the Bulge, the Battle of the Rhine River with the Engineers, and at the Blue Spoon River. I was the first-aid man with the 1303 Engineers and the Third Army. The bridge the Third Army built over the Rhine River was 1,900 feet long, and while we were there the Germans shot an 88 machine gun bullet through one of our ambulances. It took about 19 days to build that bridge.

I helped pick up the dead behind the battlefield. The dead were placed on a large semitruck, which drove in between the graves. The bodies were stacked up like cords of wood, and as the truck got to a grave, you took one and placed them in it. One dog tag was nailed to a wooden cross, another sent home. It made a man wonder whether the next one could be his grave. I have picked up dead men in all kinds of shape. Some were shot to death; some were burned. It really makes a man angry to see his fellow man all shot up and dead.

We took all our medical training during basic training. How to set minor broken bones and minor first aid. We learned how to help the doctors. They were captains. It never prepared us for what was in store in combat. They always told us to take care of our boys first, then the Germans or Japs. I treated a few wounded Germans, but no Japs.

The first thing I saw when I got to the Philippines was a Jap head with two corn husks on each side of it staked to a pole. It had a sign that said, "THIS IS THE WAY WE DO THEM IN THE PACIFIC."

I had not been in the Philippines long when they sent me to get this colored man out of an army truck who had been run over by a tank. His head was as flat as a pancake. When I pulled on him, his brains ran all over my clothing. Some men said that the first-aid men had it easy. Some of the men standing around who saw me said they could never have done that. They would never say we had it easy again.

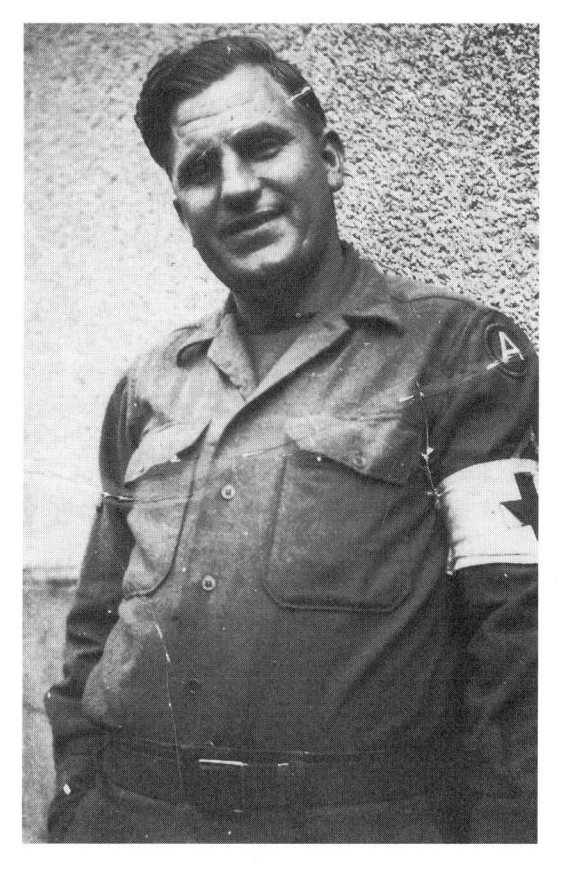

Grady Forsyth. *Courtesy of Al Castillo.*

I was never wounded, but I got too hot in basic training and passed out. We went on a 35 mile hike, and I stayed in the hospital for nine days.

I was 35 years old when I came home. My homecoming was great. I rode a taxi from Rome [Georgia] and just when I got near home, we drove behind a school bus, and some of the children on that school bus happened to be my nieces and nephews, and they recognized me, and they commenced screaming and waving at me. But the sad thing was, my baby girl did not know me; she was afraid of me. She was six weeks old when I went in the service, and she was about three years old when I came home.

What stands out the most in my memories? Well, the atomic bomb in Japan and the Rhine River and the Battle of the Bulge. The worst battle I can remember was the Battle of the Bulge. But after it was all over, I was glad I served in both theaters of war, Germany and the Philippines. I have seen a lot to make me be proud to be American. I am glad God carried me through all of it.

Chapter Twelve

The Miracle Day
Desmond T. Doss

Desmond T. Doss was a member of the Seventh-Day Adventist religion which allows participation in the duties of citizenship, such as military service, but encourages its members to be noncombatant.

When I was drafted into the army on April 1, 1942, I asked for a noncombatant classification, but the admitting officer said there was no such classification and that I would have to go in as a conscientious objector. The reason I didn't want that classification was that the conscientious objectors in those days were putting on antigovernment demonstrations, and they wouldn't salute the flag or do anything else for the war effort. But when the officer explained that if I went in under any other classification I could be court-martialed if I refused to do ordinary work on God's Sabbath or refused to use a weapon, so I decided that I must choose to be a conscientious objector.

Assigned to the 77th Infantry Division as a medic, Doss was the victim of harassment, which he continued to endure until the division landed on Guam. Gradually, however, the harassment stopped as the men of the 77th realized Doss's commitment to the unit. They knew that he would risk his own life to come to their aid.

The 77th Division went on to Leyte in the Philippines, then on to the battle in Okinawa.

I would like to tell one story of something that happened on Okinawa on the day before I let approximately 75 men down the face of the Maeda Escarpment, for which I received the Medal of Honor. This is an experience

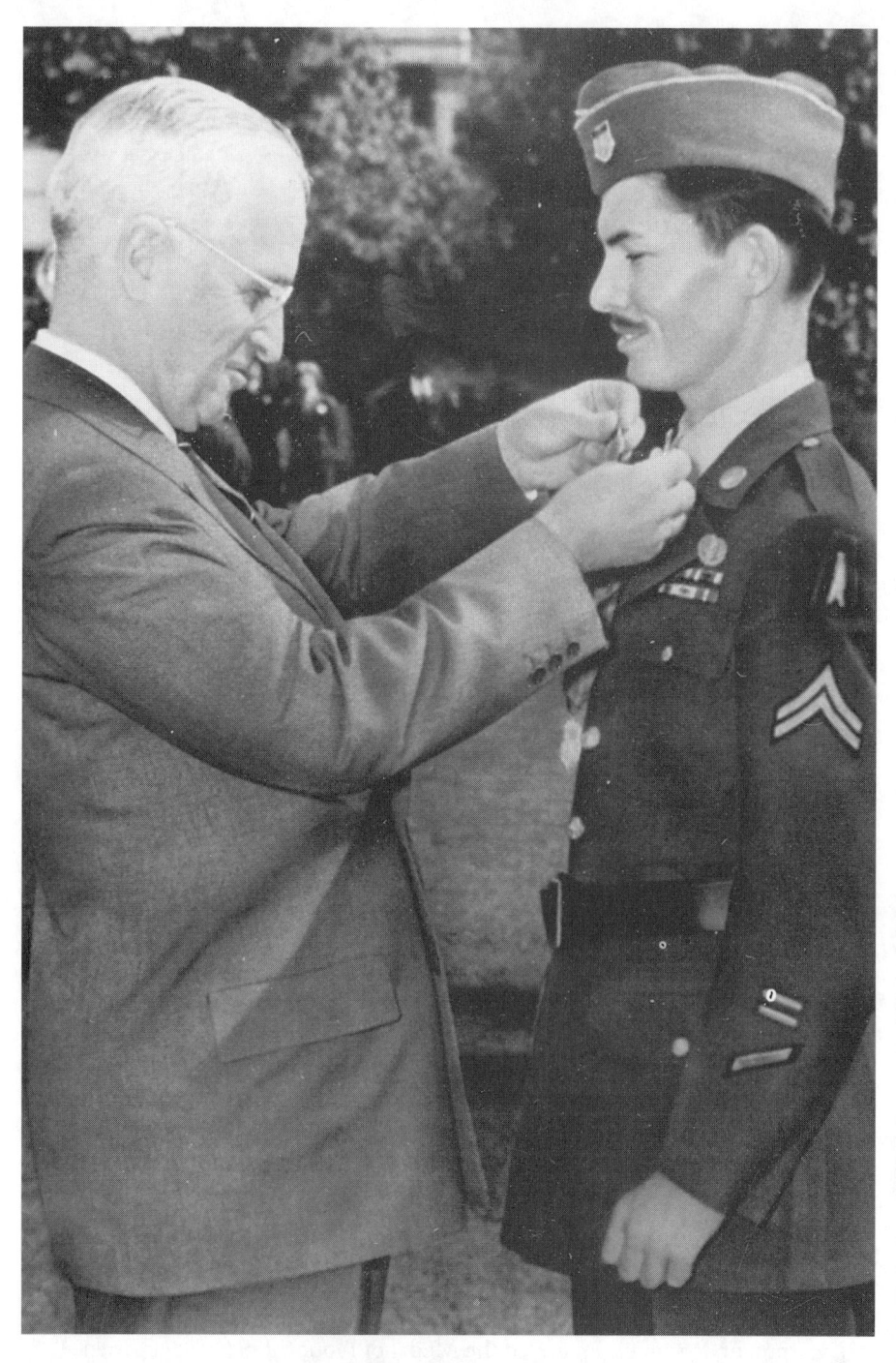

Desmond T. Doss receiving the Congressional Medal of Honor from President Harry S Truman. *Military Archives Photo.*

12. The Miracle Day

I like to call the "Miracle Day." We had been fighting for the escarpment where the cliff was about 400 ft. high. The last 35 feet up extended out so that it was about five feet further out at the top of the escarpment than it was 35 feet below. We had put up a cargo net to climb up that last 35 feet. We had been fighting for the escarpment for four days. The Japanese were dug in on top of the hill in caves and hollow places that looked like natural terrain, and it was hard to fight them.

On Miracle Day morning we were to go up on the escarpment again. I mentioned to Lt. Gornto that I believed prayer was the greatest lifesaver there was and I thought the men should pray before they went up on the escarpment. He quickly called the men together and said, "Doss wants to pray." Now that wasn't what I had in mind—I meant each man should pray himself. But I did pray that the Lord would help the lieutenant to give the right orders as our lives were in his hands and that we all would use all safety precautions, that each man would make his peace with God before he went up the cargo net, and that we would all return safely.

With that we went up and almost immediately got pinned down. Company A was fighting on our left, and they were badly shot up so we were ordered to take the whole escarpment by ourselves. With that we started forward and knocked out eight or nine Japanese positions. The amazing thing was that no one in our company was killed and only one man was injured—by a rock that hit his hand.

It was such an outstanding happening that our headquarters heard about it and sent the signal corps up to investigate it. How would you like to hear the report that went back to headquarters and even further?— "It was because of Doss' prayer."

The next day we didn't pray—figured it was an easy mop-up job. That was when our men had to retreat, leaving approximately 75 wounded men on top of the escarpment. They were my men and I couldn't go off and leave them even if it cost me my life. So I stayed there and let the men down by rope about 35 feet to the place where they could be taken by litter to the aid station.

For the next five hours Doss lowered the men from the edge of the cliff. He had only one rope, which he tied around each wounded man, one at a time. He used a double bowline knot that he had worked out one time in the States—a knot that he says God brought to his mind that day. The bullets passed by him again and again, close enough to feel them go by, but again he felt that God protected him, for he didn't get hurt that day on the escarpment.

Doss was wounded not long thereafter and brought back to the United

States. After recovering from his wounds, he received the Congressional Medal of Honor from President Harry S Truman on October 12, 1945.

I feel that I received the Medal of Honor because I kept the Golden Rule that we read in Matthew 7:12. "All things whatsoever ye would that men should do to you, do ye even so to them."

Note: Desmond Doss's wife, Francis Doss, also contributed to this chapter.

Chapter Thirteen

Stateside
George S. Barnes, M.D.

Some of us never heard a shot fired in anger, but we did what we were ordered to do.
—George S. Barnes, M.D.

Dr. Barnes describes life in the Army Air Corps on the home front.

I graduated from Tulane School of Medicine in 1942. We were the last class in medical schools to get a 12-month internship. Subsequent classes got only a nine-month internship.

During our internship several of my class requested that we be assigned to the U.S. Army Air Corps [the USAF was formed in 1947]. Some eight or ten of us from Charity Hospital, New Orleans, Louisiana, were sent to Carlisle Barracks to learn about the army and military ways in six weeks. My only military had been the Boy Scouts. Carlisle did a good job. On completion of Carlisle some five or six of us were assigned to the air corps general hospital at Kearns, Utah, for six months learning about military medicine. We were ward physicians.

At the end of six months those of us who had a superior rating were sent to Randolph Field to learn about air corps medicine. After three months we became Aviation Medical Examiners (AMEs). Following this we were assigned to a replacement depot in Lincoln, Nebraska, from which we were reassigned to various air bases in the United States.

I was assigned to Pyote, Texas, Air Base along with a fellow Tulane graduate. Pyote was a training base where combat crews for B17s were formed, and they learned how to work together as a crew. As AMEs we held sick call, did flight physicals, and also would fly with various crews who had some crewmen who complained of airsickness. We found a few men who definitely did not have motion sickness, but the great majority of the crews were anxious to maintain flying status. After six months being active AMEs we qualified to be flight surgeons ("I wanted wings till I got the d____ things").

Most of our crews went to the Eighth Air Force and were assembled at Kearney, Nebraska. The flight surgeons rode troop trains to Kearney, but we had to turn around and go back to Pyote.

It was a great disappointment to us that we didn't get to the Eighth Air Force. We continued to train crews at Pyote which switched to B29s in late '44 or early '45. We saw V-E Day at Pyote, then the B29s were being trained for Pacific duty. I was reassigned to a B29 base in Sioux City, Iowa, where I remained till V-J Day.

Since I was a single officer with no "points for discharge," I was reassigned to go to Europe with the occupation forces. I was assigned as Deputy Surgeon for the European Air Transport Service headquartered in Wiesbaden, Germany. We had bases all over Western Europe.

In June 1946 I had acquired enough "points" just for length of service to be discharged. Coming home on a converted hospital ship, we got home in two weeks. I was discharged in August '46.

Chapter Fourteen

From the States to Down Under

SAMUEL E. WARSHAUER, M.D.

Dr. Warshauer saw service in Australia and New Guinea and on Biak Island.

War was raging all over Europe in 1940, and finally I was told that I would be called for active duty unless I had a good excuse. Since I had not earned any money in practice, I figured there was nothing to lose by becoming a medical officer. A physical exam was required, so I went to Fort Moultrie, an army post near Charleston. They said my pulse was too rapid and advised me to return daily for three days to recheck it. After spending the night in Kingstree, my pulse was normal on arising. So without smoking or eating, I returned to Fort Moultrie and passed the exam. Soon I got a telegram ordering me to report to the commanding general, Camp Shelby, Mississippi. The only trouble was that neither I nor anybody else knew where Camp Shelby was. Julius Levine, a veteran of the First World War, said that it was near Hattiesburg, as he remembered the name of this post when he was in the army.

It was a two-day trip to the camp by car. I spent the first night in Columbus, Georgia. Fort Benning, a large infantry post, was nearby, and the city was full of soldiers. The next afternoon I arrived in Meridian, Mississippi at lunch time. A store on the main street had military uniforms in the window. It appeared that this would be a good time to buy a uniform, so I purchased a blouse, "pink" pants, a shirt and tie, a Sam Brown belt, a campaign hat and a regulation army officer's cap. I also got some insignia. When I arrived in Hattiesburg the town was full of soldiers milling around. I checked into the hotel, put on my new uniform, and walked out onto the street, feeling very odd in this peculiar outfit. The next morning I drove to the camp.

Camp Shelby was a very cold, muddy place. I immediately started to look for the commanding general. The first person I asked said: " The only general we got is at the division headquarters." From there I was sent to the headquarters of the station complement, which had charge of the hospital. They assigned me to the medical service and gave me a small-wall tent with a cot and nothing else in it. It was very cold and, of course, there was no heater in the tent. November 10, 1940, was then the beginning of my military career which was to last until September 1945.

The 30th Infantry Division (Ohio National Guard) was encamped here, and our hospital served the 30,000 soldiers in training. The chief of the medical service was Major Brewer, a regular army officer, who was a competent, knowledgeable doctor with whom all of us had a good relationship. There was a Doctor Milton Saslaw from Miami (he later became the health officer there). Also there was I.C. Sharon from Cincinnati, a bridge player, and a dentist, Cohen, from Jackson, Mississippi, also a golfer. We frequently played bridge at Saslaw's house (he had rented a house in Hattiesburg) and golf at the local golf course. Sharon and I would take weekend trips to New Orleans and once went as far as Texas. One could go fishing in the gulf at Biloxi, where there was a fine resort hotel and golf course. One Sunday in June 1941 while in Biloxi on a fishing trip, we learned that Germany had invaded Russia.

During the summer of 1941 a few of us were sent to Camp Polk, Louisiana, where the army was conducting large-scale maneuvers. We helped run the temporary hospital there. Once I accompanied a trainload of patients to the army general hospital in Fort Sam Houston, San Antonio, Texas. My chief said to be sure to get some fritos and guacamole salad, my introduction to Mexican food. I flew back to Polk in a commercial airplane, another first.

My term of service was to end in one year, November 1941, but I elected to sign up for another year, which was a wise decision, as the Japanese bombed Pearl Harbor on Sunday, December 7, 1941. Cohen and I were playing golf that day. When we finished, the attendant gave us the news. We said, "Where is Pearl Harbor?" All personnel were ordered back to the base and were to stay in uniform at all times. The army really got busy. President Roosevelt made his speech to Congress, describing the attack as "a day which will live in infamy," and the country was at war!

There was accelerated mobilization of draftees. All the men were required to be processed, which included receiving a physical examination.

14. From the States to Down Under

An examination team was organized of which I was a member. We went to New Orleans, stayed in the Jung Hotel, and examined a few hundred men in Charity Hospital each day. We sometimes finished in time to play golf in the afternoon. After a few meals in the celebrated restaurants, Antoine's or Arnauds, I generally ate in the hotel. We worked New Orleans for two weeks, then went to Gulfport, Mississippi, for a week and to Pensacola, Florida, for another week. We then went back to New Orleans to start over again. Pensacola was the site of a navy aviation-training base where they practiced landing seaplanes. Once or twice I rode in a plane during this exercise.

After this tour of duty outside the camp, I was sent to Camp Livingston in Alexandria, Louisiana, to join the newly organized 250-bed, 171st Station Hospital. We knew that we would soon be sent overseas, the destination and length of stay unknown. Miriam Miller and I had been going together since I started practice, and I did not want to lose her. When I sent her a telegram proposing marriage, she accepted. Our families traveled down to Alexandria, and we were married in the Temple there on May 4, 1942. We planned to go to Monroe, Louisiana, a town near Alexandria, for a honeymoon, but were informed that we would not have time, so we were offered the house of Betty (Goodman) Rosenthal. The next day we all departed for San Francisco, the military personnel in a special train and the dependents in a regular train. About four days later we all arrived in San Francisco and stayed in the Roosevelt Hotel. This was a run-down relic of the last century, but we managed to tolerate it for about ten days before we sailed to Australia in the naval transport *West Point*. This was the largest and fastest passenger ship in the navy. Before its modification as a troopship, it was the *America*, the finest and fastest ocean liner in the United States.

Six officers were assigned to a small stateroom on the boat deck which was furnished with two double-deck bunks. We drew lots and rotated around, with two different men sleeping on the floor each night. After 11 days we arrived in Auckland, New Zealand. That evening they let us go ashore—we found a hotel and had steak and eggs. The ship refueled and left late that night for Melbourne, arriving two days later. It was very cold in Melbourne—we were housed in tents. But after a few days we went north about 30 miles to Seymour, Victoria, the site of a small Australian army post, and set up a working hospital.

I entered the army as a first lieutenant, the lowest grade of medical officer. Soon I discovered that by taking correspondence courses one could qualify for captain. As I had over four years in grade (Reserve), the promotion soon came through. This fact, and the four years of training in internal medicine, enabled me to become Chief of the Medical Service in the hospital, which was the best job I could have hoped for in the army.

We were a close group and enjoyed our stay in Seymour. Leo Kohn was on my service, a bridge player, and on one occasion we played with Australian officers on an adjacent installation. Kohn and I had a good partnership and through the years made a small, but steady income from bridge.

Our patients came from New Guinea, where the 42nd and 31st Infantry Divisions were engaging the Japanese. But soon the flow of patients dried up so we were transferred to Port Moresby. The island of New Guinea, the second largest in the world, was divided in half. The western half was a Dutch colony (part of the Dutch East Indies), and the eastern half was divided between Australia in the south and United Kingdom in the north. These areas were German until after the First World War when they were given to the Allies. During World War II, New Guinea was invaded by Japan, and a large Japanese force remained in the interior until September 1945.

We packed up our supplies and entrained for Brisbane, where we embarked on an Australian hospital ship. This was a very pleasant voyage. The ship, with green crosses on each side, was brightly illuminated by flood lamps. No patients were aboard, so we were assigned the very comfortable patients' beds. Six good meals were served: breakfast, morning tea, lunch, afternoon tea, dinner, and supper. Liquor was plentiful and cost one shilling (17 cents) per shot. We arrived just before Christmas 1942. In anticipation of the holiday the CO had us buy gifts in Australia, so I bought a good many souvenirs, which were distributed to the people. Port Moresby was a very small place. It had one dock, a small "hotel," a police station, and a store. We went a mile or so out of town and set up our tent hospital adjacent to an evacuation hospital (about 1,000 beds) which preceded us, and we remained there until late 1944.

A word about the commanding officer. The CO of the 171st was Lt. Col. Charles Wilkinson, a National Guard officer who did general practice in Wake Forest, North Carolina. His wife and small sons traveled across the country in the same train as Miriam and the other wives. His sons became doctors; one of them ... now practices surgery in Wilmington.... After we had been in Port Moresby a few months, he wanted me and the Chief of Surgery, Horace Thomas, to be promoted to major, which was the standard grade for our position. After the recommendation for promotion had been returned a few times, he asked me to write it myself, which I did and within a week was promoted to major.

The American Board of Internal Medicine was founded in 1936. I thought it a good idea to take the examination, so I wrote the secretary and he agreed to send the written questions to the colonel. Under his supervision I completed the exam in his tent and some time later was informed that I had passed. The exam consisted of two parts, written and oral. The latter could not be given overseas, so I was told to take it when I got back to the United States....

Port Moresby was not an unpleasant place to be. There were some mosquitoes, but no malaria. Each officer had his own small tent and canvas cot. I had an inflatable air mattress and a mosquito bar and had no trouble sleeping. The food was poor, mostly dehydrated things. Dried eggs not very palatable, but hot cakes were good. There were various canned meats and vegetables, and no one got hungry, but none gained weight. We had frequent movies; a large screen was placed at the end of a field, and we were seated in front in the open air. We could sometimes play bridge in front of a tent and watch the movie at the same time. Occasionally an entertainer would visit the hospital. I remember Ray Bolger coming with a small troupe. We decided to build a tennis court, but we moved away soon after it was completed.

The medical service was either very busy or very idle, depending upon the receipt of casualties. There was fighting in central New Guinea. This island is divided by a high range of mountains, and the terrain is very rough. Much of the land is covered by a tropical rain forest, but there are also some areas of high grass. In the forest men contracted malaria, and in the grassy areas they were bitten by a mite, the vector of scrub typhus fever. Bacillary dysentery was also common. We published a paper in the journal *War Medicine* reporting a great many cases of scrub typhus or tsutsugamushi fever. This disease was caused by a rickettsial bacterium, and we had no curative drug. The mortality was about 20 percent. Malaria was treated with Atabrine or quinine. We had no specific treatment for dysentery. Not infrequently, a patient had two or more of these diseases at the same time. Besides infectious diseases we had the usual medical illnesses. I can recall a case of coarctation of the aorta, one of myasthenia gravis, and other serious ailments which required evacuation to a general hospital in Australia. Leo Kohn had a ruptured lumbar disc which was removed in Australia. He was offered a chance to return to the United States but preferred to come back to us, much to the astonishment of the doctors in the general hospital.

About every six months we could go on leave to Australia. I went to Sydney with a companion, and we decided to go to a lodge in the Australian Alps, where one could ski. We had no reservation and were kicked out the next morning, but we did see the snow and rode on a slow, unheated train back to Sydney and Bondi Beach. My companion had been at my wedding in Louisiana. I remembered him when he was a surgical resident in the James Walker Hospital the year after I left to go to Richmond. He was unmarried but had a few girlfriends at home who sent him food packages. These were very much appreciated, especially the cans of tuna fish. After the war he married one of the girls, settled in Hendersonville, and practiced general surgery until he retired some years ago.

My office was in the front part of a large hospital tent. The rear two-thirds was occupied by the hospital laboratory, in charge of a lieutenant, a parasitologist. I often played chess with him in my office. One day he came in with a .45 caliber automatic pistol. I asked him how it worked. He proceeded to demonstrate the weapon and, in so doing, accidentally discharged it. The bullet traveled through the tent next door, where a dentist was busily engaged in some type of dental surgery. It passed between the patient and the dentist. Very fortunately no one was injured!

After about two years in Port Moresby, patients stopped coming, and the war moved north. The regaining of the Philippines was about to begin. We closed the hospital, packed up and boarded a Liberty ship, the *Howell Cobb*, to go to Biak Island. This small coral island was part of Dutch New Guinea, and off its northern coast, at about one degree south latitude. The colonel was ordered home, and we became integrated into the 2,000-bed, 132nd General Hospital. I was appointed Assistant Chief of the medical service. There was a hospital group on the island. It comprised three, 2000-bed units: one came from Harvard, one from Johns Hopkins, and our nondescript outfit. Luckily for me I was in the 132nd, as I would have been very low on the totem pole in one of the other two. The Chief of Medicine was a pediatrician-public health officer, a lieutenant colonel, who was really neither interested nor trained in internal medicine, so I had a free hand to manage the clinical side of the service. He took care of the administrative details, which was an ideal arrangement for me. We then prepared to receive casualties by air from the Philippine campaign.

En route to Biak, our ship remained anchored in the harbor of Hollandia, Dutch New Guinea, for about a month. We had nothing to do except eat and sleep. The food was poor, and the quarters were very hot, but Kohn and I managed to get up a bridge game with some of the newly arrived officers of the 132nd. They had an exaggerated idea of their bridge talent, so we accumulated lots of Dutch guilders. There was nothing to spend money on in New Guinea. My salary as a major was about $450 a month. Miriam was allotted $400, and I kept the balance. Like almost everybody then, I smoked, but cigarettes were 50 cents a carton (five cents a pack), so I really couldn't spend the 50 dollars left over from my pay.

While we were stranded at Hollandia, the invasion of the Philippines began on the island of Leyte. We heard the news by radio on the ship's public-address system. Jack Brams, my mother's first cousin, was stationed in the army hospital in Hollandia. One day I paid him a visit and spent a good night in the officer's ward of his hospital. I had a fairly good meal, took a shower in fresh water, and then returned to the ship. There must have been over a hundred ships at anchor. They all looked alike, but by semaphore signals our ship was identified, and I rejoined my friends.

Biak, a coral island, was north of Dutch New Guinea at its eastern end, one degree south of the equator. An airstrip was created by scraping off the surface soil; the underlying white coral resembled cement. There was a cold, freshwater spring leading into the ocean, and one could go swimming at this point. The fresh water would be on the surface, and the warmer salt water below. It was an interesting experience.

When we set up our hospital in Biak, we received casualties by air from the Philippine war zone. The troops waded through freshwater streams which were infested with snails carrying the larvae of schistosome parasites, the cause of schistosomiasis japonicum, a disease which affects the liver. Our hospital made the first diagnosis of this disease in a live patient. We had a case of a very sick soldier with fever and an enlarged liver. A diagnostic laparotomy was done which showed little white nodules throughout the liver; inside each nodule was a schistosome parasite. Treatment consisted of giving an antimony compound, which resulted in his slow recovery.

After about six months on Biak, it became my turn to go home. The Chief of the Service and consultants offered to promote me to lieutenant colonel, but I elected to return to the United States. The group of returnees boarded a freighter, a C1 cargo ship, in Hollandia. I was assigned a small interior cabin with another major, named Zimmerman. The cabin was stifling hot, so we stayed inside as little as possible. I think it took about two weeks to get to San Francisco. During the voyage we received the news that President Roosevelt had died; none of us really knew much about the vice-president, Harry Truman.

Upon arrival in San Francisco, a few of us went to the Saint Francis Hotel and had a drink. I went to the maître d' and told him that we had just arrived and hadn't had a good meal in three years. I asked him to give us the best he had. We gorged ourselves with this treat.

In the meantime I called Miriam in Wilmington, telling her that I would be home as soon as possible. The next day I was ordered to get on a troop train headed for Fort Bragg. The train consisted of a number of old nonair-conditioned Pullman cars. My car had one drawing room, which I occupied as the only officer, and 12 sections with soldiers in each of the two beds, upper and lower. There was a kitchen car attached; the meals were brought through the cars on a trolley from which the food was ladled out. It took four nights to get to Atlanta. Cars were detached as we moved across the country, and by the time we got there the food was exhausted. I remember buying all the sandwiches in a station food cart, and giving them to the men in my car. We were then attached to a regular train to Florence. I had some meal vouchers, so we had breakfast in the station café in Florence. We all got off in Fayetteville the same afternoon. After a perfunctory exam at Fort Bragg we were free to go home. Miriam met me at a hotel in Fayetteville where we spent the night, and we drove to Wilmington the next morning. I had orders to report to an R&R outfit in Miami Beach and was assigned to the Shelbourne Hotel.

I had passed the written half of the American Board of Internal Medicine in New Guinea, so I applied to take the oral part. The board assigned me to Philadelphia, but this was out of the way for Florida, so I requested permission to take it in New Orleans. In those days gasoline was rationed, and we had only enough coupons to get to Miami. So Miriam and I drove to Atlanta, parked the car there, and took an overnight train to New Orleans. The examination was given in Charity Hospital. Two cases were presented: one was syphilitic aortitis (then a very common disease), and the other sickle cell anemia and a stroke. In due course I was notified that I had passed.

Away we went to Florida. The Shelbourne was a fine hotel. It cost me nothing, but Miriam's bill was one dollar a day. The bar served drinks for 25 cents, the food was good, and there was plenty of entertainment. We told the army that any assignment in the United States would be fine, but much to our dismay, I was sent to Camp Butner, near Durham [North Carolina]. We spent the hot summer of 1945 there and made some friends among the officers. The camp was occupied by soldiers from the European Theater of War, many of whom suffered from frostbite, and we examined them prior to their discharge. While we were in Durham the Germans surrendered, the atom bomb was dropped on Japan, and the war ended. I was released from active duty, but remained in the Army Reserve. Since December 7, 1941, I had not worn civilian clothes and had none. I bought two Hickey-Freeman suits in a store in Durham and set out to find a place to practice.

Chapter Fifteen

Into Enemy Fire
ARTHUR V. O'CONNELL

Arthur O'Connell was 21 years old when called into active service. He was the recipient of the Silver Star and the Combat Medical Badge.

I was a combat medical corpsman throughout World War II in the Pacific Theater of Operations, serving in major campaigns on Guadalcanal, and in the Solomon Islands, New Guinea, and the Philippine Islands. I was attached to the 118th Combat Engineer Battalion and the 172nd Infantry Regiment. Combat medical corpsmen are always the first to render medical aid to wounded soldiers and are always in exposed, unprotected, dangerous situations. We are recognized by being awarded the Combat Medical Badge, as infantrymen are awarded the Combat Infantry Badge—both coveted and cherished recognitions.

The 43rd Infantry Division was a National Guard division composed of men from Maine, Vermont, Connecticut, and Rhode Island. We were called into active service in February 1941, 11 months before Pearl Harbor. We were sent to Camp Blanding, Florida, to start regular training. I was sent to Fort Sam Houston, Texas, for advanced medical training at the Brooks Army Hospital.

After being stationed at Camp Shelby, Mississippi, and Fort Ord, California, the division was shipped overseas in the late summer of 1942.

After spending a few months in New Zealand, we were shipped to New Caledonia, thence to Guadalcanal, where we relieved Marine Corps units and experienced our baptism of fire. Then we were shipped in June 1943 to the Solomon Islands; in 1944, to New Guinea; and in 1945, to the Philippine Islands.

I was extremely lucky never to have been a casualty. Casualties among combat medical corpsmen were very, very high.

The following account from the Providence, Rhode Island, Sunday Journal *(Feb. 1945) describes the action that won Arthur O'Connell his Silver Star:*

Staff Sergeant O'Connell, while an aid man with the engineers on Luzon, received the Silver Star when he crawled into enemy fire with three companions in an unsuccessful attempt to save his company commander. As he crawled through the grass, a machine gun opened up on him. Slugs flew all around him; some kicked up dirt in his face, and three passed through his jacket. Two Japanese carrying a machine-gun came running toward him. He leaned back and threw a grenade, wounding one of them and then killed him with his rifle, while the other took cover. Then, disregarding his own safety, he crawled farther into the path of enemy fire to the aid of his three companions who had all been seriously wounded. He found one of them dead but administered aid to the other two and evacuated them to safety.

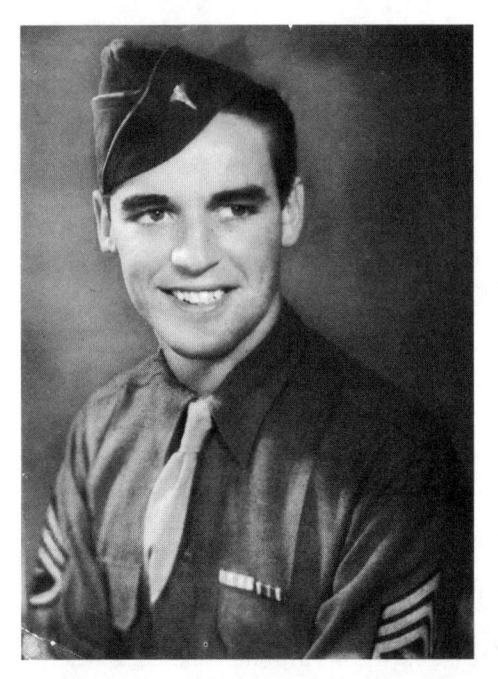

Arthur V. O'Connell. *Courtesy of Arthur V. O'Connell.*

Chapter Sixteen

ASTRP and an "Opportunity"
DANIEL SEFTEL

Daniel Seftel is now a retired physician.

At the age of 17 in (1943) with the written consent of my parents, having graduated from high school, I enlisted in the U.S. Army and joined the Army Specialized Training Reserve Program (ASTRP). I was sent to Princeton University. The group studied basic engineering for two semesters, and at 18 we entered active duty (1944).

We were sent to Fort Bragg, North Carolina, for basic training in the field artillery. Following this training the army decided they had trained too many men for the artillery, and we were sent to Fort Leonard Wood, Missouri, for training as combat engineers. Volunteers were requested for a medical detachment to this unit (1292 Combat Engineer Battalion). I volunteered.

During that period of time most of us "college recruits" took and passed an exam for Officer Candidate School in the infantry. Most of my friends opted for this "opportunity" and left. I decided to remain with the medical detachment of the combat engineers. Soon after OCS they were all sent to England and participated in the Normandy invasion on D-Day (June 6, 1944). I understand most of them are now buried in the American cemeteries in France.

After completion of this training we were designated to leave for the European Theater, but the Germans surrendered in May 1945, and the plans were canceled. We were then shipped to the Philippines in July 1945 to prepare for the invasion of Japan. Shortly after our arrival in the Philippines our medical officer called me in (I was still a private in rank)

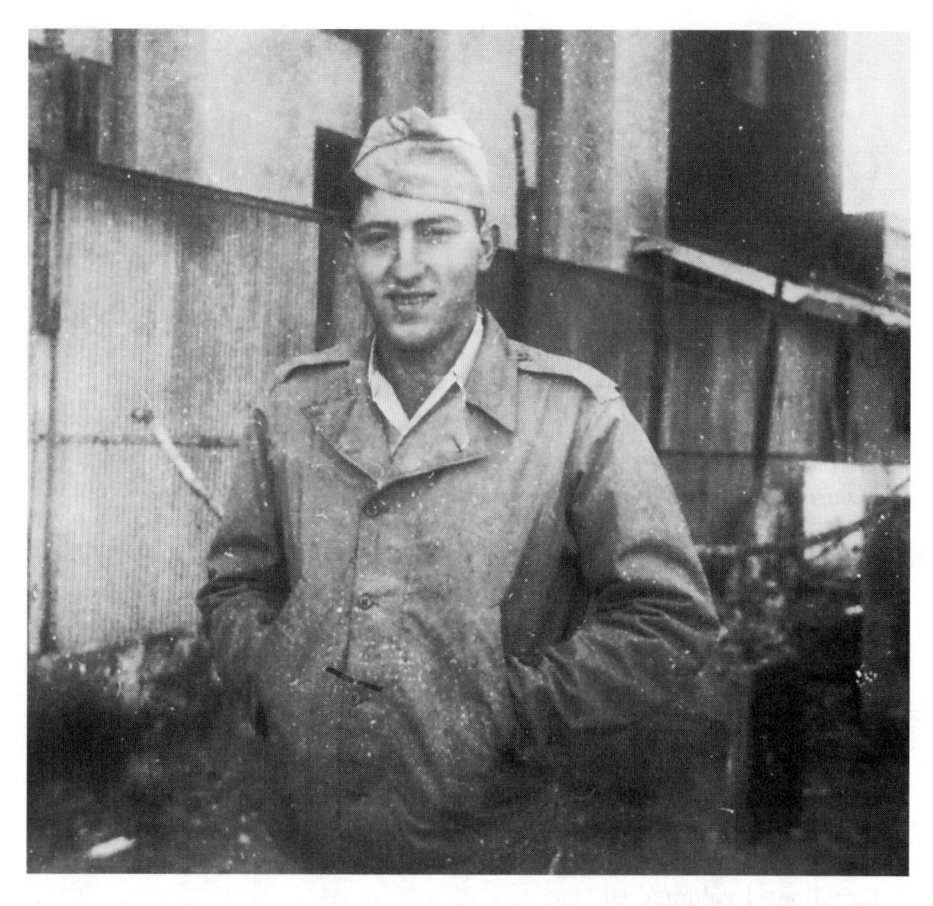

Daniel Seftel in Nagoya, Japan. *Courtesy of Dr. Daniel M. Seftel.*

and informed me of the invasion plans. However, since I was the youngest I was to remain on the ship with him for ten days (D plus ten) to take care of the wounded on the ship and then go ashore. Several days later he called me in again; he had changed his mind since a certain sergeant had a wife and three children back home. I was to take his place and go in with company A of the combat engineers on the third wave on D-Day. About one week later the first atomic bomb was dropped and a few days later the second, and we knew it was all over. We did go to Japan after the surrender in September but as occupation troops.

Following my discharge from the army, I completed my undergraduate schooling and then went on to medical school. I consider myself very fortunate in deciding not to go to OCS . I am currently living a healthy, retired life at 73 years of age.

Chapter Seventeen

A Physician Scientist in the Army

RICHARD J. BING, M.D.

Dr. Bing is currently Professor of Medicine (Emeritus) at USC, Director of Experimental Cardiology at Huntington Medical Research Institutes, and Visiting Associate in Chemistry at the California Institute of Technology. German by birth, he left his native land for the United States in 1934.

To recall one's past is bittersweet; personal history is wrapped in the loneliness of the survivor; where once his experience was shared by many, his voice is now a forlorn echo of times past. His joys and sorrows of the past are beyond comprehension and evoke no sympathy in a new generation. And yet, some tales, when told, can catch the imagination, because they find a resonance; they reveal the source of the stream of history which now flows by the shores of the present.

I do not have any great battle stories to tell, but my experiences are those of a medical officer during World War II who experienced the great conflict in a scientific and clinical military environment and who after the war served as an advisor to the military government in Germany.

I entered the army in 1943 when I was an instructor in the department of medicine at Johns Hopkins School of Medicine working on hypertension and serving as a part-time assistant resident. I wanted to become a member of the American Armed Forces; I had left Germany in 1934 and wanted, as a citizen of my new country, to join the American army. I was inducted into the Medical Corps as a first lieutenant, the usual rank of newly commissioned medical officers. Because of my scientific background, I was assigned to a research division in chemical warfare at Edgewood Arsenal in Maryland. This was no typical military station. Rather it was a military think tank, an accumulation of scientific excellence. Our division was headed by Major Alfred Gilman, M.D., who with Louis S. Goodman, M.D., was the author of a just-published textbook on pharmacology. Gilman had come to the army from Yale where he was one of the first to attempt chemotherapy of cancer by means of the use of nitrogen mustard. In this division there were also Karnofski, M.D., from the Sloan Kettering Cancer Institute in New York, who was one of the first to classify cancer; George Koelle, M.D., Ph.D., an authority on cholinesterase; and Oscar Bodanski, Ph.D., a biochemist, who with his brother had just published a textbook on biochemistry of disease. There were other scientists in the department of pharmacology, toxicology, and biology.

As a newly commissioned officer, I received basic training in chemical warfare by taking an obstacle course in chemical warfare and by attending classroom teaching. In the obstacle course we were exposed to chemical agents; we had to climb over obstacles and through barbed wire, and we were even sprayed with chemical agents. I was assigned to a research project: the effects of the newly discovered insecticide DDT. In animal experiments I produced severe ataxia (inability to coordinate muscular movements) with oral ingestion of DDT. I was fortunate to do research despite army restrictions. Fortunately, chemical weapons were not used by either side, probably because both the Germans and we had large stockpiles. After a year I was promoted to captain, and in 1945 Alfred Blalock, Chairman of the Department of Surgery at Johns Hopkins Hospital, got me discharged from the service, and I was appointed assistant professor of surgery at Johns Hopkins Hospital to work on the physiology and diagnosis of congenital heart disease.

This was, however, not the end of my army service. In 1947 I received a call from the Surgeon General's office to report on the progress of German medicine during the war years. I took a military plane to Berlin, from there to Frankfort, Nuremberg, and Munich with visits to both German and American hospitals. I visited the American 97th and 98th General Hospitals in Frankfurt and in Munich. I was amused at the efficiency of the American army hospitals. They were run by career medical officers and had excellent specialists drawn from civilian life. I was also surprised at how interested the American medical officers were in helping their German colleagues. In many instances the American physicians became teachers for their German colleagues. The services certainly ran a variant of managed care. Today, however, in managed care in civilian practice, the patient's right may be challenged, and the obligation of insurance companies to the stockholders can erode patient needs. But I observed in military hospitals that excellent care made the question of patients' rights superfluous, a lesson to be learned for civilian medicine.

Today when I have to pass through the gigantic Frankfort airport, I remember the shack which served as the air terminal. It could accommodate no more than 60 passengers, then mostly military personnel. In Frankfort at the university, I demonstrated before a large group of German physicians the first clinical use of the cardiac catheter. The patient was a young soldier. When I inserted the catheter into the vein and turned on the fluoroscope, I saw to my horror that there was a bullet in the right ventricle moving with each heart beat, but the catheter did not dislodge the bullet, and the procedure went smoothly. Twenty years later when I lectured again at the University of Frankfort, a physician recalled this event. Catheterization of the heart, although introduced by Werner Forssmann, M.D., in Berlin in 1928, had not been used in Germany during the war. While in Germany I tried to locate Werner Forssmann, M.D., but there were rumors that he was in Russian captivity. After I returned home to Baltimore, I received a letter from him from a town in the Black Forest, where he apparently had begun to practice urology. Later, Werner Forssmann, M.D., received the Nobel Prize for his pioneering work.

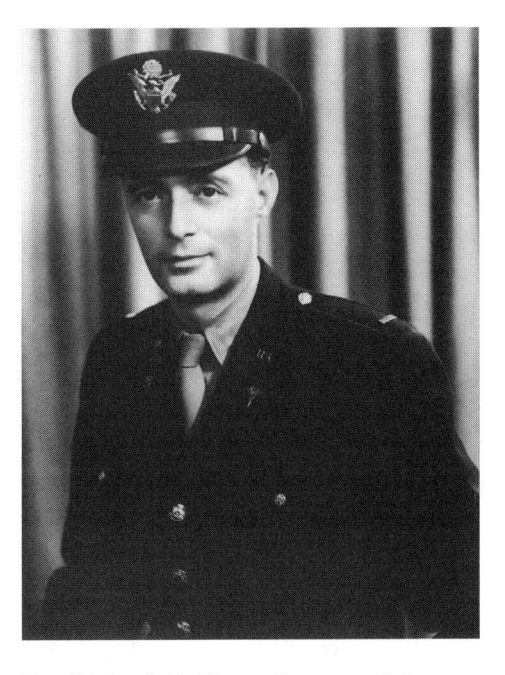

Dr. Richard J. Bing. *Courtesy of Dr. Richard J. Bing.*

Berlin, Frankfort, Nuremberg, and Munich were in a shambles. Berlin was leveled to the ground. But despite the destruction, Berlin still had an active opera; with the city destroyed, the performance of a Mozart opera which I attended was a moving example that art can survive anything, and can even be a necessity like food and shelter. Despite Berlin's total destruction, the opera was crowded, and the performance was deeply moving. In Berlin I had a meeting in one of the few intact houses in the suburb of Wannsee; it had been the house of the composer of the famous World War II song, "Lili Marlene."

German physicians were eager to learn of medical advances made during the war. Alfred Blalock, M.D., the surgeon, and Helen Tausig, M.D., the pediatric cardiologist and I had worked with children with congenital heart disease. To German physicians this was a totally new discipline. There was a tremendous search and thirst for medical information; in Germany medicine had to make a new start.

While in Germany I had to present myself to the commanding general in Heidelberg and was promoted to lieutenant colonel. When I returned to civilian life, I got involved again in the physiology and diagnosis of congenital heart disease at the Johns Hopkins Hospital. But soon my interest shifted, when the catheter, first inadvertently and later by intention, entered the coronary sinus of patients whom I catheterized for diagnostic reasons. This opened a whole new field, that of cardiac metabolism. The experience of having been in the service during this great conflict also created a common bond with other physicians returning home to resume the training at hospitals and universities across the country.

Since then much has happened to medicine. Progress in physics and molecular biology in particular has changed medicine. Its whole organization and social structure are different now. During the war there was a spirit of cooperation and willingness to serve in American medicine. It is sad that we need extraordinary situations to pull us together. The bottom line is not everything!

Chapter Eighteen

Corregidor

LOGAN W. HOVIS, M.D.

Dr. Hovis served with the 503d Regimental Combat Team (Parachute) in the Southwest Pacific Theater. He received two Bronze Stars, the Purple Heart, the Qualified Parachutist Insignia, the Combat Medical Badge, the Presidential Unit Citation, and the Meritorious Unit Citation.

Some time early in February 1945 we learned that the 503rd RCT [Regimental Combat Team] had been selected to lead the assault to recapture Corregidor. We were briefed for the mission in small groups inside a well-guarded tent which contained a large relief map of Corregidor. It was all very exciting, and we felt that this would be a very special mission.

The Third Battalion under the command of Lt. Col. John L. Erickson was designated to make the initial parachute assault. There were to be two lines of planes that, because of the small sizes of the drop zones, would discharge sticks of only eight men on each pass. One line was to release parachutists over A zone (the old parade grounds, an area of about 300 yards by 200 yards) and the other line over B zone (the rubble-strewn remains of a small golf course, about 350 yards by 150 yards).

I was assigned to the first stick to jump from the second plane over B zone, and my fellow medical officer in the battalion, Capt. Robert McNight, was similarly assigned over A zone. As officers we usually led sticks out of planes during jumps, but on this mission we were placed near the middle of our sticks to improve our chances of landing in the drop zones and thus be able to serve those who would be injured or wounded. A high percentage of jump casualties was anticipated.

The flight from Mindoro to Corregidor was uneventful. We jumped

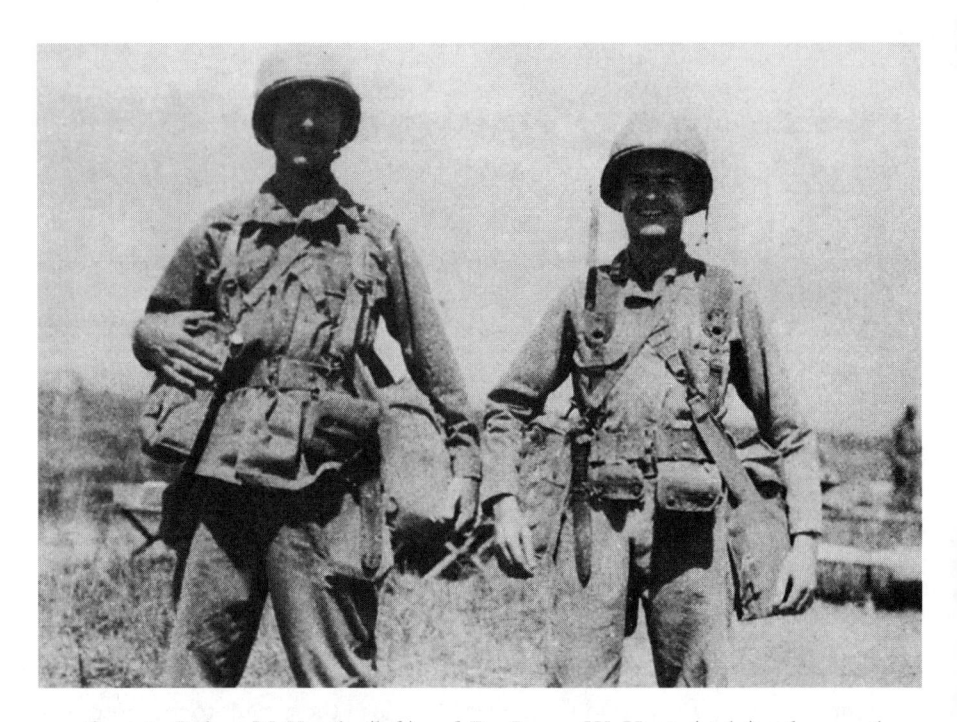

Captain Robert McKnight (left) and Dr. Logan W. Hovis (right), taken on the island of Mindoro, P.I., the day before the parachute assault of the island of Corregidor. They were the combat surgeons for the Third Battalion that led the assault and were among the first 24 soldiers to land on Corregidor. *Courtesy of Dr. Logan W. Hovis.*

at an altitude of about 400 feet above "Topside" in the face of a strong ground wind of 20 to 25 knots. The attack began about 0830 on February 16, 1945. I weighed only about 120 pounds at the time and carried roughly 40 pounds of equipment and supplies in addition to my chutes. My main chute functioned properly, and I landed close to the center of B zone. The wind caught my chute, and I was dragged across the rocky terrain. I made no effort to collapse my chute for fear of injuring my hands. Finally, my chute was fouled in the remains of some trees at the edge of the field. Meanwhile, I had become so entangled in cords and lines that I could hardly move. I was helpless until Lt. Bill Ziler came along and cut me free. He still has my heartfelt gratitude.

As previously planned I proceeded to the nearby lighthouse, located on the highest point of the island, and set up a front line aid station with the help of medical soldiers. We were soon very busy caring for jump injuries and battle casualties.

Although suffering from severe bruises and contusions himself, Captain

Hovis treated a total of 140 casualties during the first 24-hour period, displaying a willingness to work for often twenty-four to thirty-six hours without rest in order to care for the wounded—Bronze Star Citation.

Transportation of the injured and wounded was difficult because the equipment chutes loaded with litters drifted into the bay. The medical soldiers improvised by using blown-out doors, blankets attached to poles, direct carry, so on. Several medical soldiers evacuated casualties while subject to enemy fire.

Sometime during the morning I learned that Capt. Bob McNight had sustained a severe fracture of an ankle on landing, had then been pinned down behind a fallen tree trunk for a time by enemy fire, and, of course, would have to be evacuated.

Both of the regimental chaplains sustained jump injuries. I received word that Chaplain Herb was out on B zone in severe pain and unable to move. During a lull I went out with some medical soldiers, splinted his fractured leg or legs as best I could, and helped to bring him in on a door.

Sometime during the first day I was ordered to move my aid station from the lighthouse to the ruins of one of the homes in what had been officers' row. The lighthouse became a command post, a logical decision. The aid station remained at this second site until February 20. During this time I made daily visits, when sniper fire was minimal, to the morgue which had been set up in the ruins of Topside theater for the purpose of helping to identify bodies and to keep an accurate record of the losses of my battalion. Most of the bodies were covered by parachutes. I turned back one parachute to reveal the body of Capt. Emmet R. Spicer, Battalion Surgeon, 462nd Parachute Field Artillery. It was my first knowledge of his death. While I was a student in the Army Field Medical School at Carlisle Barracks, Pennsylvania, during August 1943, Captain Spicer had visited the school as a recruiting officer for the Parachute Infantry and had persuaded me to volunteer for this service.

On February 20, the Third Battalion Headquarters and my aid station were moved to the vicinity of the ruins of Topside hospital. Diarrhea was a common ailment in the Southwest Pacific Theater. On Corregidor it could be fatal. On several occasions afflicted soldiers left their foxholes at night to relieve themselves and were riddled by friendly fire. Many new replacements were understandably trigger happy.

On February 24, we filed around the north side of Malinta Hill and past the eastern portal of Malinta tunnel. A tank was stationed at the portal and protected our passage by steady machine gun fire into the tunnel. A new headquarters and nearby aid station were established in depressions on the central ridge of the tail of the island about one third the total distance of the tail from Malinta Hill. That afternoon we came under sniper fire. The bullets were almost spent and sounded like buzzing bees. Several of us slapped at them reflexively. We were unable to locate their source, but assumed they came from our front. Then a trooper standing no more than ten feet from me was hit in the leg. With his cooperation and while dressing his wound, from the course of the bullet through his leg we were able to determine that the sniper was behind us and probably on Malinta Hill. A patrol was sent out and the sniper was soon eliminated.

The First Battalion led the attack down the tail of the island and the Third Battalion followed. On February 26, I was on a road with an ambulance several hundreds of yards from Monkey Point when that point exploded. I was tending to a medical soldier who had joined our unit only a few days before the Corregidor mission. He had been hit in the center of the chest during a firefight down over the hill from the road. His life was rapidly ebbing away, and I felt very sad and helpless. When the explosion occurred the air above us was filled with debris. A falling rock penetrated the hood of the ambulance and destroyed the carburetor. Fortunately, no members of the ambulance crew were seriously injured.

We ran up the road to the site of the explosion. I found Capt. William C. McLain and worked with him in caring for the casualties. Captain McLain was very shaken; the edge of the crater produced by the explosion was only a few feet from where he had been at the time. The debris had been forced up and over him, and he had escaped physical harm.

The explosion had literally shattered the First Battalion. The Third Battalion moved through the area to continue the mop-up of the tail of the island. We were still so engaged when General MacArthur visited the island for the formal flag-raising ceremonies. Prior to his visit, the island was sprayed from the air with DDT to control the multitude of flies that were breeding in decomposing Japanese bodies. At the time DDT was considered to be relatively harmless to humans.

One of the last casualties that I treated was a trooper who tossed a phosphorus grenade into a high cave on Hooker Point on the tip of the tail of the island. The grenade was promptly returned in his direction and exploded in his face. His wounds included phosphorus burns of his eyes that I lavaged with water and copper sulfate solution. I have often wondered what the final outcome of his unfortunate experience was.

We remained in the vicinity of Monkey Point until March 6. After active fighting died down, the mortar crews directed many rounds at nearby Caballo Island where many Japanese had sought refuge.

On March 6 we returned to Topside and soon thereafter were transported by sea back to our base camp on Mindoro.

The following are excerpts of letters written by Captain Hovis to his parents during the Negros campaign. During the campaign he was serving as the Senior Surgeon of the Third Battalion of the 503rd Parachute Infantry Regiment.

April 15, 1945   We are in combat again and have been for about a week. You will probably never read or hear anything in the news about this mission. We are engaged in the least spectacular but most grueling and dangerous type of warfare—"mopping up." The scene is another island in the Philippines. I am very busy again—many of our men are being killed and wounded. The Japs that we are fighting are clever, well entrenched, and well armed.

A few days ago I went forward just behind the assault line to help evacuate several casualties. Was attending to a wounded trooper when I suddenly heard "crack-crack-crack," the familiar and ominous rhythm of a Jap machine gun sounded in my ears and "bees" whizzed by uncomfortably close. I hit the ground and flattened out. About ten yards from me was a brigadier general [BG Robert Shoe] and a group of his subordinates who were in the area observing the action. Unfortunately, three machine gun bullets found the general's left shoulder. I bellied over and administered first aid. We were not able to evacuate him for the better part of an hour. The machine gun had us "pinned down" until somebody took care of it. The general was the only man to be hit. He was a "good patient"; he stayed calm, and he did not interfere with our treatment and evacuation of him.

The fighting during this mission will probably be as bitter and costly as Corregidor, but the living conditions are better. This is a beautiful fertile island. When viewing the surrounding land and sea scapes it is difficult to realize that war has blighted this land. But the planes overhead, the rumble of artillery, and the sharp cracks of gunfire prevent even temporary escape from reality.

The news of President Roosevelt's death saddened us.

April 27, 1945   I have not been able to write to you for about two weeks. In the event that you have not yet received my last letter, I shall review the situation. We are again in combat and have been for several weeks. This mission will not make the headlines. We did not jump. We are engaged in so called "mopping up" work on another Philippine island. But, it is the roughest mission we have yet had and it is far from over. We are up against well-armed, well dug in, well organized numerous Japs who are using smart defensive tactics with the terrain in their favor. We are gradually pushing them back and killing them off, but we are paying a high price. More of my friends have been killed and more of my aid men have been wounded. So, once again I am extremely busy. And once again, like Corregidor, I am alone [the only medical officer for the battalion]. Lt. Pierce was sent to another sector temporarily. Fortunately, living conditions during this mission have been better than previously. We are receiving fresh bread, some fresh eggs, and much better field rations than in the past. The present C-ration is much better than the C-ration of six months ago. Even the K-rations have been improved. I'm afraid the Japs are far from being licked. Even when they are finally thoroughly defeated, I doubt if they will realize it. For example, there is absolutely no hope for the Japs we are now fighting. Yet they fight as though they are the personal guardians of the Emperor. My letters will probably continue to be infrequent. It is unavoidable. All too often night falls before I realize it. And, of course, we use no lights. Sometimes I hope this mission will soon end. Other times, it doesn't seem to matter. The sooner this one is over, the sooner the next one will start. The present tempo of the war is terrific. No combat outfit sits very long these days. With each new mission I become more and more proud of my aid men. They have guts and stamina and are cool-headed under fire. It tears my heart out every time one of them gets hit. One was killed on Corregidor. During this action, one of them lost a leg as the result of wounds. He was hit while working his way under fire towards a wounded rifleman. Despite his wound, he reached the rifleman and treated him. He is an example of the kind of men I have in my section.

May 13, 1945 (Mother's Day)   I am woefully behind in my letter writing. But we are still heavily engaged in this campaign and it continues to be rough fighting. As we advance the terrain becomes more rugged and the Japanese defenses more obstinate. Several more of my aid men have been wounded, but none seriously, for which I am very thankful. Received a letter from the medical soldier who lost a leg. His spirits are good and he is facing his misfortune with an admirable philosophy. The news of Germany's surrender was exhilarating to us. However, we won't fully appreciate it until more men and material are sent to this theater.

This current mission has progressed into mountainous jungle warfare—just like old times. The 503 troopers are experienced jungle fighters. Nevertheless, jungle warfare is eerie and we have been having considerable rain. This mission will probably be our longest to date. As before, the Japs insist on being killed off to the last man—and there are a lot of them.

I was not pleased to learn that Harry [a brother-in-law] had debarked at Okinawa. I have often been thankful that I arrived overseas prior to the time that it became necessary to send replacements fresh from the States immediately into the battle lines. I was introduced to combat gradually. Each new mission has been on a yet larger scale.

Combat medics have finally been authorized a combat badge similar to the Combat infantry badge. However, they will not draw the extra $10 a month. Congress decided that would violate the Geneva Convention. But now that the European part of the war is over, Congress may change its position. Japan definitely does not observe the Geneva Convention. We do not wear Red Cross insignia because they draw Japanese fire. Rest assured that my foxhole is deep and I am not taking any foolish chances.

May 30, 1945 We are still engaged—it won't be long until we reach the two month mark—a new record for continuous combat time for us. We have spent 3½ months in combat during the past six months. We keep hoping that the Japs will realize their situation is hopeless and surrender. We have them isolated with no chance of escape or relief. Yet they fight on forcing us to kill them off in toto. This we are more than willing to do, but it costs us too many men.

Since my last letter another of our medics was killed by a Jap land mine. He was an excellent soldier, married, and the father of three children. It is depressing to live in the constant presence of potential sudden death. We are still fighting in jungled mountainous terrain and we are still having frequent rains.

June 1, 1945 [I was transferred from the Third Battalion to Regiment to prepare to assume the assignment as Regimental Surgeon in place of Major Stevens who had acquired enough points to return to the States.]

Tonight, for a change, I have *good* news to relay to you. Today I returned to the job which was my first assignment in the 503—Asst. Regimental Surgeon. However, the circumstances are different this time. Major Stevens is scheduled to leave within a few days. Then I will become the Regimental Surgeon. This is something I never expected. Somehow I remained healthy, intact, and on the job through five missions while rotation, injury, illness and death claimed all the medical officers senior to me.

August 8, 1945 The topic of conversation over here is, as it undoubtedly is in the States, the atomic bomb. It should shorten the war.

Now have a medical laboratory. The last group of medical replacements included a well trained laboratory technician. I gave him the use of the Japanese microscope I obtained on Corregidor. We have a lab capable of running all the routine tests, including dark fields (for early syphilis). It helps us make more accurate diagnoses. The technician is very dedicated and conscientious. He works long hours when necessary. Equipment that we can't obtain doesn't bother him—he improvises.

August 17, 1945 It looks like it is just about over. We won't believe it until our troops occupy Japan. We don't trust the bastards.

The remnants of the Japanese garrison here have not surrendered and have not given any indication of doing so. They are completely cut off and may have no knowledge of the peace proceedings. We are dropping leaflets by the thousands hoping that they will believe the message.

August 21, 1945 The dilly-dallying over the surrender continues—and it irritates us considerably. Our particular group of Jap antagonists have given no indication of giving themselves up. Occasionally, single soldiers or small groups turn themselves over to our custody. We know that there [are] several thousands in the mountains. We have no desire now to go in after them. The war is over and we have already lost too many good men.

September 4, 1945 The formal surrender of the Imperial Japanese Forces of Northern Negros occurred Thursday, August 30. Lt. Col. Lawrie and his immediate staff (including myself) accepted the capitulation of the Japanese Commanding General (Lt. Gen. Kono), his staff and his forces. The two staffs lined up facing each other. The climax of the ceremony was the presentation of sabers by the Japanese to us. I was opposite a Japanese captain. He stiffly approached, presented his saber, and ceremoniously bowed from the waist. The ceremony took place in foothills near the base of the largest volcanic mountain on the island. The Japs had marched down from their strongholds in the mountains. We rode out in jeeps and trucks to the end of a road to meet them. All went smoothly in strict accordance with the rules of warfare. General Kono fainted at the end of the ceremony; heat exhaustion on top of debilitating illnesses. I revived him and supervised his transport to our hospital in Bacolod. He was a cooperative patient.

The surrender produced many medical problems. The Japanese number in the thousands and many are in foul shape—wounds, starvation, deficiency diseases, dysenteries, malaria, skin diseases, etc. We have established a POW hospital utilizing Japanese medical officers and technicians who care for their sick and wounded under our supervision.

Once they became convinced that their Emperor had surrendered they became very passive. We have had no trouble with active hostility. The healthy ones are in stockades. We had to teach them how to use our type of latrine. Initially, they got up on the latrine boxes, squatted, and frequently missed the holes.

September 20, 1945   Not too long ago we were anticipating parachuting onto Honshu island ahead of an amphibious assault. Thank God it is over.

We have collected over 8,000 Jap prisoners on Negros, which means that during the past three months they outnumbered us on this island about 8 to 5. When the 40th Division left Negros their G–2 estimated that only 1,500 effective Japs remained on Negros. We arranged the surrender of all these Japs without the aid or interference of higher headquarters.

During the war the 503 has now killed or captured over 15,000 Japs— three times our standard strength.

Addendum: I recall one very sad day fairly early in the campaign when the Third Battalion sustained 14 KIA [killed in action] losses, ten of which were due to what is now called "friendly fire." These losses included my dear friend Capt. Murphy. A short artillery round (ours) landed in his company headquarters.

Chapter Nineteen

Medical Supply

GLEN A. FOOKES

The following account is from interviews conducted by Amy Sandberg of Alma College with Glen A. Fookes of Alma, Michigan. Mr. Fookes was 90 years old at the time of the interviews. He died in June 1999.

Well, when I got my notice to report then I got on the train here. They picked us up on a train. There were a lot of men on there who were just going in like me. And this train went to Fort Custer, Michigan. And they got us off of the train there at Fort Custer. We stayed there for a few days. And then they started shipping them out from Fort Custer. They put quite a lot of us on one train and then they all didn't get off at the same place. They got off at different camps, see.... I got off at my place where I took my medic training. That was Camp Robinson, Arkansas.

Well, we had some training, like the infantry does. Exercises and long marches maybe once a week. Ten miles, 15 miles, maybe as high as 25 miles. And then every afternoon mostly we had outside classes, you know, [on] just like ballgame seats. You sit out there and then the doctors come and face the crowd and talk about the body and different things and the heart and so forth. They had several doctors there. Some of them were quite smart doctors, too.... We had other kinds of exercises we had to do. Keep us busy doing something. I remember one Sunday there they got us going. We had to change our fatigue uniforms to our dress uniforms and we had so much time to get back to our cabins. Then they'd blow the whistle, and we had to run down and get into formation. When that whistle'd blow you were supposed to be there.... Then they'd go back, and they'd blow the whistle a little later on and tell you how many minutes you had to get back down to the fort. It's crazy the way some of the army things happen. It don't make sense.

Well, maybe it made sense to a certain extent. To me it didn't. And to others it didn't, either. Like when we was in Fort Jackson there. There wasn't much to do, but we had to be there in that camp. They had a lot of boxes there. They had us pile them boxes over here. Then the next day pile 'em back over here, and stuff like that. Don't make no sense.

Course we had the other work there to do. Guard work and KP and that kind of work. Other than that we didn't have much to do while we were there.... Later on ... we activated our company there in Fort Jackson, South Carolina, and ... I and a few other guys went to Atlanta, Georgia, for further training. See now I'm in the, well, depo stuff, supplies, when we get down there. Some of our guys out there went to hospitals, and some of them went to other places, and they didn't all come from the same place. So I was down there in Georgia for I think about four or five weeks. Then I came back to Fort Jackson, and I was back there a while. Then they sent a sergeant and ten of us guys, and I was in the bunch that went, I was one of the ten, and we came to—they had another medical place in Toledo, Ohio. So we went there for I guess, oh, maybe a couple weeks. Then we went back to Fort Jackson.

So it was getting along towards March then we loaded up, and we got a train. We had a train all of our own. They had a mess car on there. You'd eat and cook and everything on that one car.... Of course, we had other cars to sleep in and like that, but they fed us and everything right on the train. We didn't stop anywhere. We arrived in the desert, out in the Mojave Desert in California. That's where we set up our depot.... This place out there, as I get it, was a holding and a consignment point for supplies to go to the South Pacific. But at one time they trained troops ... in the desert.... They had about 300,000 men there. And they had some big warehouses. So that's where we set up our depot ... in one of them big warehouses. So when things got slow out there, they took all these medical supplies. They took quite a lot of medical supplies for so many soldiers. They took that with trucks and took it all back to Los Angeles. Then when we set up our depot, they trucked all that stuff back to us. It was all mixed up. They just threw it in the truck. So we had to sort it out and repair what we could of it. Then, that was sent to the hospitals in the States. I guess it couldn't go overseas because it was used stuff. It took us, March—I think we left there about the first of July. It took us that long to take care of that stuff. Some of it we couldn't do nothing with.... But ... we repaired all we could repair, and boxed it up and inventoried it. You had to tell how many of this and that was in each box.

About that time we were ready to get leave out there. And the desert was getting pretty warm. It was getting up to 110 or 115 degrees in the daytime. But the desert's kind of a, to me, I can't hardly explain it to you. It's hotter than the dickens in the daytime and dropped way down cool at night. I used to put a couple blankets on me at night. In the daytime like I say it might get up 110, 115 degrees. We were right up close to a town called Yermo. There wasn't much there. A couple miles from where we had a warehouse deal set up. So, like I say, we got that work all done [and] they sent us back to Fort Knox, Kentucky.

Well, like I say, that was long about July sometime. So actually, we didn't have nothing to do, either. We just exercised. That's about all we done each day. We exercised. They would give us exercise in the morning and in the afternoon, too.

Well, like I said, we didn't have any regular duties there. We were more or less just waiting to be shipped overseas. When the time come later that summer, just before Thanksgiving, they shipped us over to New York. We waited in a convoy. I'm not too sure, but it seems like we were about 12 or 13 days before we landed in Southhampton, England....

So we stayed there for, oh, probably a couple of weeks. There was a hospital there, so we, all of our company, they fed us there at the hospital. We got all of our meals from them. We had another place where we had a room. Course when the time come, why, when we got on the ship, this was another holiday, Christmas. I traveled on the holidays. Got on the boat Christmas morning. We didn't leave the harbor until about midnight that night. We crossed the English Channel over into France. So we were in France for a while, not too long. Then we got a train over there, and I think we went into Paris and stayed there overnight. Then we traveled on to where we were going to set up our depot, a little town called Carrington.

The village was empty, some warehouses. So we set up our depot in those buildings right there. We were close to the Normandy Peninsula. That's where we done all our work. When the war ended, the Germans surrendered, we moved the supplies, as I told you. They spent all that money to inventory all of them, and what did they do with them? They give the whole thing to the French people. We had stuff in our depot so we could make up a whole hospital and ship it out. Beds, and everything they needed. That was the kind of stuff we had. We stayed in Carrington until the war was over with. The rest of our company went, and I don't know where they went. I suppose to the South Pacific.

Now I'd seen something strange over in the Normandy Peninsula, and the boys that was with me, they figured the concussion from a big gun is what caused this. There's a big tree, quite close to the road; way up in the top of that tree there's a cow up there. The boys were thinking a concussion ... from a shell caused that.

I've always remembered that.... And the Battle of St. Lô there; we went through [it] with our train, going where we was to set up our depot. That town—there wasn't anything that looked like it was over four foot high. Everything—they just mowed it right down. I think that a lot of our own men, our aviators with the airplanes, killed a lot of our men to get to the Germans because they were up on the high land, and we're down here, see. St. Lô there. They ... bombed it so bad, they just bombed everything. Like I say, they killed a lot of our own men, because they couldn't get things "up." That town of St. Lô, they just wiped it right out. You couldn't believe there wasn't anything over four foot high out of a town.

We stopped there and looked around a little bit. There were still people that survived that, or got out of there and come back. I don't know where they were staying. Maybe they had little shacks, I don't know. They come along by the cars, and they had pails, and they had dippers in them, and they had cider. And they were giving us the cider. That's quite a drink over there, cider for them. And they had a lot of cognac, which is similar to our whiskey here. Of course, I guess some places you can get cognac here. I never bought any cognac; I bought whiskey. Ain't much difference. They claim in Paris that when the Germans went through there they took all the good cognac.

Two or three French homes I been in; one place where they did the washing. I was there at some mealtimes, and they had cider to drink. They got this old song they sing, "Apple Blossom Time in Normandy." You ever hear that? They had great big barrels [of cider] on two-wheel carts, and the horse pulling.... Lots of strange things over there in the old country. Not so strange now as they would have been years back. Like I say when I was a kid living up in the jungles, the woods of the north, I couldn't see how they survived up there, but that was the same way with some places in France, too.

The government had a box factory at Bordeaux, France. That's where the boys landed in the First World War. Now and then there had to be so many GIs there. The French run it and everything, but they just had to be there; I don't know why they sent me and another guy from where we was at, down there for a week. Boy, I'll tell you, we drove out to the slummy part there, and I don't see how people could even live at all in that slum. That would be just awful. One place, Carrington, where we was at, you couldn't hardly walk the way we was supposed to go, along the canal—...they throw the fish and everything into the river—oh, man, talk about stink, you can't even believe it. In town there, when the people live upstairs, that's when I see guys in town, GIs walking down the middle of the road, and people up there are opening windows and throwing their dishwater down, right on the sidewalk. I seen that.

We had some French women working in our depot; they come over with their great, big purses when they come to work. We knew what they was doing; they were stealing stuff. Nobody bothered them. No, they didn't bother them at all. A lot of them people wanted bed sheets. See, that was one of our items in our depot. We made up a complete hospital, you know what I'm talking about; just like a complete house. And we had all that stuff. It was crazy for them. You could get a fortune for them in French money. They had the money, but they couldn't buy nothing with it. They'd give you a fortune if you get a sheet and take it and sell it to them.

Another thing they were crazy about—once in a while we used to [get] hold of blankets come from England. That wasn't government issue, so we could sell them or give them away or whatever if we could get a hold of them. They went crazy for that kind of stuff. They made coats out of them. They were blankets with all different designs and some of them were quite pretty, if you know what I mean. You've seen Indian blankets, maybe? Something … [those lines]. They'd give you a fortune for it, too. They wanted it cause they could make a coat or jacket or whatever. A lot of the French had a lot of money, but they couldn't buy nothing with it. Only on the black market, that's the only way they could get it. Now I sold a lot of stuff on the black market over there; well, not a lot, but a few clothes I didn't need that had been government-issued to me. The guy used to come from the black-market place, and he use to come to our camp a couple of times a week at night and see if there was anything that we wanted to sell him. They'd buy most anything, no matter what it was.

Like I say, most of the women and the kids, they were crazy for the chocolate bars. That's always one of the big items that they wanted to buy. Chocolate bars and cigarettes, too.

I don't know [if the war changed me]. I can say that it probably did some men that were in the war, because there was time they'd send back ten or 15 men and put them in our company, and they were the guys that got off in the head. Couldn't stand the infantry fighting anymore. So it does. It did affect some people, but it didn't affect me. You kind of get to thinking about home and like that, you know. But other than that, I don't think about it any, too much. Like I say, we weren't in any danger any time, just the one time that I told you, when they thought the Germans were dropping paratroopers back of the front lines. And that's where we was, back of the front lines.... [I saw] the Battle of the Bulge there. They took them big six-by-six trucks, and they loaded guys in there; they didn't know whether they was dead or alive. They got them out of the front lines, back to the first-aid station, and just piled them right there. Some of them were dead, and some of them were still living. That was quite a deal over there especially, that Battle of the Bulge. Of course, that was the final battle. There was other battles; a lot of men was killed there. Anyhow, the Allies had to come in on the lowlands and the Germans up on the top, and they couldn't get them out of there. The only way they could do it was bomb them. They say a lot of our men bombed our own guys in order to get to the Germans. They couldn't get to them otherwise.

Chapter Twenty

An Unbroken Chain
JEREMIAH HENRY HOLLEMAN, M.D.

Selecting the title "An Unbroken Chain" for these writings was somewhat of an afterthought. When hope of continuing my education seemed so fragile and appeared on the brink of disruption for lack of financial resources, time after time, a Godsend or unexpected event would occur and add another link to the chain of events that allowed me to continue my studies.
The thought often occurs to me, if the chain had been broken and never mended, how different my life would have been regarding people, places, and achievements.
—Jeremiah Henry Holleman, M.D., F.A.C.S.

From An Unbroken Chain: Memoirs by Jeremiah Henry Holleman, M.D. *(pp. 119–144). Dr. Holleman's book, a private publication for his family and friends, was published in 1997. Dr. Holleman served with the 89th Division, Combat 314th Engineer Battalion, all the way into Germany, liberating a concentration camp.*

Time was nearing for the end of my internship and induction into the army. Dr. Linberry, Chief of Medicine, offered to get my military commitment deferred if I would sign up for an internal medicine residency. I thanked him and declined. It was not a hard decision to make.

A letter came from Agnes with good news. She was going to be the first student in the history of the University of Tennessee School of Nursing to be allowed to get married and stay in nursing school. The old ironclad rule had been broken. Miss Nell Ruth Murry was Chief Nurse and it was her decision. I am sure her decision was influenced by the exigencies of the military, but Agnes accused me of being her pet when I was in Medical School.

The date was set for June 12, 1944. It was to be in Greenwood. I had picked out a small diamond ring and paid for it on the "lay-away plan" for some time. I took the ring to Memphis and plans were finalized. All I had to do was show up June 12, 1944, with the wedding band. Agnes, Mrs. Smith and Effie would make all of the plans. I left Memphis and went back to Birmingham with a slight sense of apprehension, which I reasoned was probably due to the newness as well as to the finality of the situation. I had the feeling of being on the fast track and for a while had difficulty concentrating on my work and studies. I was distressed to see Papa had suffered a slight stroke, although he was recovering. My parents were excited about the wedding....

I asked Dr. Ben Carraway for a week off around June 12. I knew it would be okay, but first he had to do a lot of teasing. The Greyhound bus from Birmingham pulled into the Greenwood Station about noon on June 11, 1944. In that era most events were dominated by the demands of the war effort. The rationing of gasoline and the restrictions on travel ruled out having a full wedding rehearsal. The best man and other participants were from out of town.

The hotel I checked into was near the Methodist Church. That evening I attended a dinner for the wedding participants who were in town. Mrs. Smith and Agnes gave me instructions on the proceeding to be followed at the wedding. Effie was to be the Matron of Honor, my friend Dr. James Bailey from Memphis was to be the Best Man and the minister was Brother Shed Hill Caffey. That night at the hotel I unpacked my new officer's uniform with the First Lieutenant silver bar on the shoulders. I had received confirmation of my commission two weeks prior.

The reception was grand and elegant, but I was ready to get my bride and get out of there. We left Greenwood with a destination of Jackson, Mississippi just as the sun was setting....

Time flew by. It was time for Agnes to go back to Memphis to finish nursing school. I received orders to report to Carlisle Barracks in Pennsylvania for basic military training. It seemed the whole world was in a state of flux, but when you are young, you know it will all come together some day.

Carlisle, Pennsylvania, is remembered by most people for its native son, Jim Thorpe. He was a native of the Black Hawk Indian Tribe and was one of the greatest athletes of all time, excelling in football, baseball and many Olympic events. Carlisle is remembered by me and most World War II physicians as the site of Carlisle Barracks. That was where physicians were sent for indoctrination in military courtesy, customs, and other traditional military lore. We had classes in writing letters military style. There were classes in writing and interpreting military orders. We had a course in map reading, which was important to know. There were lessons in military law, proper wearing of the uniform, how to salute, and who to salute. We learned the insignia of rank for the army and the navy. We had lessons on food service and sanitation. We learned which injuries and illnesses were considered "in line of duty." There were classes on "Table of Organization" which describe every army unit from a squad, platoon, company, battalion, regiment, division, and corps in the army. Besides all of these things, we had to march. The course lasted about five weeks and concluded with a fifteen mile march. One segment of the march was over a small mountain called "Coronary Hill." All of these lessons were essential to performing in the military, but it was not a fun place to be for a new groom.

From Carlisle Barracks, I received orders to report to a large Army General Hospital in Tyler, Texas. In Tyler, I was actually in a pool of doctors, awaiting permanent assignment to an army unit. The wait was short. I was assigned to the 89th Infantry Division. The 89th Division was training for overseas deployment at Camp Butner near Durham, North Carolina ....

I arrived with an acute tonsillitis and temperature of 103 degrees. I found a room in a cheap hotel.

The next morning I felt some better and caught a bus to Camp Butner, and went to the 89th Division Personnel Office for my assignment. An infantry division consisted of three regiments of riflemen, an engineer battalion, an artillery battalion, and a medical collecting company; a total of about eighteen thousand men. The division was commanded by a Major General. Medical Officers in the military were called "surgeons" even if their chief responsibility was inspection of the mess halls or latrines. I was assigned as surgeon of the combat engineers battalion and commander of their medical detachment. I had 12 medical technicians "medics" under my command. Our charge was to attend to the medical needs of the eight hundred officers and men of the 314 Combat Engineer Battalion. My designated title was Battalion Surgeon. We were issued steel helmets and mess kits. I pasted a small photo of Agnes in my helmet liner. The helmet would go with me through my tour of duty and eventually home. The photo is still in place....

Training to go into combat was serious business. Everyone, including me and the medical detachment, had to crawl through the "infiltration" course with live machine-gun fire just overhead. We also had to go through gas chambers with real toxic gas, wearing gas masks. We knew the call to go overseas was coming, but did not know when or [in] which direction we would be sent....

After a short time, I had learned the names, the capabilities and the attitudes of the twelve medics who were under my command. Sgt. Ossana, a second generation Italian, was dedicated and knowledgeable. He was my right arm. Our place of operations and sick call was called the "dispensary." We usually finished sick call at noon and spent afternoons seeing emergencies or doing some training exercise—bandaging, splinting, etc.

On one occasion, we finished sick call at about 11:00 A.M. The medics were drinking coffee, reading the newspaper or just relaxing. Into the dispensary stepped a tall, stern, scowling officer wearing an eagle on one shirt collar and a caduceus on the other. Someone spotted him and yelled "Attention!" We all stood up in attention mode. No "at ease" was spoken.

"Lieutenant!" he finally spoke.

"Yes, sir," I replied.

"Why in the hell haven't you got these men out training?" he asked me in a vicious tone.

"We just finished sick call and were taking a break," I answered.

"I'm Col.——, 89th Division Surgeon. When I come back I expect to see some training going on!"

He walked out the door to his waiting jeep and driver. I never saw him again as long as we were in the United States. I related the incident to my battalion commander, Col. Elliott. He assured me he was satisfied with my performance and intimated the division surgeon had an ego problem.

To the best of my memory, it was in October of 1944 that events occurring suggested we were about to make a move to go overseas. In mid–November, the order came to move out. I said good-bye to Agnes and promised to write as soon as I could. The entire 89th Division, eighteen thousand officers and enlisted men, along with trucks, jeeps, half tracks, and artillery pieces boarded a train at Camp Butner. The next day we arrived at Fort Miles Standish near Boston. Fort Miles Standish was a "staging area" where final preparations were made prior to boarding ship for overseas. It was now obvious we were headed to the European Theater of Operations. That evening General George C. Marshall addressed an assembly of all officers of the 89th Division.

The next day, we boarded ship just as the sun was setting. With all aboard, the gangplank was raised. As darkness was settling over the harbor there was a lurch of the ship followed by a sensation of slowly moving. We were going out to sea! I stood on deck and watched the lights of

Boston. As we moved away they became dimmer and dimmer, then just a faint halo above the horizon, then total darkness. There were no sounds except the waves of the ocean and the chugging of the ship's engine. There was a slight feeling of eeriness as we moved further out to sea. I wondered if Agnes had gotten home to Greenwood.

At first light the next morning, it was obvious our ship was part of a huge convoy. In every direction there were troop ships and cargo ships traveling in the same direction at the same speed. Moving in and about the convoy of troop and cargo ships was the very welcome presence of the U.S. Navy. Approximately twelve destroyer escorts were weaving about in search of German U-boats. They were very graceful and agile warships. They dropped numerous depth charges on real or imaginary targets. Huge spouts of water erupted skyward from each detonated depth charge.

The first morning aboard ship we set up the 314th Engineer Battalion aid station. It was located mid-ship on a lower deck so when lighted it would not be visible at night. Conditions on ship were tolerable, but not elegant. The officers' quarters had triple deck cots, two to each small state room. Many of the enlisted personnel slept on swinging hammocks. The ship was grossly overcrowded. Officers were assigned to tables in the Officers' Mess. A good officer and a good friend of mine named Harold Grinstedt ate at my table. He had a horrible cold and coughed incessantly through each meal.

The North Atlantic Ocean has a reputation for being rough and stormy in the winter. This year it was living up to that billing with a vengeance. The winds howled, the rolling, crashing waves and swells were often twenty or more feet high with deep valleys between each wave. The ends of the ships frequently cleared the water. Sea sickness abounded. The motion finally got to me. It's no fun to try holding sick call holding onto a barf bag. After days of tossing at sea, what a relief it was to anchor in the still waters of the Azores Islands while the ships took on fuel and supplies. The remainder of the trip was smooth sailing.

Our ship was named the U.S.S. *Excelsior*. She, along with three other ships, broke ranks with the convoy and anchored in the harbor of Le Harve, France. As our ship lay at anchor, we waited overnight for orders to go ashore....

We were aware we were going into the combat zone. Motivation and morale of Armed Forces personnel during war time are roused and deeply intensified when individuals have a strong belief in the cause for which they are fighting. It is also a morale booster to have the goodwill and support of people on the home front. The will to fight and endure is enhanced

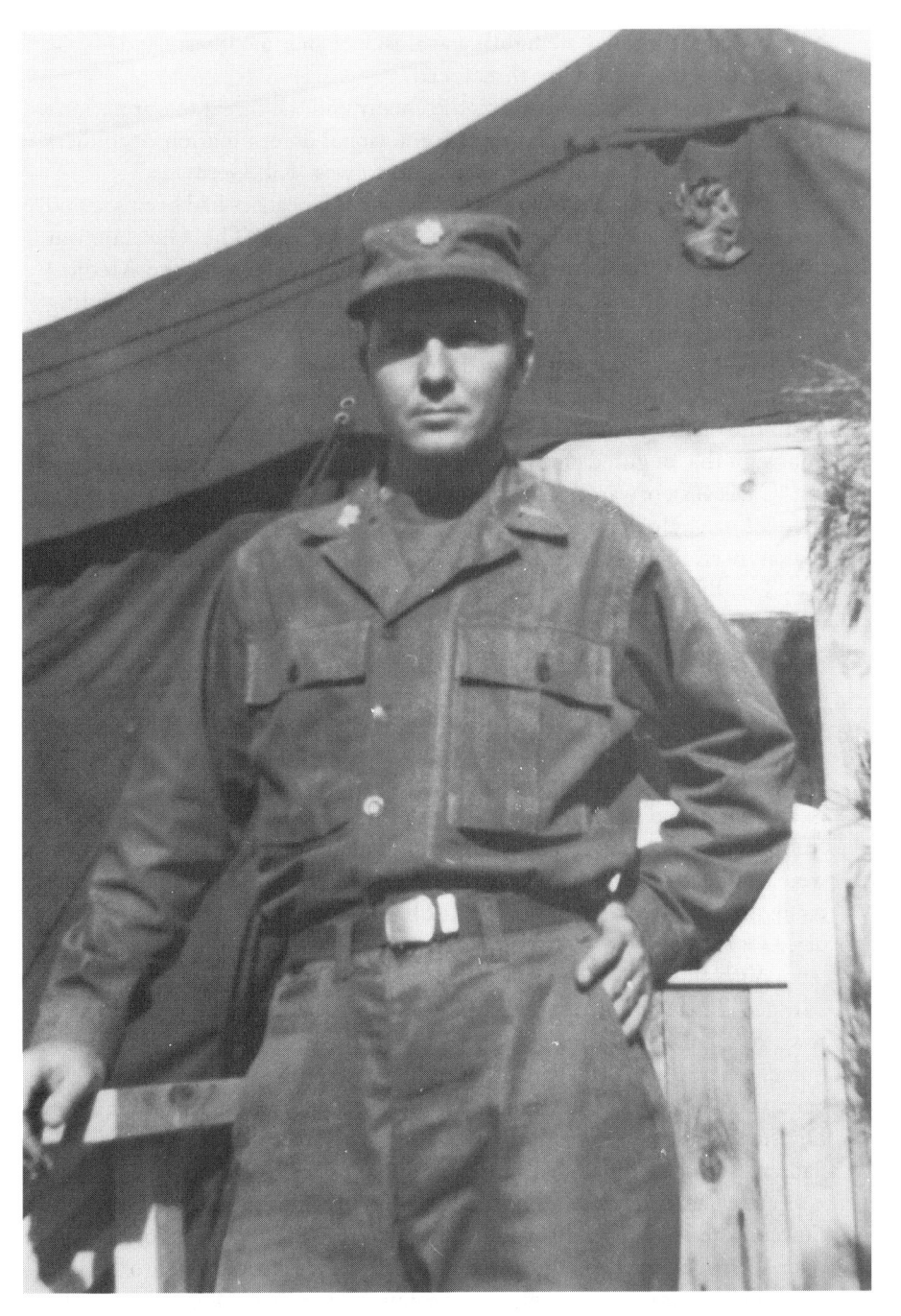

Dr. Jeremiah H. Holleman. *Courtesy of Dr. Jeremiah H. Holleman.*

by knowledge that they are fighting against evil and that liberty and justice and even the homeland are threatened....

The atrocities committed by the enemy and the threat to our nation's security were sufficient to create the emotional determination of soldiers of the 89th Division. The Division's motto was "Kill Germans."

When the 89th Division joined the war, the beaches had been secured and fighting was inland in France and Germany. The German war machine had been wounded, but was far from defeated. The Medical Detachment had two vehicles. One was a jeep for the Commanding Officer and a driver. The other was a truck for carrying men and equipment. Our entire Division moved slowly forward as a unit. There was a reconnaissance team ahead and on each flank to look out for enemy troops. With the onset of darkness we continued to move forward. The first ominous sign that augured entry into the battle zone was a roadside sign reading "Cat Eyes Forward." This meant turn off head lights—turn on cat eye lights. Each vehicle was equipped with "cat eye" lights, a small dim light that showed the road but was not visible from afar.

The 89th Division was integrated into the 3rd Army under Command of General George Patton. Our advance across the French countryside and through villages went unchallenged except for an occasional sniper and the occasional straggler from the German army. The baptism by fire came as the Division approached the town of Metz in the Moselle Valley in southeast France. This engagement lasted about two days. The Graves Registration headquarters was near our aid station and was located in an abandoned warehouse. A walk through this warehouse provoked a feeling of sadness and a heavy heart. Lying side by side, still in uniform were a large number of young American soldiers, lying still in death. One young man with a heavy mop of thick blond hair still lingers in my memory.

With this first engagement over, the Division resumed the forward advance. The next encounter with the Germans was at the small French town of Boulay. Our aid station occupied the ground floor of a private home. The 314th Combat Engineers were standing by, but had not yet been used as infantry men. After Boulay was cleared of the enemy, the Division continued moving eastward into the areas called Saarland. We had crossed the French-German border and were in Germany!

After crossing into Germany, resistance stiffened and progress was slowed. The 314 Engineers were called on to replace a bridge across a small river so trucks and artillery pieces could advance. In the town of Hamburg and the surrounding fields, a ferocious and prolonged battle occurred. While in Hamburg, I witnessed an awesome sight. I heard a drone overhead and looked up. The sky was filled with airplanes. There must have been over a hundred bombers flying in formation. They were escorted by fighter planes. Hours later my medical detachment drove through the town. The American dead had been removed, but the streets and fields were filled with dead German soldiers. It was an eerie feeling. I had my jeep driver stop long enough for me to jump out and retrieve a German Mauser rifle. (I still have it.)

Agnes and I were communicating almost daily by mail, but on some days I was unable to write.... Censorship prevented me from writing about the war. I was required to read every letter men of the medical detachment sent home and cut out any information that may have been useful to the enemy.

After about seven weeks on the front, the entire 89th Division was pulled out for a week's rest and relaxation. We went as a unit to Luxembourg City and everyone had a shower—the first in seven weeks. From Luxembourg we went to Paris. For four or five days I saw the sights of that city. I saw the Arc de Triomphe, the Champs Élysées, the Eiffel Tower and Notre Dame Cathedral. In the cathedral there were piles of hay the German soldiers [had] used as beds when they occupied the city. I ate at a sidewalk café and on the last night in town saw the Folies Bergère and the CanCan dance.

Back on the front, Paris was just a memory. The American lines were approaching the mighty Rhine River. The 314th Engineer Battalion, in concert with some engineers from the corps level were to build a pontoon bridge across the Rhine, capable of supporting trucks, tanks and artillery. The town of St. Gore was selected as the site to build the bridge. St. Gore is three miles north of the treacherous shoals and the Lorelei. This was the opportunity for the engineers to have their day in the sun. There were two large medieval castles on a high bluff overlooking the river thought to be occupied by Germans. Our artillery hurled shells against the castles. They bounced off with no notable damage. It was fascinating to watch the bridge take shape. Large, inflated rubber pontoons joined together side-by-side bridged by parallel runners were in place within twenty-four hours. Infantry men crossed the bridge on foot followed by trucks, artillery and tanks. The engineers had come through. Part of the 314 Engineer Battalion remained in St. Gore for maintenance of the bridge.

Later in the day it was interesting to stand on the west end of the bridge and watch a large contingent of German prisoners of war march across the bridge. Though herded by armed American soldiers, the German prisoners strutted as if they were in charge.

By far the most repugnant ... [sight] of the entire war was a concentration camp at Ohrdurf, Germany. As our division approached, the Germans abandoned the camp. As they abandoned camp they ... lined up and machine gunned twenty-eight inmates. They were laying in a row each in a pool of his or her own blood. They were in dirty prisoner garb. They were emaciated with sunken eyes and cheeks; their arm and leg muscles were wasted in atrophy of starvation. Their bodies were lying in grotesque contortions. Entry into a shed revealed human bodies stacked like cords of wood laminated with layers of lime and layers of bodies. Many of the bodies appeared to be well-nourished persons. There was a furnace type structure with piles of charred bodies and body parts. It was hard to realize we were looking on the remains of human beings who were once fathers, mothers, brothers, and sisters of loving families. They most likely were once the butcher, baker, postman, merchant, physician, teacher, innkeeper, craftsmen, all respected citizens.

The Ohrdurf Bürgemeister (Mayor) was ordered to tour the camp accompanied by an American officer. He denied any knowledge that the camp existed. That night the Bürgemeister committed suicide.

The 89th Division continued to advance eastward. I was sad to learn my friend and dining companion aboard ship, Lt. Grinstedt had been killed by the Germans. That same day a German POW was brought into our aid station. He had been shot in the left arm with an M1 rifle. The arm dangled by a lone tendon. One snip with the scissors completed the amputation.

On orders from General Patton, our division pulled out of the frontal attack and made a large half circle maneuver to entrap and attack the German army in a pincher movement. We arrived at and occupied the city of Zwickau near the Czechoslovakian border, after a short skirmish. Here I learned I had been promoted to the rank of Captain. It was here we received news of the death of President Franklin Roosevelt. He died April 12, 1945.

We were at the rear of the main German force and were prepared to attack. The attack was placed on hold. We encountered an unfriendly unit of the Russian army. They did not wish (were probably ordered) not to fraternize with American soldiers.

On May 7, 1945, we received the news that Germany had unconditionally surrendered. This war was over! It is estimated that approximately five hundred officers and enlisted personnel of the 89th Division were killed in action and twelve hundred were wounded.

From Zwickau, Germany, on the Czechoslovakian border our destination was Rouen, France. The 89th Division was being splintered. The 314th Engineers were slated to clear fields of land mines along the French coast. The battalion traveled across countries in a convoy made up of trucks and jeeps. The war was over, but hazardous duty was still ahead.

The 500 mile trek across central Germany and northern France vividly revealed the destruction and ruin of war. Frankfurt was the first major city we passed through. Not one building was standing; The city was totally deserted. The streets were filled with rubble in a vast sea of destruction. The bombers and artillery had done their job well. The findings in other major cities were similar. In villages and smaller towns, destruction was less severe. Along the roads were burned out German and American tanks and trucks. Hugh stacks of ammunition littered the road sides. Villagers we encountered showed mixed reactions. Some waved as we passed through, others were glum and sullen. The fields lay fallow, overgrown ... with weeds. Bodies of decaying horses and cows lay in the fields.

At one of our rest stops, we found a large stack of heavy ammunition. Lying beside it was a German helmet. Closer observation showed the helmet was attached by a wire to a large shell. It was a booby trap. The engineers defused it and probably saved some souvenir hunter from being blown to bits.

At Rouen, France, we were assigned quarters in a large chateau just outside city limits. One afternoon, I took a group of the men from the medical detachment into town for sightseeing. We parked the truck and walked around town. The next day our battalion C.O. Col. Elliott called me to his office and handed me a citation from the Military Police. When I asked why I had received a citation, he said it was for leaving our vehicle unguarded on the streets of Rouen. I had no idea the natives had been stealing army vehicles or that it was unlawful to leave one unguarded. Col. Elliott took care of the ticket.

We were moved out of the chateau and officers were billeted as paying guests in the homes of French natives. I was lodged in the home of an old couple, Monsieur and Madame Auguste Mongouar. We enjoyed a warm relationship. At a later date I sent them chocolate candy and a canned ham from the U.S.A., items not available in Rouen. While in Rouen, I visited the old market place where Jeanne-d'Arc was burned at the stake.

I desperately wanted to come home. I was afraid of being stuck in the Army of Occupation in Germany, so I volunteered for the war in the Pacific. This assured me a three week leave in the United States before deployment to war against Japan. The United States was gearing up for the invasion of the Japanese mainland.

For transport home, I was temporarily assigned to the 28th Division from Pennsylvania. On arrival in New York, I had orders to proceed to Camp Shelby, near Hattiesburg, Mississippi. I telephoned Agnes to meet me there. On the train out of New York, I saw a newspaper with big black headlines "U.S. Drops Atom Bomb on Japanese City...."

At the end of my leave, I expected to receive orders to [go to] the Pacific Theater, but to my amazement I was ordered to Camp Butner, near Durham, North Carolina, where I had trained with the 89th Division.

In spite of the massive destruction of Hiroshima by a single atom bomb, Japan refused to surrender. The first bomb was dropped August 6, 1945. A second bomb dropped three days later on August 9, 1945, destroying the city of Nagasaki. On September 2, 1945, Japan surrendered to General Douglas MacArthur aboard the Battleship Missouri....

From my own personal sense and being, I was satisfied with my contribution to our country's effort in the war. The 89th Division Combat 314th Engineer Battalion was an essential element of the division and the execution of the war. I was proud to be part of this unit. We were placed in harm's way many times and performed well. Our battalion had only one fatal casualty in the war.

In retrospective reminiscence, if I could have made any change it perhaps would have been to be assigned to an Infantry battalion. It may have been slightly more hazardous, but to me the men who wear that combat infantry badge are the real heroes of this war.

Chapter Twenty-One

Minefield

GREGORY S. KIRCHNER

Gregory Kirchner served in England, France, Belgium, Luxembourg and Germany as a member of the Medical Detachment of the 417th Infantry Regiment of the 76th Infantry Division.

On October 29, 1942, at the age of 24, I was drafted into the United States Army. I left the Pittsburgh area from the East Liberty train station not knowing just where I was headed. I remember we made our first stop at an army camp at Indiantown Gap, Pennsylvania. Some of the men left the train at this point. I remained on the train for what seemed a lifetime until we reached Camp Picket, Virginia. It was here that I had my basic training as a medic. Quite a change from my civilian job in a carpenter shop. At the end of basic training, I was sent to Fort Meade, Maryland, for further training. Eventually, the 76th Infantry Division was activated, and I became a member of the Medical Detachment of the 417th Infantry Regiment of the 76th Infantry Division.

The scope of our training became more intensified and included ski training in northern Michigan. At this time we were based at Camp McCoy, Wisconsin. Before leaving there for our trip overseas, I had occasion to use my medical training on two occasions. The first occurred at the camp while we were on maneuvers. Due to an error by a forward observer, artillery was directed into an area occupied by men. I was called on to give medical treatment to a man who was injured by the artillery. Shrapnel entered his leg just below the knee and blew away four inches of bone. His leg had to be amputated at the knee.

I again rendered medical service at Camp McCoy while on our way to Mass on a Sunday morning. It was snowing quite heavily as I was riding in back of a 2½-ton truck. The truck slowed down then crashed into a car that skidded across our path. As the truck came to a halt, I saw an infant in the snow near the truck. The crash had knocked the baby, the parents, and another woman out of the car. As I picked up the baby a large lump formed on the baby's temple. The baby died in my arms. The father, a soldier, had a leg broken in four places. The mother received injuries to her left hand. The injuries were severe. The other woman had one eyelid severed by flying glass.

My travels took me across the Atlantic Ocean to England, France, Belgium, Luxembourg, and Germany. While in combat I served with Company I of the 417th Infantry Regiment of the 76th Division. Normally there are three medics assigned to each infantry company. I outlived the first two plus eight replacements. When I made sergeant I was taken off the front lines. The man who took my place was killed the next morning.

During my term on the front lines, I experienced many gruesome times; the worst being when in 15 minutes I had seven casualties, five of whom had all or part of a leg blown off.... In regards to the minefield incident, I offer this explanation. An infantry company consisted of three platoons plus a headquarters section. One medic was assigned to each platoon. Just prior to the minefield incident, one medic had been killed and another wounded. This left me as the only medic with the company. The company commander ordered me to stay with the headquarters section where each platoon had radio contact. That way if I were needed I could be contacted quicker than if I stayed with the platoon I normally traveled with as we advanced.

In our advance the entire company passed through a field without incident. It was later we learned that the field was mined. The first platoon had crossed a road into an area that was also mined. The headquarters section remained on the road. An explosion took place, and a man came from the field that I had just passed through. He said there was a casualty. I returned to the field I had just came through. The last man in the line of advance had stepped on a mine. The front of his foot was blown off. This was the first we learned that the field was mined. As I treated him, I discovered another mine about a foot away from the injured man. I told the injured man of this second mine. I marked it with a streamer of gauze tied to a stick. I told the injured man to warn the stretcher bearers about the mine. The other men from this man's platoon were still stretched out in single file toward the road. As I moved forward I explained to each man that the area was mined. I told each man that he marked the

21. *Minefield* 113

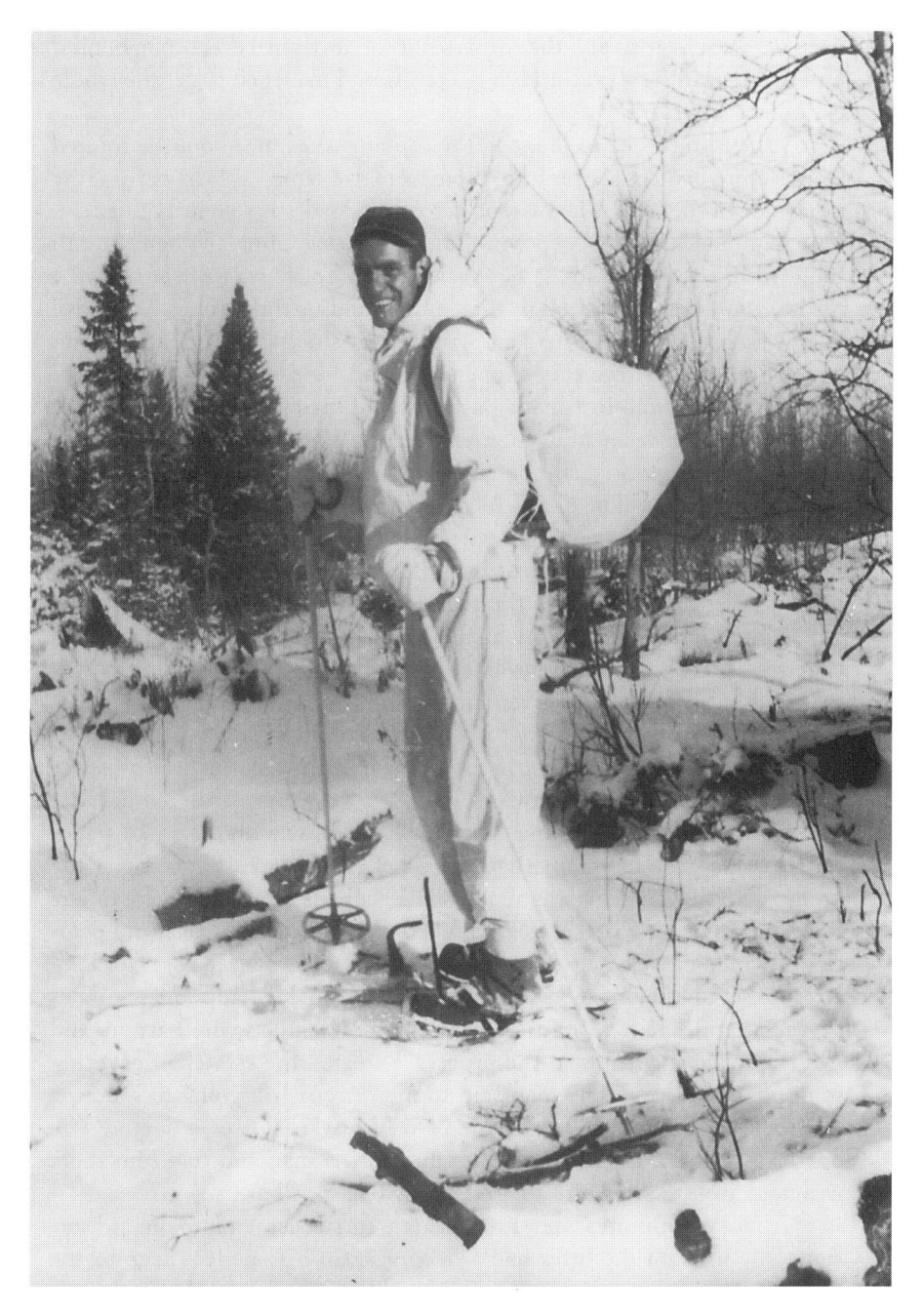

Gregory S. Kirchner, 76th Infantry Division, ski training at Waters Meet, Michigan, in the United States. *Courtesy of Gregory S. Kirchner.*

"safe" trail to the road and that he was not to move until every man behind him had moved forward through his position. I managed to get the whole platoon to the road.

When I returned to the road the captain asked me about the injured man. Before I could answer him, there were five rapid explosions from the other side of the road. The platoon across the road was also in a minefield. One man had kicked a "trip wire" and set off five mines. When the call came for me, the captain said, "Wait, if you get hurt, we won't have a medic; you have been through the field behind us three times." The five men were brought to the road and laid side by side, where I treated them.

Three days before this happened, I had been walking side by side with the fellow who lost his leg at the hip. Our mail had been brought up to us, and he was reading a letter from his wife. He said to me, "Well, Doc, by now my wife could be entering the hospital for our first baby. I hope to God she will be okay." As I treated him in that minefield, he said to me, "My God, what will my wife say." Here was a man almost blown in half, and he was thinking of his wife, not himself. It was when daylight arrived that I saw that the end of his nose was blown off. At that same time I could see that my hands, arms, and the front of my uniform were red with blood. Two days later he died in an ambulance on the way to a field hospital. We had given him plasma, but he needed whole blood. I have tried for over 50 years to reach his family without success. [Mr. Kirchner did make contact with his widow in 1999 with the help of newsman and author, Tom Brokaw.]

As the war was winding down in Europe, our division had penetrated deeper into Germany than any other Allied force, but being as the linkup with the Russians was already politically determined, we got orders to hold fast where we were. We were left in what was like a neutral position. As medics we set up a first aid station in a German house. Not long after we set up the first aid station, a man came in. He had some scratches on each hand. He had been dismantling some barbed wire barriers and had scratched his hands in the process. I treated the scratches, covering some that needed it. The man said to me, "Aren't you going to send me to the hospital?" When I told him "No," he asked to see a doctor. The doctor was in the next room and examined the man and told him there was no reason to send him to a hospital. The man left us.

About ten minutes later, litter bearers carried a man into our aid station. The man on the litter had a deep gash in his one leg, deep to the bone and extending almost the full length of the limb. We could not understand how or where he could have sustained such an injury. As the doctor and I were treating him and applying a "Thomas leg splint," I

21. Minefield

noticed the man's hands. He was the same man who had just left the aid station. How in the name of God did this happen? We questioned others to learn just how. The town we were in was under control of the army, and an order had been issued to the German civilians to surrender any weapons they had. A woman had a rifle and gave it to our patient. Without checking the rifle the man held it by the barrel end and slammed it against a tree. The gun exploded and hit the man's leg. He got his trip to the hospital.

Shortly after this happened, a man came to me and said, "Sergeant, get your gear together and come with me."

"Where are we going?" I asked.

"You are one of 20 men of the whole division whose name was drawn for a five-day furlough to London."

He had to convince me that it was indeed true. We rode in a truck across Germany into France where the trains were operating again. By train we traveled to Le Havre from where we crossed the English Channel. We reached London the day the war ended in Europe. All furloughs were extended to ten days. The celebration in London could be a book in itself. Trafalgar Square was so crowded you couldn't have fallen over even if you wanted to. At one time I was at Number 10 Downing Street. As I stood near the gate in the iron fence, Winston Churchill came out of the house and passed within arm's length of me. Later that day I was at the gates of Buckingham Palace where the Royal Family appeared on the balcony. Sir Winston was with them.

At the end of the ten-day furlough, our return to our outfit was delayed because every mode of transportation was being used for the transportation of prisoners of war. When we finally arrived back to our headquarters, my first sergeant said to me, "Where the hell have you been? We've all been to Switzerland. Do you wanna go?" I left with a buddy the next morning for ten days in Switzerland.

With the war ended, the need for some type of laundry service became apparent. This was solved when a German woman laundered our clothes, and we repaid her with a meal from our mess hall. On one occasion a woman returned a shirt to a fellow much quicker than he expected. The mess hall wasn't open to give her a meal, but he had just received a package from home that included about a dozen packets of the newly discovered fad Lipton's Noodle Soup, so he gave the woman several packets. She could not speak English; he could not speak German. She had no idea what the packet contained. Several days later the woman came to us when we had a GI who could speak German. The German woman was laughing when she explained this to the German-speaking soldier. She explained that she was mystified as to what the packet contained. She saw the word "soup" on the packet and thought it was "soap." Because the packet was so small, she thought it must be a very good grade of soap—she washed her hair with it! As the water ran down her face, she tasted it and learned what it was. She really laughed at herself. We did get her a meal from the mess hall.

Reverting back to the story of the minefield. On Valentines Day in 1998 I received an out-of-state phone call. The man calling went through directory assistance to reach me. On the phone he said, "Doc, I don't know if you realize it, but it is 53 years today since you treated me on the battlefield in Germany and saved my life." He was one of the men who had had a leg blown off. He lost his between the knee and ankle. We have since met for the first time in over half a century. We still correspond.

Two years ago while visiting my son in Chicago, I met up with an army buddy with whom I served. We spent a day with him and his wife. Next month we will be in Chicago again. We will again be with him and his wife plus two more buddies from the state of Wisconsin. I'm really looking forward to it.

The good Lord has brought me through recent open-heart surgery for quadruple bypass. At 80 years old I have much to be thankful for. With ten children and 19 grandchildren, I get lots of prayers coming my way.

Chapter Twenty-Two

"Young and Foolish as We Were"

DANIEL E. DiIACONI, M.D.

Dr. Daniel DiIaconi served as a Lieutenant in the Third Army.

My experiences during service in the ETO with George S. Patton's Third Army ranged from frightening to annoying. One day as I led my medical platoon convoy on the road to Orléans, a drunken driver in a convoy truck almost crashed into my jeep. When I pulled him over and advised him to sleep it off a while, he became abusive and pushed against my chest— that was too much for my driver, a native of Georgia, who knocked the drunk Negro out with a massive right hand to the jaw. We laid him in his truck and drove off feeling we had done a good deed getting [him] off the road in his condition. A few minutes later he came roaring up to us again and attempted to force us into the ditch. Failing at that, he roared off ahead of us and ambushed us in the narrow streets of the next village, firing at us with his M-1. We escaped and reported him to an MP further down the road....

One day before we crossed the Rhine, my driver and I decided to copy George Patton's caper of peeing in the Rhine. As we stood exposed on a bombed-out bridge approach over the river—exposed literally—a sniper from the far shore missed us closely. The jeep made a fast 180 degrees, and we got out of there, buttoning up as we fled.

During the severe winter weather of '44, the army decided to bring in dogsled teams to help evacuate casualties because the roads were causing much trouble for our ambulances. By the time the dogs arrived, however,

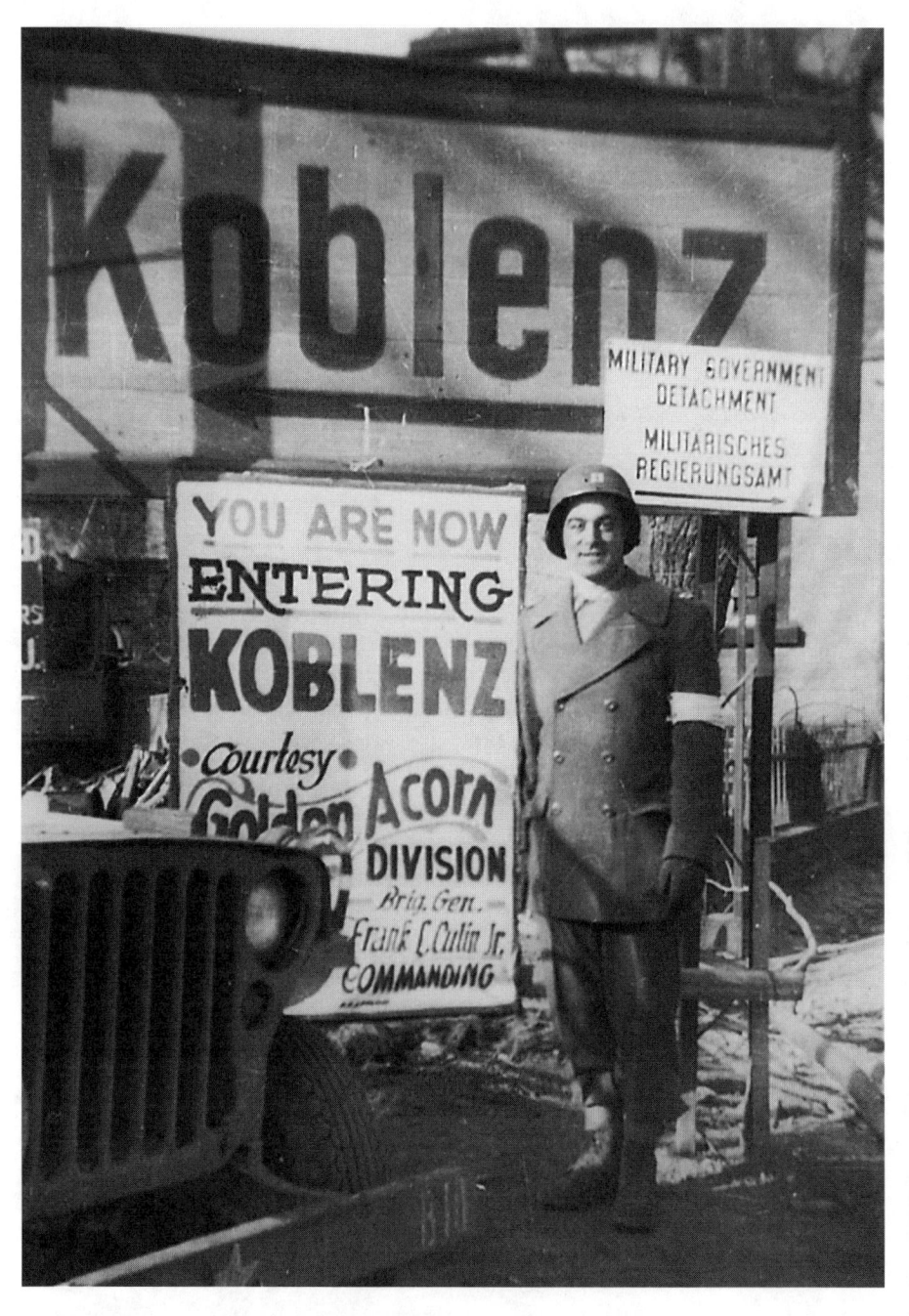

Dr. Daniel E. DiIaconi entering Koblenz, Germany. *Courtesy of Dr. Daniel E. DiIaconi.*

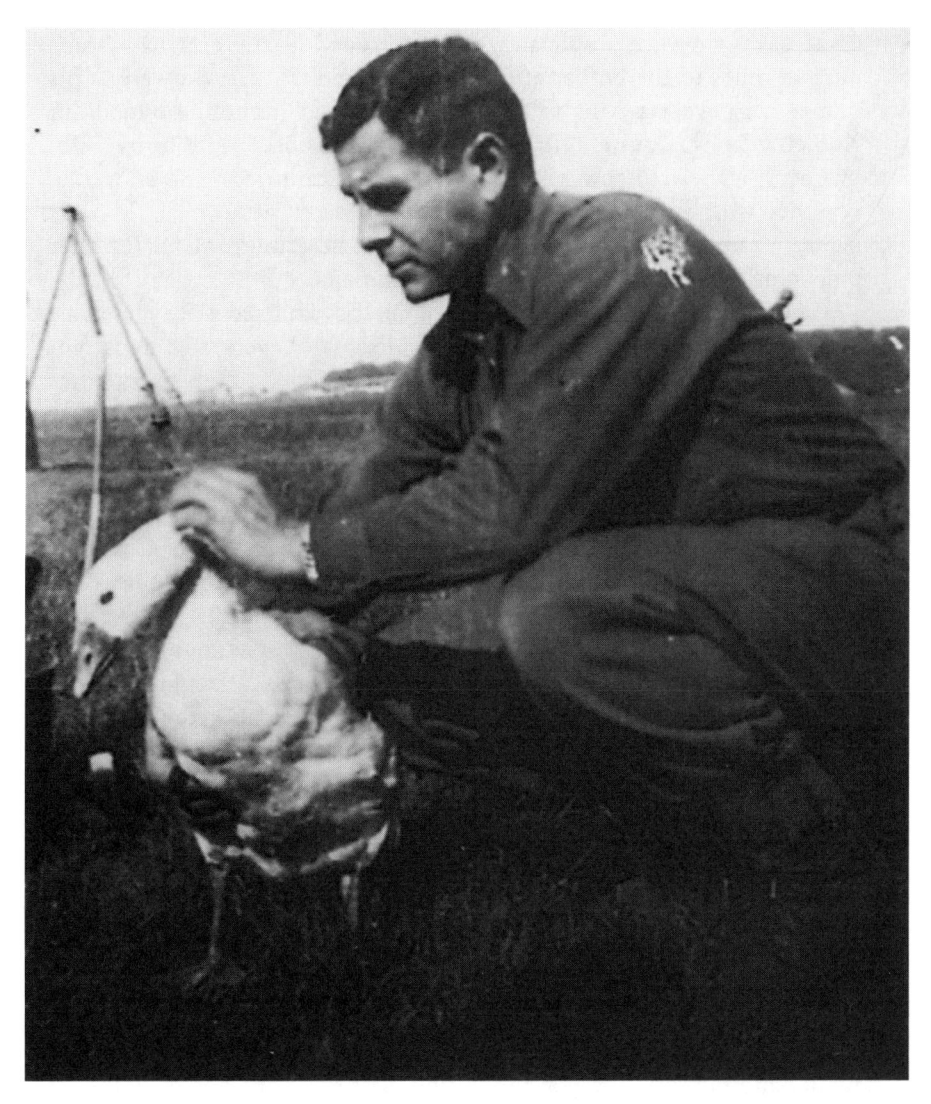

Dr. Daniel E. DiIaconi with mascot. *Courtesy of Dr. Daniel E. DiIaconi.*

the snow and ice were gone. We enjoyed playing with the dogs, riding the sleds over the wet grass, and noting how the dogs behaved. On the picket line, if it broke, a serious fight would erupt, but the next morning when in the traces those very same dogs would sleep cuddled against each other. That was business—no fooling around!

During the Battle of the Bulge all our vehicles were requisitioned to transport fighting elements to the battle front north of us. One of our doctors was a Jewish physician who had escaped Nazi Germany by running 18 miles to the border after he was warned that the SS were at his home. He never saw his folks again. As we sat immobile outside of Koblenz, he was quite agitated. When I tried to console him—"Oh, Werner, they won't know who you are if we are captured"—he said, "Oh, yes, they will. They have my fingerprints, pictures, etc., on file." Fortunately, we were not captured. He continued to be a runner all his life after practicing 50-plus years in Terre Haute, Indiana.

In the spring we picked up a stray, domestic, white goose ... and made him our company mascot. Young and foolish as we were, that goose got Company I food and liquor to excess, and we laughed to see his attempts to fly after having lapped up some booze. He went missing after a few weeks; I'm sure he made a tasty dinner for someone.

While we sat on the airfield outside Koblenz, we had German POWs to help maintain the camp. One of them was a stonemason who built an efficient stone oven for us in the tent we used as the Officers' Club. We used the cast-iron top to warm and cook goodies sent from home. With captured champagne cooling in the snow and hot snacks, we endured well. One of the POWs told me, "Captain, you people are fighting the wrong enemy—you should be fighting the Russians." I laughed him off at the time as full of Nazi propaganda, but in hindsight—the Wall, the Berlin Airlift, the arms race—it makes one think.

Fifty-five years ago I was a prolific storyteller, and one particular joke must have made quite an impression on a fellow officer. We had a fifty-year reunion in Indianapolis a few years ago, and he said, "Dan, I want you to tell that joke to my wife." Can you believe it?—50-plus years later.

As I write this I await the annual visit of a man from Manchester, England. This person is the son of the people I was billeted with in Wales before D-Day. Our transatlantic trip ended in Liverpool and from there we went by train to Ponty Pridd, Wales. Getting off the train we lined up in battalion formation on the station platform, and I looked out onto the hillsides to see unending piles of mine tailings. My thought was, "My gosh, this is just like a scene out of *How Green Was My Valley*." Subsequent experiences living with this Welsh family reinforced just that feeling. Their son was a five year old at that time, and Lieutenant Dan must have made an impression because 30 years later his father wrote to ask if Barri might come to hunt with me in Oregon. He did, and now comes every year. We have become family; my wife and I attended his daughter's wedding in June 1998 in Britain. His mother and father have been steady correspondents since 1944. When our battalion moved out of Cilfyudd,

I bought about 15 dollars worth of supplies (food, cigarettes, socks) at our PX and left them with the family. When I visited them 11 months later after V-E Day, they were still using some of those items. Chocolate bars had been doled out in tiny pieces; cigarettes were smoked one or two a week. They had relished Spam.

After V-E Day we left Regensburg and embarked for the Good Old United States of America. The battalion had already been assigned to the Eighth Army that was to invade Japan. Fortunately I was at home in Pittsburgh, Pennsylvania, on leave when Hiroshima and Nagasaki brought the war to an end.

Recalling the Atlantic crossing to the United States brings back another memory. One of the other officers had "liberated" a dachshund, which he said was purebred, and he intended to breed it at home. He smuggled it aboard, having drugged it into silence and carried it in his musette bag. The second day out the ship's PA system announced all dogs were to be brought to the fantail at 1600 hours. We thought sure the dogs were to be sacrificed, but, no, the captain had had kennels built, and the 50-plus dogs rode home in luxury.

I carried two bottles of champagne in my musette bag (which now serves me in hunting). Those two bottles were to be used to celebrate either the birth of a son or 25 years of marriage. My wife and I had three girls, so on the 25th anniversary the bottles were uncorked—and poured down the sink. They were undrinkable.

Chapter Twenty-Three

Ambulance Driver in the Italian Campaign
DES BALL

In the winter Italy was very cold with snow, rain and lots of mud. We seemed always to be muddy ... in summer it was hot and dry and we always seemed to be covered in dust.

We normally slept on the stone floors of farmhouses, etc., or [in] holes in the ground. I am not writing about the other Field Ambulance personnel, those medics and doctors who worked at dressing stations sometimes under fire and generally in rather hazardous conditions ... someone else will have to tell their story.
—Des Ball

The following account is taken from Des Ball's personal history, Field Ambulance, The Italian Campaign: Recollections of an Ambulance Driver, *recorded by his daughter Shirley Ann Fairest.*

1941–1945

I was 19 years old going on 20 when I joined the army, and after basic training was sent to an Ambulance Unit where I was driving an ambulance which was originally a delivery van commandeered from some firm or other. The NZ [New Zealand] Army at that time was so run down that the military were then allowed to commandeer trucks and cars, whatever vehicles were needed from private companies.

After months of training and going on maneuvers, etc., I, amongst many others, was pleased to find myself on a ship bound for the Middle East.

23. Ambulance Driver in the Italian Campaign

We were escorted most of the way by an Australian cruiser, and at one stage by a Catalina Flying Boat. On the way we stopped at Fremantle and then on to Aden where most of us saw for the first time how the really poor of this world lived and worked as we watched the coaling of a boat at the dock near us. The local men carrying baskets of coal on their heads while walking up a gangplank dumping the coal in the ships bunkers and then walking down another plank for another load. The air was full of coal dust and they were covered in it. No dirt money and long hours for very little pay. From Aden we headed up the Red Sea for Suez and Port Tewfik and it was from here on that we began to feel the heat. The sky was blue as was the sea with not even a ripple, and the coast we could see was to us an amazing sight of all these bare mountains with the desert colors of reds, yellows, blues and black. There are people living there, but on what, it is so hard to imagine. On arriving at Tewfik we waited in the stream for some time before being unloaded, and it was not long before the locals came out in their boats to trade in what appeared to be mainly junk, but they had to make a living somehow, I guess. At Maadi we loaded onto army trucks and were taken to our various units, mine being Fourth Field Ambulance.

The war was ending in North Africa, and the troops were settling back to Maadi and the usual training and overhauling of equipment, trips into Cairo, etc., where all of us new reinforcements learned the language of the grim digs (the old seasoned troops of the North African Campaign). The language consisted of Kiwi-English, Arabic, and once we got to Italy it would also include scraps of Italian. We were soon introduced to Stella beer, Zibib, and other rather potent drinks which were available in the drinking dens of Cairo. We were soon also to see sights which we had never before seen in New Zealand!

After some months the division moved to an area between El Alamein and Alexandria. Here we were lucky to be camped right on the beach and so had plenty of swimming. Leave to Alexandria was quite frequent, a different city to Cairo founded by Alexander the Great and one of the old trading cities of the Mediterranean. A lot of the population of Alexandria was of Greek origin and had been there for hundreds of years. We knew the division was being readied for action somewhere in Europe; some thought Greece or Italy. Some of the vehicles were waterproofed to give the impression it would be a coast landing somewhere, just in case the information got to the enemy. At last the division moved to embark on two convoys, one leaving from Port Said and the other from Suez. On the way to Suez I remember we pulled off the road and spent the night sleeping in the back of the trucks. We were miles from anywhere, and it just seemed to be desert as far as the eye could see. We woke next morning to a heavy fog, and as we pulled out onto the road to continue our journey, out of the fog came dozens of Arabs looking for anything we had discarded.... We never could work out where they had come from.

We arrived at Suez, and after a few days camped in the desert, we were rounded up and were loaded on to the various ships of the convoy. Our convoy carried all the heavy equipment, i.e. tanks, guns, ambulances and trucks, while the convoy from Port Said carried mainly troops. The whole convoy traveled up the Suez Canal and finally out into the Mediterranean. What a great sight with ships spread out on both sides and behind us as we were in the front line of the convoy. We all had barrage balloons flying, heavy machine guns on each side of the bridge, and a larger gun at the stern. It must have been half way when we ran into a severe storm, with thunder and lightning, and then some of the balloons were knocked out by the lightning. Our convoy stopped at Siracusa on the east coast of Sicily for a few hours, and it was then that we learned our destination was to be Bari in Southern Italy. The other convoy was to go to Taranto. Not far from our destination we heard over the intercom "Enemy Aircraft Approaching." We saw no sign of enemy aircraft, but in a very short time a number of Spitfires were flying over and around the convoy. As we neared the port of Bari we could see on our left the fields and houses of Italy, and on our right rising out of the sea were the distant mountains of German occupied Albania ....

As a complete brigade of about five to six thousand men plus tanks, armored cars, personnel carriers, field and anti-tank guns, we headed off in a northerly direction. We seemed to be getting along fine until we came to a road junction and took the wrong turning which led up a no exit road into the village square of a remote village. Here every vehicle and piece of equipment had to be turned around to go back the way we had come. It must have taken almost a day before we were on our way heading in the right direction. Our destination was the Sangro River which marked the front line, and as a division it was our job to push the German forces back across the river and out of the seemingly impregnable villages and towns which they held as part of their winter line. As we headed towards our destination we could see snow on the tops of the Apennines, a range of mountains which form the backbone of Italy until the Po Valley is reached. The Sangro River is in the region of the Province of Abruzzi, probably the most backward and wild of the provinces of Italy. The mountains come down almost to the shores of the Adriatic and there are lots of forests which are ... home to some of the last wild bears and wolves in Europe. I believe some of it has been declared a National Park now.

The rumble of guns in the distance told us we were nearing our destination, and now if my memory serves me right, we took over from one of the Indian Divisions. All the buildings in Italy were made of solid stone ... [and] were good as defensive positions, and the infantry usually had high casualty rates as a result. All driving at night was done without lights especially where ambulances were concerned as we worked mostly in front line areas and a good part of the time at night. The first wounded I carried back were from the railway station which comprised the station and a number of other buildings and was being used as a battery headquarters by one of our 25 pounder regiments. They had been shelled very heavily, taking a couple of direct hits, killing some and badly wounding others. There were still a few shells landing round about when I headed back to the dressing station. On the way I had to cross a strongly built stone bridge which was often shelled so I did not waste any time crossing it. It was unusual that it was still standing as the Germans blew up most bridges as they retreated. The weather was cold with rain, and it was not long before chains on wheels and anti-freeze in radiators ... [were] the order of the day.

The order of attack was to cross the river and with our artillery firing a heavy barrage, the first since North Africa, while the infantry waded across under heavy fire and suffering casualties. This kept us busy carrying them back to the dressing stations. The Sangro River was like one of the braided rivers in Canterbury [a region on the South Island of New Zealand] made up of numerous small flowing streams in winter, but a formidable flooding river during the spring and summer melt of snow from the mountains. Once the infantry had crossed the river and gained ground on the opposite bank the engineers went into action putting a Bailey Bridge over so as to get tanks, guns, and other support equipment over. This was not a pleasant job, often up to the waist in freezing water and under fire and almost always under cover of darkness.

As the Germans were driven back to the hill town of Orsogna and various mountain villages, it became a hard slog for the infantry who were taking positions then being driven off them, then retaking them again ... almost a stalemate. For the rest of us it was an artillery battle of each side shelling one another's roads and bridges and buildings. There was one place which would be well known to all who took part in the battle of the Sangro, and that was the mad mile and the brick works which were under observation by the enemy and shelled as soon as anything was seen to move in the area. Going up that road and past the brickworks was just foot hard down to the floorboards. So while all this was going on we were kept busy. Then it started to snow and snow, so that put an end to the attack on

Orsogna and the other German positions. The front became just a holding position, so we were pulled out while some other division took over so that we could go to some area more important. After a journey of a few days we found ourselves on the Cassino front which was part of the American Fifth Army area where we were to take over from some American division that had suffered heavy casualties in the advance to, and the battle for Cassino, a town that was going to be hard to take.

My first job in this battle was working ... [out of] a dressing station set up in a former farmhouse not far from the village of San Angelo which straddled the Rapido River a couple of miles down river from the town of Cassino. We were holding one part of the village, the south side of the river and the most direct route we used from the village to the dressing station, and from the dressing station back was the original railway track. The Germans had pulled up all the rails as they retreated, and it was rough driving especially at night when you were driving by instinct and the light from the muzzle flashes of the guns. The family who called the farmhouse home ... [—the farmhouse] which we had taken over as a dressing station[—]would not move out and took the risk of living through the battle. I suppose that they had nowhere else to go. I do know that in one of the later battles for the town after we had been pulled out ... the farmhouse ... [was] destroyed. One of our chaps who ... returned to the area many months later said it was just a heap of rubble, so what happened to the family I do not know. One day when I was down at the village I walked through the labyrinth of rooms that made up the buildings our infantry were holding to see a workmate from New Zealand. We could see the movement of the odd German in the buildings on the other side of the river, and when I asked why they did not fire on them, they pointed out that there was nothing to gain by doing so. Such was my ignorance of infantry work!

Things could seem quiet, but unexpected danger was always present as was demonstrated when we were called to pick up two casualties. One of our tank regiments had been sitting in static positions and acting as artillery just back a little from San Angelo. Seeing as things seemed quiet and [they were] bored with sitting in the tank, two of the tank crew had got out and were sitting by the tank playing cards when a shell or mortar bomb hit the side of the tank, wounding one and killing the other who must have taken a direct hit, as all we could do was collect the pieces and roll them in a sheet of canvas and take them and his wounded crew member to the dressing station.

At times we were called on to help civilians caught up in the turmoil of the battle, although this depended on the situation we ourselves were in at the time. This happened with the family I have mentioned who decided to stay on in the building we were using. The elderly lady who seemed to be the matriarch of the family was found dead outside the buildings one morning, killed by a shrapnel wound. She must have gone outside during the night, ... as the odd shell landed about.... I was asked to take her body, accompanied by her son, back to a village some miles behind the lines for burial in the village cemetery. We arrived at the village, and I left the son with his mother at the undertakers while I went and reported to the AMGO [Allied Military Government Officer]. This one was an American, and he invited me to lunch at the Army Mess. This was on the second floor with windows looking out onto grassy fields about a quarter of a mile away. We were watching a British pioneering regiment who were used to keep the roads in order filling in shell holes, etc. They were mostly Africans. They were putting up their little white pup tents in orderly rows and close together. Must have been a hundred or so tents, and they had just completed the operation and were being inspected by what looked like a couple of officers when away in the distance we heard a couple of muffled booms, and in a second or two what sounded like express trains passed over the building and landed with mighty bangs in the center of the tents, and there were pioneer troops running in all directions. Just typical of how stupid those kind of officers could be. Even if they thought they were in a safe area, [they still had] too much parade ground stuff.

After picking up the old lady's body which had been put into a coffin seemingly made from old boxwood, the son, a priest, and myself took the road to the cemetery about a mile from the village where a grave had been dug. After the ceremony I returned to the dressing station, and later in the day was sitting outside talking when we noticed a truck going along the road we had taken to the cemetery. It stopped, and about a mile away we could see three figures climb out of the truck and make their way down to a farmhouse just below the road. A moment or two later we heard the distant boom of a gun, and seconds later a shell landed on the side of the hill above the truck, then two more reports of a gun firing, one shell landing just down the hill from the truck and the third shell a direct hit; where the truck had been [there was] just a huge explosion and sheet of flame. The blokes from the truck were probably looking for wine and were right out of their area. They are probably still doing time in a British Punishment Center for losing the truck in that kind of situation! The road in question was reasonably safe for Red Cross vehicles but a dangerous place for any others....

Coming back to the battery headquarters late one day, I picked up

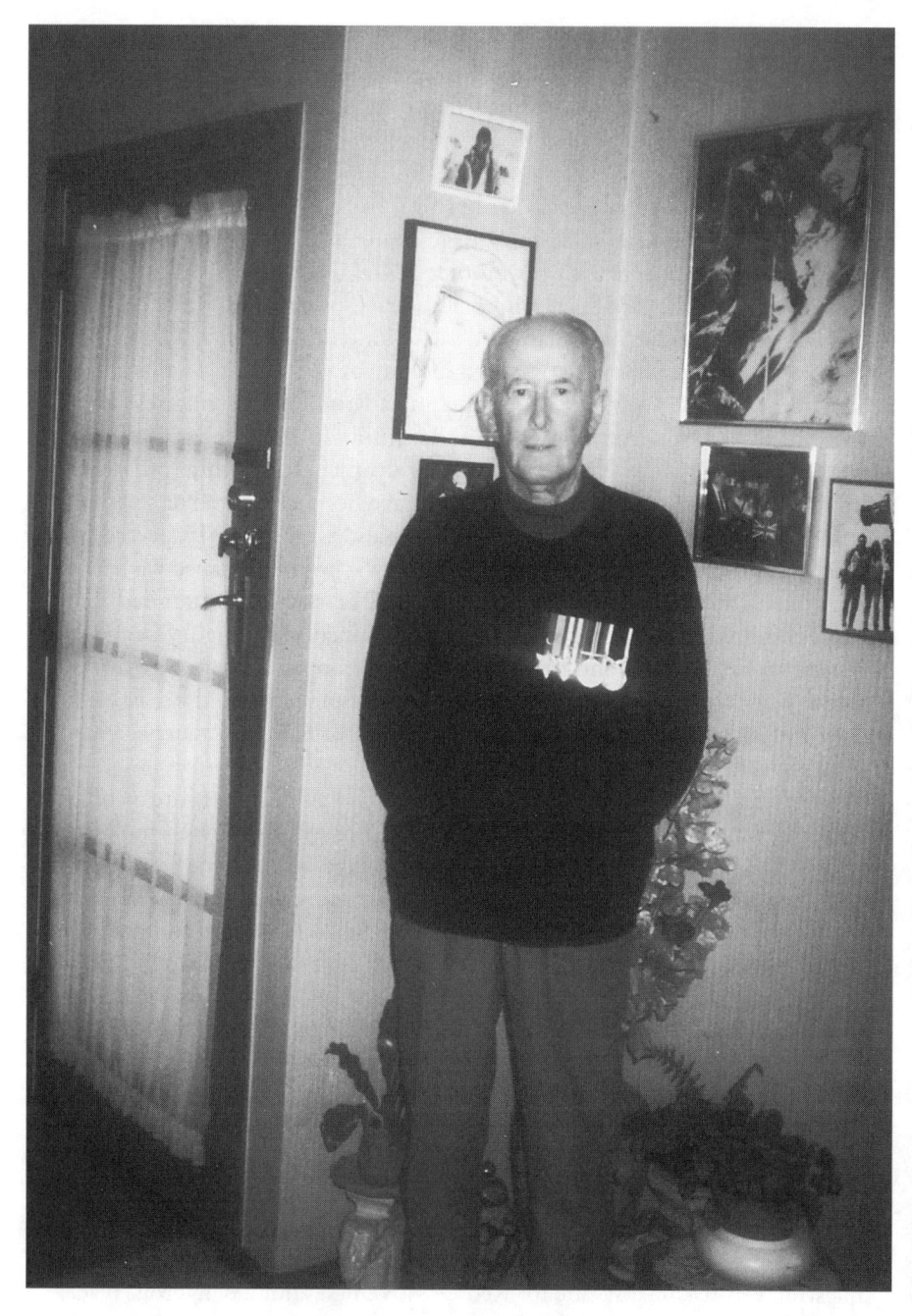

Des Ball today. The medals he is wearing are: 1939–45 Star, Italian Star, War Medal, NZ Defence Medal. *Courtesy of Des Ball.*

three NZ signalers who had been laying a cable along the road not far from the battery HQ. This was done by a jeep with a drum of cable on the back which unwound as they moved along the road. They had been shelled, with one killed and two wounded. I took them to the battery where the doctor or Medical Officer, as they were sometimes known, did his job, and then took them on to the dressing station.

It was while I was with the battery I witnessed the bombing of the Monastery. It was a fine morning when we heard the noise of a hundred or so heavy and medium bombers approaching. They came in waves as they dropped their bombs on the Monastery and then flew off home again. After the first few waves the top of the hill and the Monastery seemed to be erupting in flames and clouds of smoke. A month later the town of Cassino was given the same treatment. All this bombing seemed to do was make it easier for the enemy, as we could not move our tanks around in the town because of the huge bomb craters....

After some months the division was pulled out of the battle mainly because of the heavy casualties we had suffered. One casualty being Brigadier Kippenberger who lost both legs through standing on a mine while watching the progress of the battle from Mt. Troccio. He was one of the most liked senior officers of the NZ Division. Mines were used extensively by both sides, and you had to be wary of them at all times. Even for months after I came home from the war I would often subconsciously stop ... walking in certain places, it was so ingrained into my mind....

The last thing that stuck in my mind when we pulled out of Cassino was the view of the Monastery looking like a rotten tooth. It was surrounded by smoke from smoke shells fired by the artillery to stop any observation from the ruins. Some weeks before we had seen our planes dropping supplies by parachute to the "Gurkhas" who were pinned down on the slopes just below the Monastery ... from what I remember none of the "Gurkhas" made it back.

We next moved on to the town of Sora, a town to the east of Cassino, and before the town fell to our troops an interesting drama took place. We had a dressing station set up in a building situated among other buildings on some crossroads. The whole area was almost like a small village. One morning a horse pulling a light "gig" containing people came down the main road from the direction of the German lines at full speed. It had come through the German ... positions, which we could see at a distance up the road, without a shot being fired. They were a family of father, mother, and two teenage daughters. The interesting thing being they all spoke English with broad Scottish accents! The mother and father with still a trace of Italian, but the daughters who were Scots by birth spoke broad Scottish. The family had gone to Italy on family business just before the war and could not go back to Scotland. Not long after they arrived in our lines the Germans started shelling the place, and we quickly took cover in some of the buildings. All of a sudden the man of the family remembered his horse, and before we could stop him he rushed out amongst it all shouting "the horse ... the horse", with which he quickly then untethered it and ran it inside. He was lucky, as two of our blokes had been killed the day before in the same place. ... It was summer now, and the roads were very dusty, and if a tank or any large vehicle went past you ended up covered in white dust. Most of the big attacks were put in at night which was a sight to behold. Haystacks on fire from our infantry setting them alight with incendiaries as German snipers often hid in them, and bad luck for the Italians who would hide valuables, even the odd tractor or car under them to stop the Germans carting them off....

The dressing station at this time seemed to be in a rather hazardous position as it was situated amongst a lot of our guns, and guns always drew enemy fire. I had delivered some wounded and was standing talking outside the dressing station which was situated in a strongly built stone farm building. Dug in around about were a number of our 25 pounder guns, and now and then we could hear German shells going over but landing well back behind us. We happened to be watching three gunners climb out of the gun pit about a hundred yards away and put on a Bengazi Burner to make a cup of tea. Next thing there was an almighty bang, and we could see that a shell had landed almost on top of the three gunners. We grabbed stretchers and ran down, but could do nothing but pick up the pieces. Two of the three were just a heap of mangled flesh, and the third did not have a single scratch but was in total shock.

One quiet day while sitting in the aid post, the door opened, and in walked a soldier in just shorts and a singlet; it was summer at the time and very warm. The front of his singlet was covered in blood, and he calmly asked was there any chance of getting a dressing done. He had been hit by a piece of shrapnel from a German hand grenade which had hit him in the rib, but not gone any further. He must have been just out of range of the full force of the blast. He and two other signalers had been laying a cable from the back of a jeep and had taken the wrong road, and next thing they had found themselves in the German lines ... a very easy thing to do at times. One of the enemy had come from behind a tree and thrown a grenade at them.... [The signaler] ... dived into a ditch by the side of the road and crawled back until he came to one of our tanks, who pointed him in the direction of the aid post. We did not know what had become of the jeep or the other two men. The doctor took out the shrapnel, put on a dressing, and I took him back to the dressing station from where he would be given a few days to recuperate, probably back at his unit's headquarters.

One day we were surprised to see a middle aged, Italian woman accompanied by a young, German soldier and two partisans. These were the first partisans we had seen so far, but we were to see more of them as we moved north. The partisans had brought her and the young German through the lines, as he had just had enough and wanted to defect to us. He was 19 years old and in a bad way. He was crying and very frightened. The woman spoke English and German fluently and looked like what we used to call a countess, well-educated in a number of languages, and they were usually big landowners. After some questioning by our two intelligence sergeants, she and the two partisans left to go back through the lines, leaving the young deserter with us. I heard one of the sergeants remark that if we happened to be shelled badly after she had gone, then he would make it a personal quest to catch up with [her] and shoot her.

We came out of this position for a rest, and an American unit was taking over from us. The change over took place at night which was a very vulnerable time for any army. The Germans somehow got wind of it and gave us a rough time, sending patrols through our positions as well as [heavily] ... mortaring and shelling ... the battalion HQ, which included the aid post.... The ambulance was knocked out by a piece of shrapnel through the petrol tank, and by the time a replacement ambulance got to us, the aid post was overflowing with wounded. It was a noisy night with the German shelling and mortaring and our heavy mortars behind us firing flat out, as well as a number of our Vickers machine guns situated on a hill to the front of us working overtime. We were glad when the change over was completed, and we were out of it for a while.

When out of action we still had plenty to do helping to bury the dead, digging graves in a temporary cemetery, and going through the pockets of the dead and giving the contents along with one of the identity tags (one was left on the body) to the intelligence section. We would then roll the body in a blanket and tie it with cord, one around the neck, one around the body, and one around the ankles. The same procedure was carried out on any German dead as well. We then lowered them into the graves, and the Padre said a few words before we covered them up. It was during one of these periods I was sent back to help uncover the bodies of three of our anti-tank blokes who had taken shelter in a building one night, which unbeknown to them had been made ready to be blown across the street. The Germans had had to retreat before they could set the explosives off. A shell had come over during the night. It had hit the building setting the charges off and burying our anti-tank blokes under tons of rubble. We had an engineer on a bulldozer moving the rubble while a couple of anti-tank blokes, another engineer, and myself moved along with the blade moving the odd stones, etc., until we came to a body. The smell was terrible as it was mid-summer and over a week since they had been killed. We tied pieces of cloth across our faces, but it did not make much difference as the smell seemed almost solid. We rolled them in canvas sheets and loaded them into the back of the ambulance. As we drove down the road to a temporary cemetery, the smell and blowflies like a swarm of bees followed us all the way. We dropped them off and left them to be buried. I then drove back to give the ambulance a good clean out with disinfectant!

After about a week I rejoined the battalion I had been with, as they were going into action. It was during this period that I had just dropped off wounded at one of the dressing stations, when the Germans started shelling hell out of it. The wounded were lying on stretchers under a big tent, some under trees, and in a small farmhouse. Most had no protection from the shelling, so we were told to evacuate the wounded. Myself and two other ambulances that had arrived in, started with the aid of some of the medics to load up as many as we could fit in as quickly as possible and get them out of it. The shells kept on coming in, but we just had to keep working and could not take cover. We never found out why the shelling took place as the dressing station was well marked with red crosses, and the enemy generally respected the red cross. A couple of pieces of shrapnel went through the back of the ambulance but did not hit any of the wounded lying on stretchers in the back. The holes were easily patched up as the ambulances were mostly made of canvas. As we drove up the road we passed infantry walking down the side of it. They would occasionally duck into the ditch that ran along by the road, so we knew the shelling was still going on but could not hear it above the noise of the ambulance motor, as we were well loaded and going up hill in low gear. When I returned after dropping off the wounded, the shelling had stopped and things were back to normal. Not long after this I had 14 days light duty at the Main Dressing Station with a small shrapnel splinter in the leg....

After a period of rest we occupied Forli, a town on the road that links Rimini on the Adriatic coast with inland towns such as Bologna. We were now in the Po Valley. A very flat country bisected by rivers and canals, which was a change as up until now we [had] had to contend with mountainous and hilly conditions. For a short time Forli became filled with our guns, trucks, tanks, and troops as we prepared to attack and occupy the town of Faenza a few miles up the road from Forli, and this drew [the] attention of the few planes the Germans still had in operation on this front. Just as it was dusk they would send one or two planes over on sneak raids to have a go at the concentration of equipment in the streets and squares of the town. Unfortunately, one evening a bomb missed its target and hit a church in which a confirmation service was taking place. All who were in Forli will remember this incident as just about every soldier in the town was organized into shifting the rubble to rescue the survivors who were trapped under the ruins.

Faenza was like all towns that had a railway or river running through it[. It had] been pattern bombed so as to destroy the bridges, which meant a part of the town had been destroyed with the bridges. Once our engineers had a bridge over, we moved in [and] established a dressing station. German snipers were still at work in the town, and they still occupied the railway station and a few other buildings around it. The afternoon of the day we moved into the town I was asked to take an ambulance jeep with a couple of wounded back to Forli. I set off in the direction of the bridge out of the town.... [C]rossing the square the jeep stalled, and after a couple of attempts to get it going I realized some telephone cables had got wound around the drive shaft as there were wires, broken glass, and all kinds of rubbish strewn around. The day was very cold, and I was dressed in great coat, jersey, balaclava, and tin hat, but as I lay under the jeep getting rid of the cable the sweat poured off me ... whether it was from fear or exertion I don't know.

The square was deserted with just a building on fire and the sound of rifle and machine gun fire in the distance, as well as the odd "crump" of mortar bombs. I set off again, and as I came to the bridge I put my foot down as I had been told they were still sniping at the bridge, and although the jeep was well marked with a red cross flag flying on the roof, I took no chances. A couple of dead civilians were lying near the bridge, killed by a sniper, I presumed. Once across the bridge I was in the cover of some buildings, and without further incident was soon back at Forli where I stayed the night as I had to bring back a Medical Sergeant who would not be ready to go until the next morning.

When he and I left Forli the next morning, a dense fog covered the whole area, which is not uncommon at this time of year, and of this we were very thankful as it meant it would give us some protection from observation as we approached Faenza. The night I was away at Forli the blokes I had moved into a building in Faenza with, because of the intense cold had broken up some furniture and lit a fire in the fireplace, and next minute had attracted a number of mortar bombs on the roof; they were lucky that it was a two-story building. The Germans had evidently poured smoke creating fluids down the chimneys....

The battle for the Senio started late in the afternoon with our fighters strafing and rocket firing Typhoons shooting up enemy positions on the stopbanks, as well as houses, tanks, and trucks in the rear area. This went on for a number of hours, the planes flying so low they seemed to disappear below the fruit and olive trees in front of us. Then the heavy and medium bombers came over and bombed all along the German lines for a considerable time; the air became thick with smoke and dust. The noise was tremendous, but not to the same extent as when the artillery started up. When the last bombers had flown off, the guns behind us opened up, all our 25 pounders as well as support from larger guns of British units. The air and ground just seemed to be rocking and shaking with the noise of the barrage which went on for hours. All of a sudden the guns would stop and everything would be silent just to let the enemy come out of his cover to see if our infantry were coming. Just a minute or so, then down the barrage would come to catch them out in the open. After some hours of bombardment the guns lifted a couple of hundred yards, with our infantry crossing the river and following close up to the barrage and cleaning out any troops who had survived; those who had were mostly too dazed and just surrendered. It was amazing ... [how] few German wounded left for us to pick up; their ambulance boys must have done a good job getting them back out of the way.

Once the infantry had consolidated the area across the river, the engineers who had been clearing paths through the minefields started to put a bridge over the river. This had to be done quickly so tanks could get across and support the infantry against counter-attack by German armor, as well as to let ambulances and other support vehicles over. The bridge would not be built where the old blown-up bridge had been, but a little way along the river to make it hard for the enemy to pin-point the place. With the assistance of a bulldozer they would build a branch road off the main road, then trucks would bring up a prefabricated Bailey Bridge and bridge the gap to the other side.

All this was done at night and under fire with the Germans mortaring, shelling, and machine gunning all along the riverbank trying to find them. After heavy fighting the enemy fell back to prepared positions on the Gaiana River. The division was now preparing for the attack which was to be put in across the river in conjunction with all the other divisions along the Italian front. This we were told was to be the last major battle of the war in Italy in which we would have more air, armor, and artillery support than we had ever had at anytime in the war. The idea, we were told, was that the German forces in front of us were not to be pushed back but destroyed as an organized fighting force so they could not fall back on the Po River, which if defended would take almost a D-Day landing to cross. We were to find that the paratroopers were put into the line to oppose us and that the NZ Division was to be used as the spearhead and make the breakthrough up the Po Valley. The paratroopers opposing us were no doubt the best regiments in the German army, but as Freyberg [Sir Bernard Cyril Freyberg, Commander in Chief of NZ forces] pointed out the best troops in the world would fold under intense and prolonged artillery bombardment, and it looked as if they were going to get plenty of that. About 80 percent of casualties during the war were caused by shrapnel from shelling and mortars and 20 percent from small arms fire. While things were being organized, we on the ambulances were kept busy with casualties from German shelling, mortaring, and the other injuries of war. I had just come in with some wounded and was talking to one of the other ambulance drivers who had just come up the same road as I had. He told me that when he had tried to come out from behind the farmhouse containing the First-Aid post, some paratroopers with a machine gun ... [had opened] up on him. The ambulances were well marked with red cross flags and red crosses painted on them. They had to send an armed party to clean them out, but once he got onto the main road back to the Dressing Station they opened up with a mortar, but luckily mortars are not that accurate. I was at an Aid Post on the other side of the road to where he was and was coming up the road about the same time as he was and received the same treatment. I think the paratroopers could see that Germany had nearly had it and were willing to take anyone down with them.

An example of the Dressing Station in action was ... the one mentioned above. As there was no building handy they had put up a marquee [an open-sided tent] amongst some fruit trees just off the road. The wounded were lying on stretchers under the trees and under canvas.... [A] couple of doctors with the aid of medics had put up trestles and were working on the most urgent cases as well as attending to the others lying around on the ground. Across the road about six of our 25 pounder guns were firing intermittently and the odd German shell was coming into them in reply, but the doctors and medics were just carrying on as if nothing was happening. The doctors were mostly just young blokes not much older than myself and probably not long out of Medical School and learning their trade the hard way.

The battle of the Gaiana River started in the afternoon with our fighters and rocket firing Typhoons strafing the German positions on the stopbanks as well as buildings, guns, tanks and vehicles. In the rear areas they kept this up for an hour or more flying so low as to almost seem to be below tree top level. Before this our infantry had moved back from their positions on the stopbank so as not to incur any casualties from our own guns. After the fighter planes had moved on, the heavy and medium bombers came in and continued to bomb the German positions along the river. This must have gone on for an hour or so, but I can't quite remember how long. The air became thick with smoke and dust. It was just starting to get dark when our artillery opened up. The whole horizon behind us seemed to catch fire with the leaping flames and flashing of the guns, and then the noise and blast of the guns caught up with us. The air and ground seemed to shake and rock with the noise; you could not talk to the bloke next to you. It was the most gunfire the division had ever had in support in any of its battles ... [in] Greece, Crete, North Africa and Italy. I would ... [have] hated to have been on the receiving end, but as they said, we were only just getting our own back.

The barrage went on for four hours, I would say, often stopping to let the paratroopers put their heads up to see if our infantry were coming, then ... [starting up] again to catch them in the open. The barrage then lifted a couple of hundred yards while Crocodiles and Wasps (Churchill tanks and Bren carriers converted to flame throwing) drove up to the stopbank and started spraying the German positions with flames. From where I was watching we could see the arc of the flames hosing through the trees ahead of us. While this was going on the odd shell was coming in but not causing many casualties....

Although the German army had ceased to exist as an organized fighting force, we had not seen the last of the German air force or what was left of them, as one night before we reached the Po River they must have put all the few planes they had left into the air dropping butterfly bombs. They seemed to be flying around most of the night. Butterfly bombs were about the size of a hand grenade and had a propeller attached which turned as they fell, priming the bomb so they could roll into a slit trench, under a truck, or just be touched and then explode. They were packed in a canister, which when dropped burst open, scattering scores of bombs all over the place.

We were the first division to reach the Po River. The NZ engineers put the first bridge over, a pontoon bridge as this was a large, wide river. The division drove on, being welcomed all the way by cheering Italians and welcomed with flowers and wine. Venice was liberated, and on we drove to Monfalcone, a ship building town not far from Trieste, and it was at Monfalcone we had our first contact with elements of Tito's Yugoslav army, and it could be said, experienced the first taste of what was to be known as the Cold War....

With the fall of Mussolini and the defeat of the German army, all the class and political hatreds that had been suppressed and lay simmering under the surface now became active and sometimes violent as I saw in a town on the way up the Po Valley. We were resting for a few days and someone said there was a town not far from us, the name of which I can't remember, [that] had been by-passed and that no Allied troops had been in the town. I was driving the ambulance jeep at the time and got permission to go and have a look at it. Three of us set off and soon reached the town and made for the first bar we came across. The Italians were making a great fuss of us with free drinks all around, and we were getting a bit "full" when we heard a great commotion out in the street, a street that was crowded with people celebrating what was for them the end of the war. Next moment, we saw about two dozen people escorted by a few partisans being marched up the road and the bystanders hurling abuse, as well as other odds and sods at them. I asked one Italian who they were, and he said Fascists, but I think at that stage of things anyone you had a grudge against was labeled a Fascist. We watched the goings on for a few minutes and were just about to go back to the bar when what sounded like a shot rang out, and one of the labeled Fascists fell to the ground, and not wanting to get embroiled in the local politics, we breasted the bar and continued our celebration. I managed to drive back to the unit okay, but woke in the morning with a hell of a headache!...

New Zealanders made friends with anyone and were always well liked by the peoples of the countries they ... found themselves in. All the peoples of the Trieste area got on well with us and looked on us as liberators. Most of them were not happy with the thought that Tito's army might occupy the area and would have been happy to see us stay forever. We had tried to make friends with Tito's troops, but had always been given the brush-off or ignored. They were taught that we were just a part of the war mongering, capitalist West's, imperial forces....

After some weeks in England and Ireland visiting and staying with various relations, I was on my way back to join the division in Italy, this time by rail. It was amazing how quickly the peoples of Europe, after all the destruction, were getting things moving again. We boarded the train in Calais (hard seats) and traveled through France, Switzerland, and Italy, where we left the train at Bologna after a journey that lasted five days. From Bologna we were then taken by army trucks to Taranto to where divisional base camp had been established. After a couple of weeks of boredom, we boarded the troop ship which would take us back to New Zealand....

A short stop in Australia, and New Zealand next stop, and what a great feeling to see the coast of home looming on the horizon. First stop Lyttelton to let the mainlanders off, then on to Wellington where we boarded a train for all stations north, and finally Auckland.

The New Zealand we came back to seemed to be a greatly changed place, or maybe we had changed. We felt somewhat like strangers in a strange land where the trivial seemed to take on great importance. A thing we missed most was the comradeship which born in war was not explainable to those who had no experience of war. Still seeking something that had now faded into history, we were inclined to congregate in bars and clubs to relive it all again.

Some are still seeking [it], as you can see on any afternoon you choose to visit an R.S.A. [Returned Servicemen's Association club].

Once young lions, now men grown old.

Chapter Twenty-Four

"I Was Doing Something Good"
Daniel Goolsbee

Daniel (Dan) Goolsbee was 17 years old when he left high school in Texas to join the U.S. Navy in 1942. He excelled as a navy corpsman and took on responsibilities far beyond his years.

I was sent to San Diego for boot camp. When we were given an opportunity to choose what we wanted to be trained in, I decided that the Hospital Corps was what I wanted. Other than an uncle who was a veterinarian and who took me with him sometimes to treat animals (which I didn't like), I had no reason to be inclined toward the Hospital Corps. We studied anatomy, physiology, pharmacology, and so on. I made good grades; I had a 90 average. There were pharmacists, morticians and the like in the class who didn't do as well.

The San Diego Zoo surrounded the training area. We woke up to zoo noises every morning. The Museum of Natural Sciences, which the military had taken over and where we had classes, had a dinosaur skeleton on display in one of the rooms where I had a class.

After Hospital Corps school the navy let us pick where we wanted to go based on our grades. Another corpsman said that I should choose to go to Treasure Island if I wanted to be assigned to a ship, so I did. Treasure Island Naval Hospital gave me further training as a qualified assistant in operating room technique. I was picked for this because of my grades in Hospital Corps school. I assisted in many different types of surgery, such as orthopedic, general, and brain surgery. I learned how to set up the instrument trays, to sterilize, and to prepare for surgery. I loved the work and thought it was great. I wasn't killing somebody, not shooting anybody. I was doing something good.

The badly wounded patients coming back from the battle areas began to arrive. They were in bad shape. The worst I ever saw. One time I worked 36 hours without stopping. I was finally told to go get a shower and something to eat. I sat down on the tile floor in one of the scrub rooms and fell asleep for three hours! I woke up about noon.

I stayed at Treasure Island as an instructor another six months. I taught the class that came after me. I was 18 years old then.

I moved across the street to the general dispensary, the emergency room for 100,000 people stationed there. We worked 12-hour shifts. I had been in the navy almost two years then. I was teaching sterile technique and set-up for simple surgery. My students were navy corpsmen on ships. By now I was a pharmacist mate 2nd class.

I had one class that didn't care about learning. One day I said to them, "I might as well go overseas." Right after that there was a knock at the door, and a navy Wave [Women Accepted for Volunteer Emergency Service] said my orders were in for overseas. The Marine Corps needed corpsmen.

I went to Camp Pendleton in San Diego to take further training. I couldn't understand what the classes I took had to do with the navy. I learned how to deliver babies and other odd things like how to determine medicine for a child according to its weight.

At Tan Farine Race Track near Los Angeles, which the navy had taken for its use, we had classes in amphibious training: how to get off a ship onto the LCMs [Landing Craft Men] and onto the beach.

We finally got on a ship for Guam. It took 31 days to get there. We stopped in Hawaii for recreation. Next we went to the Marshall Islands and sat there for several days. As far as the eye could see there were ships. We sailed for Guam.

I have never seen so many ships in my life. So much confusion. Everyone getting shot. It was terrible.

I carried two bandoleers of ammunition to the beach when we landed. We had nothing to eat. They should have given us C rations to stick in our shirts, but they didn't. We got into the LCMs, landed on the beach, and dug in. The ships pulled off with the food. We had nothing to eat for 24 hours.

The Japs were shelling us. We could see a silver object floating in the water. Joe was from Kentucky. Old Joe said he was going to get the object. I said, "No. They told us to dig in and shoot at anything that moved." Finally the waves brought it in, and he told everyone he was going to get it. He rescued a shiny can of food with no label. He opened it, and it was diced beets. We ate them. They were bland with no seasoning. I liked spiced beets. I couldn't eat beets for some time after that.

We eventually went inland and established a military government hospital for civilians. There were 100,000 civilians on Guam, with villages scattered around. We were operating in tents at first. We got to the capital city and took over the old naval hospital with its operating rooms which were out of date. We cared for the civilians on Guam and the Japanese POWs. Some of the prisoners were very appreciative of the care while others were arrogant. One pinched me when I tried to wake him up. I gave him a slap, and he woke up. I knew he wasn't asleep. I spent six months there.

Repatriation of prisoners had begun. The Japanese released some civilian nurses. Maria was one of them. She was sent home to Guam and was the surgery nurse before the war. When she came back to work in the operating room, I felt I wasn't needed there anymore, so I finally asked to run a dispensary at Baragada village. Price School was there. I stayed there for eight months. It was challenging, but enjoyable. It was like a public health department. The civilians were appreciative of our care.

At first I was in a tent, then a Quonset hut. My living quarters were there, also. The first night the marines, who were on one side of the road and I on the other, chased a Japanese straggler down between the tents and shot him.

Next door was the Foreign Economics Administration which had been sent out there to operate a farm to send food to the military hospitals. I ate with the 75th Seabee unit for meals.

They were going to bring a dairy to Guam. The cows got there, but the processing equipment never made it. We figured out how to filter and pasteurize the milk. I had a small walk-in cooler at the dispensary and we kept it in there. We could produce about ten gallons of milk a day. We also figured out a way to make money from it.

Two cousins of mine were stationed on Guam. One was a B-29 pilot, and the other was a civilian who developed the radar system for the B-29. They were brothers. On their day off they would come to the village to watch me hold sick call and inspect sanitation conditions. I was ten years younger than they, and they were fascinated by our milk production. They would trade a fifth of whiskey for a fifth of milk (we put the milk in empty whiskey bottles). We would sell all the whiskey they could get, then use the money to buy other things.

The Navy-Army Medical Research Unit (NAMRU) came out to the

village and did "stool cultures" on the natives. The cultures were all positive. Everyone had parasites. We had to deworm everybody! Castor oil was given with all the treatments. I had a terrible time trying to give this to all the school kids. I finally devised a method: I would put on shorts, lay them down on a bench on which I was sitting, hold their heads between my legs, and pour the castor oil down their throats.

Many of the civilians had "Yaws" or tropical syphilis. It is known as "lazy syphilis" because under a microscope it doesn't move as much or as fast as regular syphilis.

I delivered a bunch of babies. We had two native nurses trained to be midwives. We delivered about 70 babies during my eight months in the village. The native people reproduced a lot, especially after the war.

I could diagnose pneumonia, abnormal heartbeats, and such like. A doctor was following along once when I was diagnosing patients. He said, "I'll tell you the truth. You do better than most young doctors diagnosing." I had a habit of saying, "possible this or possible that." He said that I did better than "possible."

After eight months they didn't want to leave us in the village until we rotted. So I went back to the civilian hospital on Guam and became Acting Chief Master-at-Arms. I was now pharmacist mate first class. I made up the personnel schedules. I visited the dispensaries in the villages. Once I found that one of the men had shot himself. To this day I don't know why. He was in his middle thirties and had been a schoolteacher before the war. He knew my schedule and obviously wanted someone to find him. He was very isolated from everyone.

We weren't supposed to take pictures (I don't know why), but we had X-ray film, made a camera, and took pictures anyway. They wouldn't let me take them home, so I destroyed them.

At Christmas, our second Christmas on Guam, the Red Cross ladies in the States made ditty bags for patients at the hospital. Some were for men, and some were for women. They decided to give some to us. I was one of the fortunate ones; I got a man's ditty bag. On Christmas morning the men who got the women's ditty bags took out their gifts of women's pajamas or nightgowns and put them on! We had a good time anyway.

I did this work for six months until the war ended. I had a great time. I was out of the navy in February 1946 and didn't turn 21 until August of that year.

Two things I learned from this experience. One, age made no difference if you were willing to learn and accept the responsibility. Two, surgery could be performed under very crude conditions with acceptable results.

Chapter Twenty-Five

"You Did What You Had to Do"
Julia Parrish Sadler

In Korea we wore fatigues and combat boots on duty and off. We were like a family as there was none of our own people around. Too, I have washed my hair or taken baths in an army helmet. You did what you had to do. The first mail that was brought to me was in a large mail bag and some who were with me read my letters, too. Most of the people I was with called me "Rebel" or "Grits."
—Julia Sadler

Julia Parrish Sadler joined the Army Nurse Corps at the age of 21. Headed for the European theater, she ended up in Korea instead, after surviving both a shipboard appendectomy and a plane crash.

I was born in Quitman, Georgia, in 1923 and during the Depression about 1929 moved to my mother's (Hattie Pittman's) farm in Austell, Georgia. My grandfather J.A. Pittman was born in the house where we children grew up. We lived there until 1941 when my older brother Billy joined the air force [U.S. Army Air Corps]. Billy was an MIA [missing in action] while I was a student nurse at Crawford Long. We thought that we would never see him again, but somehow he got back to us. James, my other brother, was a sergeant and tail gunner in the air force in England. All three of us were away from home at the same time, and I know now that my parents must have been devastated. At the time my daddy was working at Dobbins in Marietta—they called it then the "Bell Bomber plant." I remember him buying "war bonds and Mama using stamps to buy groceries."

After graduating as a student nurse in March 1945 from Crawford W. Long Hospital in Atlanta, Georgia, my roommate, Kathryn Duvall, and I joined the army—mostly because the paper kept printing these stories about drafting nurses. We went to Ft. McPherson and joined and were sent to Ft. Rucker, Alabama, for basic training. We met so many people, good and otherwise. I had never been associated with so many women. It was a time of segregation, and I remember one very nice, black nurse who was sent there by mistake and immediately shipped to another post. I worked for a short time at an army hospital in Hattiesburg, Mississippi. Then my roommate and I signed up for overseas. We were sent to Ft. Jackson, South Carolina, for more training, such as going through the gas chamber (with a gas mask), rope climbing, and many classes, and two-, five-, or ten-mile marches. After this we were sent to Ft. Dix, New Jersey.

Earlier though, I was selected to be a supernumerary (one who goes if somebody else gets sick and can't go). The enlisted men took our baggage from our barracks at Ft. Jackson—they took everything I had but left me! All of the girls I had known went to the Pacific area. I was left with a group of northerners from Indian Town Gap, Pennsylvania, and I was quite an oddity. From Ft. Dix, New Jersey, we were put on a hospital ship, the St. Mihiel, which was a converted luxury liner (Dutch). We thought we were going to Europe, but the war ended before we could get there. Around August '45, we went down the east coast, through the Panama Canal, and on to the Pacific. Our ship would need repairs everywhere we stopped.

Oahu, Hawaii, was the first stop where we spent a month, and then on to Saipan, and this was after the United States had gotten the Japanese off the island. I saw Suicide Cliff which many Japanese just walked off into the ocean. There we had little food and ate out of enamel bowls, and I first learned to drink coffee. The nurses who left the barracks could not go out without an armed escort. We didn't receive any of our mail until we reached Korea.

From Saipan we went to Yokohama, Japan. There a nurse and other people came on our ship with warm clothes for us. We could see Mt. Fuji, which was quite beautiful. Too, I had an emergency appendectomy onboard ship between Manila and Saipan—no relatives, no close friends. I felt quite alone. They had tried to lower me in a net to a small boat to take me to Manila but decided the water was too rough and brought me back up. We arrived, after a terrifying typhoon in the Yellow Sea, at Seoul, Korea, in December '45. We lived in old, wooden barracks which had no plumbing. We took cold showers, but there was always a guard nearby.

25. "You Did What You Had to Do"

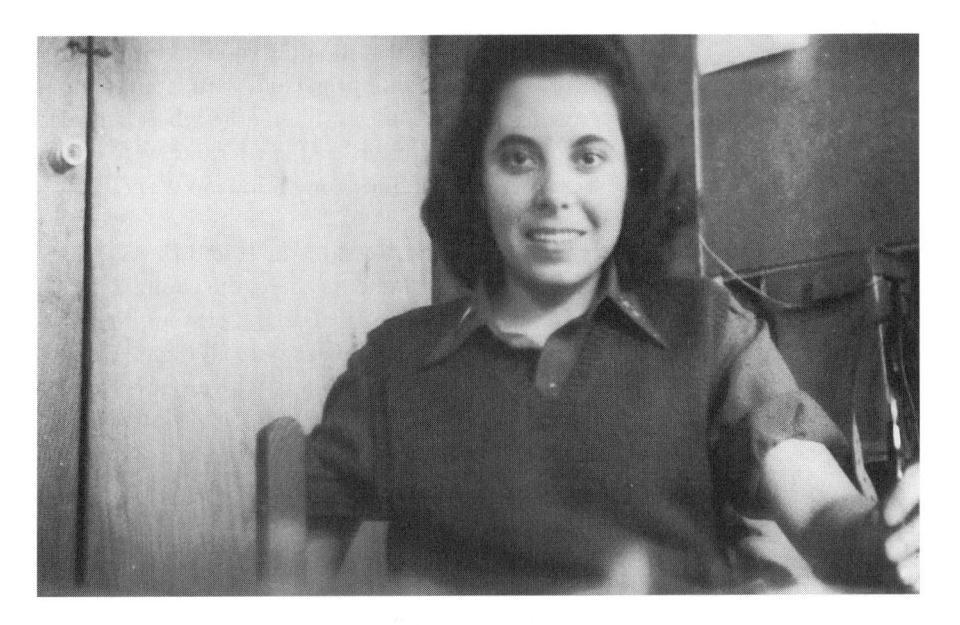

Julia Parrish Sadler on the Contagious Ward at the 377th in Taijon, Korea. She was wearing men's clothing because she had lost everything in the fire that destroyed the nurses' quarters. *Courtesy of Julia Parrish Sadler.*

The little Korean children loved us and would follow us everywhere. Thirteen of us were sent to Taejon, Korea, where we set up the 377th Station Hospital. Some of the soldiers were shot, possibly by north Koreans. One of the young soldiers had smallpox. We had very primitive conditions. My chief nurse, First Lieutenant Bertha Kellogg, was my closest friend. In fact, we still correspond.

I didn't mention our plane crash coming in to Taejon (I haven't been in a plane since). It was very cold—13 degrees below zero at one time. There was snow all over when we (13 nurses) were flown in a C-47 from Seoul to Taejon. We crashed on approach, and it was horrible. We all survived though. We also later survived when our nurses' quarters burned. We lost everything we had (for the second time).

Several of us from the hospital were invited to a banquet at the Taejon mayor's residence (he was in jail at the time), and this was one of the few good memories. When we went in the house, we removed our shoes and walked on warm mats. There was bountiful Korean food on a long, low, table which we sat at on the floor, cross-legged. Some of the food we could eat, but other dishes we knew to avoid. I remember the octopus stew and the pickled cabbage and the roasted chestnuts. A beautiful little Korean girl sang for us.

Another time one of the Korean doctors took my roommate and me on a tour of their hospital. It was a stone building, cold, with large rooms for the patients who were lying on mats on the floor—the whole family moved in with the patient to take care of them. In the lab there were horrible specimens from surgery. They begged for penicillin, and we couldn't give it to them.

When we were there it was between World War II and the Korean War. The older nurses grumbled and hated being there; the younger ones saw it as an adventure. There were different cultures and customs. There was a wonderful Korean woman, Mrs. Nahm, who sat up all night and by next to no light made a little, red "money bag" for me the night before I left Taejon. Also, I met a seven-year-old boy who could speak five languages. He was very special. He was Wong Tocinni. He may have been a spy; I'm not sure. I gave him my I.D. bracelet. He gave me his picture.

We rode horses several times—they were Japanese war-horses and were fast. Once my horse was walking on the dirt between rice paddies; he slipped, and we both ended up in the rice paddy (which had quite an odor). Once I was getting on a horse and had put my left foot in the stirrup, and he took off really fast with me hanging on and not in the saddle. I knew that if I couldn't get in the saddle I could get killed or injured. Finally, I managed to get my right leg over and knew the Good Lord was with me.

The women in Korea washed their clothes by taking them to a creek and beating them with a paddle. I think we were really "in the country" in Korea, and the northern part, especially Seoul, had more modern things. Since we were there the United States has built houses, good roads, and I'm sure things are better.

When we were getting ready to come home, we had a list of things to turn in. A flashlight was on the list, and I couldn't find mine. I remember the officer telling me that if I couldn't find my flashlight that I would have to stay there. Finally, one of the hospital staff told me just to pick one up off the ward and turn it in, and that's just what I did. Now I know that I had been intimidated and harassed the entire time of my service, but I was not aware of this then. My experience in the army was one of awe and wonderment, and I was in just long enough (16 months) to get out.

In '46 when I had enough points I came home by ship, the *Marine Devil*, which took only two weeks—going over there it took five, horrible months. I kissed the ground when we finally got to Seattle and vowed if I got to Georgia I'd never leave again, and I haven't. The best friends I had were the chaplain and my chief nurse.

Chapter Twenty-Six

The Balkan Nurses

JUDITH A. BELLAFAIRE
and DIANE BURKE FESSLER

From two excellent books on military nurses in World War II come these stories of nurses serving in the Balkan region.
  From Judith Bellafaire, The Army Nurse Corps: A Commemoration of World War II Service *(pp. 17–18), published by the U.S. Army Center of Military History:*

On November 8, 1943, a C-54 ferrying 13 flight nurses and 13 medical corpsmen of the 807th Medical Air Evacuation Transport Squadron from Sicily to Bari on the east coast of Italy, ran into severe weather. They lost radio contact, the plane's compass failed, and the pilot became disoriented in the storm. Icing finally forced the plane down in the Albanian mountains far behind German lines. The Americans were found by partisan guerrillas and taken to a nearby farmhouse. The flight crew set fire to the plane to conceal traces of their presence.

Diane Burke Fessler, in No Time for Fear: Voices of American Military Nurses in World War II *(East Lansing: Michigan State University Press, 1996), provides more information on this harrowing experience:*

After a few days they walked to the village of Berat. On the fourth morning they were there, the Germans shelled the village, forcing them to flee. They were scattered and when they regrouped, three of the nurses were separated from the others. The main body had no choice but to go on without them. These personnel wandered from village to village searching for food. One Albanian mentioned that there were British in the country.

The Americans walked to the British camp. Lois Watson Mckenzie remembered that journey. "On our way to the British camp, near the Greek border, we crossed a mountaintop and ran into a violent snowstorm with a howling wind. We were in single file on this narrow path, when suddenly the nurse in front of the sergeant in front of me slipped and started sliding down the side of the mountain. He reached down with one hand, grabbed her waist, and pulled her back up on the trail. Not a word was said, and we plodded on. When we reached the next village, the people ran out calling us heroes, and told us no one ever crossed that mountain between September and Spring. We did have a few frostbitten fingers and toes.

"We came to the British camp December 1st, and I received badly needed shoes and socks, as I had practically no soles left on my shoes. The new ones were in men's sizes, and it took several pairs of socks to fill them up. They had hobnail soles and were heavy as lead."

A British lieutenant and a sergeant joined them in their journey across the country to the coast. Twice they became very discouraged when the possibility of capture seemed imminent. They hoped to make contact with an American OSS man who had been sent to help them, but had to turn back to avoid being caught in the partisan fighting that was going on in Albania at the time.

Then a message was received that an American plane with fighter escort would be coming, but because the Germans were nearby, the British lieutenant wouldn't signal the plane. They watched helplessly as a British Wellington bomber and two C-47s circled with their wheels down, accompanied by 18 P-38s.

They finally made contact with the OSS man in early January. They traveled only at night, eventually riding in a truck he had procured. Whenever someone approached them on the road, they would jump out of the truck and hide. They crossed a mountain and were met by the British, who were expecting them.

Agnes Jensen Mangerich described their rescue. "We slept in a cave that night, and everyone was so exhausted, we just crawled over someone and found a space and fell sound asleep. I remember someone waking me up saying, 'The boat's here,' and I grabbed my shoes and coat and went to the water's edge. There were bunk beds on the boat, and two or three of us crawled into each one and went right back to sleep."

They arrived safely in Bari on January 9, 1944, after a hazardous, two-month journey covering 800 miles, although they were suffering from frostbite, dysentery, jaundice, and pneumonia.

According to Judith Bellafaire, the three missing nurses faced different hardships. They were trapped by a German unit for several months in the town of Berat. Diane Burke Fessler's book picks up the story:

Ava Maness was one of the three left behind. "We could see enemy troops were bivouacked across the street in a school yard, and a member of the family we were staying with told us the Germans knew we were there and were coming to look for us. He told us not to worry but not to try to talk to them, which we couldn't do anyway. Later I realized that our hostess knew a lot about these troops, some of whom spoke Hungarian. Her family was from Hungary, and she could hear some of what they were saying in the school yard.

"Soon I heard men talking, and two nice-looking, young soldiers came in to the room where we were. They looked at us, and we looked at them. Finally one of them gestured about our insignia, and I said the Italian word for nurse. As they left, they told our hostess that we should stay there and not to let us go outside."

They remained in the home for almost five months. Conditions were very primitive. Ava described their situation. "We had to sit on the floor, as there was no furniture. The kitchen was the room next to the one we stayed in, and I think I only went in there once. I'll never forget seeing the plates on the floor with cats licking them, but we couldn't let that bother us.

"The house had no plumbing or running water, but there was a well downstairs. The 'toilet' was in a little room that had a barrier in front of it."

In the meantime, says Judith Bellafaire, the OSS man had gone back for them. When they finally left by car in March, they were dressed as Albanian civilians and supplied with Albanian identification cards. Eventually the partisans gave them donkeys to ride and guided them across several mountain ranges. They met the OSS man who took them to the coast where an Allied torpedo boat took them to Otranto, Italy. When they arrived in Italy on March 21, 1944, they had completed a five-month journey behind enemy lines.

Chapter Twenty-Seven

POW of the Germans
RICHARD JOHN FELTHAM, M.D.

The following is from the journal of Richard John Lillico Feltham, who was a medical officer with the 20th Battalion, New Zealand Army. The journal was actually letters to his parents written when he was seriously ill with jaundice contracted in England after his release as a prisoner of war of the Germans. Dr. Feltham's material was contributed to this book by his daughter, Jenny Setchell.

...I suppose you are fed up to the back teeth with war stories but you may be interested to hear what your own little Dickey had to undergo. We were in the scrap about a month before the fatal day and it began at Mursa Matruh. After carrying out a small rearguard action to cover the engineers who were finishing a minefield, we pulled out 16 miles into the desert and joined the rest of the division. There we waited for three days till the Goons had surrounded us. This was done to delay his advance as he could not go any further down the coast with a whole division on his lines of communication. For two days they attacked but our losses were very light indeed and only because our ammunition was running low was it decided that we should have to break out of the position we were in and retire to Alamein.

What a night that was. At midnight all the trucks, cars, guns and other vehicles were lined up six abreast ready for the break through. Then the infantry went in with bayonets and carved a hole through the Goon lines. As soon as the hole was made we started the trucks up and, nose to tail in the pitch dark, we dashed through the gap. It was a terrible experience belting along in the dark with bullets, shells, grenades and what not whizzing in from all sides. I could see the tracer shells coming from a long way off. They appeared to be coming straight at me then would whiz just over the cab of the truck with a most awful crack. Tracer shells are very funny (peculiar) in that respect, they seem to be coming, very slowly until they are right up to you and then they are gone before you know it.

However, we eventually reached Alamein and spent the next 14 days in small attacks to keep the Goons busy. I won't dwell on this part very much except to say that I went in with several charges and did not enjoy them at all. The first one I went on was at night and as you can imagine was keyed up to a fair pitch of excitement in expectation of what was to come. We started off in dead silence and after a few hundred yards I began to think, "well, it will be starting in a few minutes," but the minutes passed and nothing happened. We took the objective and there was nobody there. It sounds like an anticlimax, but it was a big relief at the time.

Well, we made several more attacks (not so quiet) and on the 14th of July [1942] were told that we were to make a big attack that night and that on the following day we were to go out of the line for a rest. We went 6000 yards that night against very stiff and hot opposition. At dawn we were on our objective which was a small knoll overlooking miles of flat desert. Unfortunately the people on our flanks had not made the grade and we found that we were virtually surrounded. What a horrible day followed. We were on solid rock with no cover and no chance of digging a slit trench even, and then the Goon just belted away all day with everything he could lay his hands on. That was by far the longest day I have ever known. Our casualties were very heavy and I was in the rotten position of having large numbers of wounded with no method of evacuating them. All I had was a surgical haversack and so was not able to do much more than give morphine and put on the odd bandage. We had been told that the trucks would be up in the morning, but of course they didn't arrive.

By the end of the day we were all pretty tired and miserable. It is no fun to see your friends with legs and arms off, dying slowly, and knowing that if only they could be got to a hospital they would have a chance of living. One lieutenant I knew very well had his leg shattered from the hip right down. He knew he was going to die and asked me to give him some extra morphine. In all it was a ghastly day and I hope I never have to undergo another like it. At sunset the Goon tanks came racing up the slope and were amongst us almost before we knew it. All those wounded who could walk were marched off and I was left with about 25 badly wounded men and no water. However a Goon in a tank drove up and gave us a small can of water. By next morning several of the men were dead and I covered them with stone with the help of a man who had turned up from some where during the night. At about ten o'clock in the morning our own guns opened up and we had the doubtful pleasure of being shelled by our own 25 lbers.

At two o'clock we managed to get a goon to bring a truck and take us all to an Italian dressing station where I must say we were treated very well. By degrees we were shifted back to Mursa Matruh to a tented fly trap which was supposed to be a hospital. Once there reaction seemed to set in. I became terribly tired and washed out and to make matters worse got a bad dose of dysentery, which lasted for six weeks. When I tried to sleep I had terrible nightmares, and to top it all I began to realize for the first time that I was a blasted prisoner of war. I thought a lot about you all at home, and wondered how long it would be before you would get definite news of me. It must have been a rotten time for Bobby [Dr. Feltham's wife].

I was at Mursa for two weeks and then one day was suddenly shifted out along with a Scots padre. We were taken by lorry to Badia then to Tobruk where we spent two days without food and very little water. The Italian troops in the back areas were easily the lowest form of life it has been my lot to come in contact with. While we were there I saw two Indian soldiers shot for no reason at all. We left Tobruk on a lorry sitting on a heap of empty shell casings and had a very uncomfortable trip to Benghazi.

What a hell-hole that was. We were put into a building with a lot of other officers (most of whom had been taken at Tobruk) and the conditions were revoltingly filthy. The flies were worse than I had seen them anywhere, the food was practically negligible and the latrines defy description. The men, in a cage next door, were even worse off. Every morning a number of them were taken dead off the lavatory seats, most of them having died from malnutrition and dysentery. I was there only a very short time thank God and my next move was by air to Bari in Italy.

Bari camp was a little better than Benghazi but not much. We did have water there but the huts were dreadfully overcrowded. I still had the diarrhea and was feeling pretty low by this time. The diet was a peculiar one. The Italian camps were fed on what the surrounding country produced and the Bari area seems famous for its tomatoes, grapes and sugar beet. We had soup twice a day made from the tops of the sugar beet, not very sustaining and together with the other articles of diet, not much use to a chap with dysentery. The bread ration was very small and we felt hungry most of the day. In all it was pretty miserable and if one had no sense of humor it would have been really grim. There is always a lighter side to everything and I well remember an incident which happened one night. In a bed next to me was the secretary of the Wanganui Hospital Board (you will know him Dad, a good chap); suddenly he burst out laughing. We had been sitting round in silence, all very hungry and all feeling very sorry for ourselves. This peal of laughter made everyone sit up and take notice. When he had stopped laughing we asked him what the joke was; he said "I've been thinking, and have just remembered the old adage—laugh and grow fat—so I thought I would have my supper."

After a while we began to get Red Cross parcels and life began to look a lot more rosy. One day I saw Doug Dymock

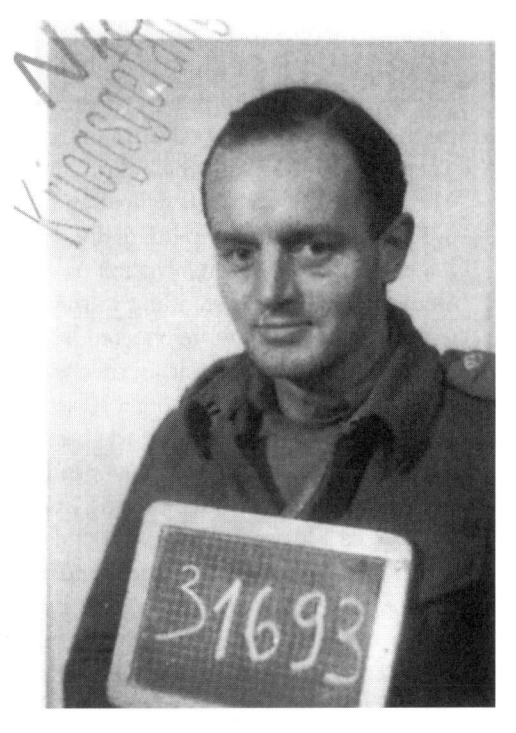

Dr. Richard John Feltham in an I.D. photo taken by the Germans while a prisoner of war. *Courtesy of Jenny Feltham Setchell.*

and had a long talk with him through the wire. I was at Bari about two months and was not sorry when I was told that I was being moved North to do some work. At this stage I was in rather a poor condition as far as my clothes were concerned. I had one shirt (almost in rags), my one pair of socks had been discarded weeks before and my boots were just about falling apart. I had a blanket that I had pinched from an Italian at Mursa and my small army pack with a towel and the shaving kit given to me by Mr. Sandford before I left Raetihi. The seat of my shorts was torn but they still held together.

So one fine morning, together with a padre and two South African M.O.s, I left Bari for good. We were told that we were going to St. Peters Castle and we began to think of an old castle somewhere in the Alps with moat, etc.—but more of that later. We had by this time got over the first shock of being prisoners and had lost the despondency of the first few weeks. In fact we were becoming a bit cocky.

We were hustled like so many animals on to the Bari station with a strong armed escort. When the train came in the guard opened the door to a crowded third class compartment. We put our luggage on the platform and refused to move, on the grounds that we were officers and as such were entitled to travel in a first class carriage. The Italians are very "class" conscious, and the guard who was a sergeant, rushed away, as we thought to get an officer who would put us in our place. He rushed back a few minutes later and hurriedly tipped a very angry crowd out of a first class compartment and pushed us in. The train was very crowded, with Italians of all types standing in the corridor. This was our first victory as prisoners, we were more cheered by the fact that we had brow beaten our keepers than because our journey was so much more comfortable. And so we arrived at our new "home," Castel San Pietro.

We were misled about the castle part of our destination. There was an old ruin of a castle near the hospital but no moat or anything as romantic as that. Actually the building was an almost new school that had been converted for use as a hospital and was everything that Bari was not. It was clean and in place of the wooden two-storied double beds of Bari we as the medical staff had hospital beds of very good quality. I think this place was a propaganda hospital, but it was much better equipped than any of the other hospitals in Italy, some of which were dreadful. When we arrived the hospital was full of British and allied soldiers, both medical and surgical cases. The hospital overlooked a very pretty valley and we felt that we would be fairly well off working there. We had arrived with some odd scraps of bread in our pockets, and were agreeably surprised when the first meal consisted of more than we could eat. However, we kept the bread just in case the first meal was a flash in the pan. But whatever else we had to put up with in "203" we always had plenty of bread to eat....

There were about 600 patients and we had plenty of work for the first six months. The trouble was that we had very little to do as relaxation and after the novelty of new surroundings had worn off we began to notice the time lagging. At first we were allowed to buy newspapers (for what they were worth) but as soon as it became evident that the Axis forces were not going to capture Alexandria then all news was smartly cut off. It was then that we were fortunate enough to contact the local communist in the shape of the electrician. He would come into our room nearly every day on the pretext of seeing if our light was working properly and once inside he would tell us all the news in very fast Italian and go as fast as he could. We made him a present of some tea on two occasions just to keep him interested. We had, for the first six months, the large number of two books, probably the worst books ever written, but we all read them and enjoyed them too. One was *The Grey Knight* by Mrs. de la Pasteur. The other was Thomas Hardy's *Tess of the D'Urbervilles*. We were taken for walks two or three times a week but there were only three routes permitted and we soon got sick of those walks.

Slowly but very surely the bogey of boredom sneaked up on us; we played bridge till we were sick of the sight of cards; for eight weeks we kept ourselves amused by running a sort of bogus medical society. We held a meeting every Monday evening, suitably dressed in white ties made from bandages. Each of us had to read a humorous paper on some alleged medical subject. Proceedings were helped by some wine we managed to get. Some of the papers were quite funny, especially two of Gru's [South African physician Captain Grusin]....

After eight weeks we ran out of ideas and the society was disbanded. Then I did a tapestry (since lost in the Russian advance) but the monotony was getting pretty bad and we all began to bicker and fight. We had been cooped up in one room all this time and without exception were getting nervy and jumpy. One day we had a real row and Fanny Lee [Captain Lee] later lost his temper with one of the Ites and was moved to a straff [*sic*] camp in double quick time. Fanny was replaced by two others, both good types. One was a middle-aged Australian "Pop" Levings, and the other an Englishman called Lancaster. Then just as we were getting too used to one another the collapse of Italy came very suddenly.

You can imagine how high our hopes rose. We were informed that we were to stay put until relieved by our own troops. Day by day we sat watching the road really believing that our tanks were just around the bend; it seems silly now but at the time we had no information and were prepared to believe anything. Anyway, our moving was out of the question as we still had about 400 patients, and many of them were unable to walk. Teste [an Italian physician] offered two of us a ride South in a car but after talking it over we decided to turn the offer down on principle.

After days of anxious waiting the Goons said that we were to be taken to Germany and our hearts dropped to our boots with disappointment. One morning, they came and gave us one hour to have all patients ready to board a hospital train. Just after that order was issued a flight of 72 Flying Fortresses passed overhead and passed Bologna to the North of us. We literally rocked the buildings with our cheers as we imagined that the Goons would not now be able to take us past Bologna, the only route they could possibly take us. We still fondly imagined that by the time that they had repaired the railway our troops would have arrived on the scene. No such luck of course. The bombers had messed up the Bologna railway station all right but there was still a double track rail which completely by-passed the city. And that is how we came to leave Italy, after I had been exactly one year at Castel San Pietro. There are countless things I could tell you but I have tried to stick to the broad outline as it were in an attempt to give you some idea what life was like in the camps I was in while a "prignionera de guerra." We were very disappointed at the turn events had taken, but that disappointment was tempered a little by the fact that we were actually moving after such a long time in one building.

...I have not even mentioned the rollcalls—those long and tedious waits in the hot Bari sun while the Ites (never a mathematical people) tried repeatedly to count us; nor have I mentioned that famous Character "Daft Demetrius"—a monk from a nearby monastery in Castel San Pietro. He wandered around the hospital in a flowing red robe, and was definitely "on our side." Every now and again he would come shuffling along the corridor, hands folded in his large bulky sleeves, looking rather like a pious Chinese mandarin. He would sidle into our room, quietly produce a large bottle of very good wine from each of his voluminous sleeves, and then shuffle out without a word. Incidentally, he was a prisoner in German hands during the last war and wore allied ribbons on his cloak. These things were amusing, and helped to pass the time, but there were other times, when, with nothing to do, one would just sit and gaze through the barbed wire and think of how things might be at home. It might sound sloppy but a great deal of our spare time was taken up with thinking of home—a habit which invariably gave rise to severe fits of depression....

The journey to Germany was interesting but uneventful. We went through the Brenner Pass and the first big town we came to was Innsbruck. I saw some women, about mother's age, literally shoveling manure from a railway truck, and thought that these Germans would be a tough bunch to defeat if their women all worked as hard as these were doing. It wasn't until sometime later that I realized that the women were not German at all, but that I had had my first glimpse of Russian slave workers. We went through Munich at night so did not see anything of that city, and finally arrived at Lamsdorf in Silesia, not very far from Breslau.

The country around Lamsdorf was flat and uninteresting, it was also the site of a big prison in the last war. I was at this camp for one month, locked in a small compound with about 20 other officers. All our patients had been taken off somewhere else and we had nothing to do, but I for one enjoyed the rest after a year's toil in Italy. After four weeks we were suddenly given one hour's notice to move, and so set off on a hectic trip across Germany to Rotenburg, near Kassel. What a hell of a journey that was. It only took 24 hours but in that time we changed trains ten times, and arrived at Rotenburg in some disorder.

Rotenburg (Oflag 9A/Z), consisted of a large three-storied building, surrounded by barbed wire and set in rather an attractive valley. After being herded through the double barrier of wire we were put into a large hall and ordered to strip. While we stood naked, the goons went through our meager belongings and then handed back our clothing bit by bit and allowed us to get dressed. The search over we were allowed to go into the main part of the building, and there almost the first people I saw were W.A.O. Canavan (Ohakune School) and Tony Johnston (Taumaranui). It was good to see someone I had known at home and they were able to give me lots of news from NZ…

When I met the two above chaps I tried to tell them the little news that I had been able to gather on our trip across Germany, but found that they were more up to date with the news than I was, the reason being that there was a "canary" (wireless) in operation in the camp. Remembering the search that I had just undergone, I wondered how on earth such a valuable article of furniture had found its way inside the "wire." I discovered later that it had been brought from another camp inside a medicine ball. This ball had been so much in evidence during the trip and subsequent search that the goon had apparently paid no attention to it at all. The German could never see the obvious. There are two very good stories illustrating this fact, and both of them are true.

The one concerns a British sergeant major who was in charge of a camp in Grauduenz (on the Vistula South of Danzig). There was a wireless in this camp and it was the custom of the operator to write out the B.B.C. news once a day and circulate the written copy throughout the camp. One morning this N.C.O. was reading the news of the day before when he was told that there were two men in plain clothes to see him at the main gate. He, thinking they were the long-overdue International Commission, put the news on his bed and went down to the gate to welcome his guests. However, they were not the expected Swiss but a couple of Gestapo. They immediately searched our friend and then told him to lead the way to his room. On the way to his room he suddenly remembered the news sitting there on his bed for anyone to see. He did some hard thinking, and when the procession had reached his room he had decided what to do. They went into his room and as soon as he had closed the door he offered them each a cigarette. They both took one. The sergeant then quickly patted his pockets in search of matches, pretended that he had none, saw the paper on his bed and hurriedly twisted it into a taper, lit it at the fire and then lit their cigarettes. The rest of the paper was thrown burning into the fire of course and the danger was averted.

The second story was told me by one of the members of the last Swiss Commission to visit us before we were released. In a small working Commando [sic] in Southern Silesia where the men went out of the camp every day to work in the fields the Germans had become a little slack in the method of searching. They would sometimes search and sometimes just ask the men if they had any contraband. On one occasion a Tommy approached the Gerry guard house with a small wireless wrapped in his jersey under one arm and three eggs in the other hand. When the Goon guard asked him if he had anything to "declare" the Tommy said "three eggs." He held these out under the Gerry's nose. The eggs were confiscated and the Tommy walked on into the camp still with the wireless in his other arm. I know that sounds a rather tall story but I was told it by a very amused Swiss and I can quite imagine it happening.

To get back to Oflag 9A/Z, I was there for about five months and managed to fill the time in quite well. There was a good library and lectures on all sorts of subjects were given every day. Although the grounds were very small, we were able to get out about once a week to a nearby field for a game of football. The monotony was occasionally relieved by some exciting event. While I was there, two men tried to escape through the wire one night. They had cut their way about half through the wire with a pair of home-made cutters when they were caught and bitten by the Alsatian dogs which were kept patrolling between the building and wire at night.

When I left Rotenburg work was proceeding on a very ambitious piece of tunneling. The tunnel began on the second floor of the building (in a lavatory) and went along and then down in the actual substance of the wall. The wall was just thick enough to allow them to burrow down it and to leave a thickness of one brick on each side of the tunnel. This fine piece of work had got down to ground level and had begun to reach out in the general direction of the camp perimeter when the Goons found it....

Well, after about five months I was sent to Thorn to work as a medical officer at Stalag XXA. Thorn you will see on the map as being about half way between Warsaw and Danzig, on the Vistula. I was posted to Fort Fifteen. When I was told that I was going to Fort Fifteen I wondered what sort of a place it could be. Approaching the fort there was not much to see except a very large solid steel gate which appeared to be set in a small cutting. There were trees on both sides of the gate as well as behind it. Once inside the gate I saw that the fort was much bigger in extent than I had imagined it to be from the outside. There was a dry moat running right round the fort....

Thorn is a small town on the river Vistula about 100 miles south of Danzig. The prisoners there were housed in three old Polish forts—British prisoners were in forts XIII, XIV and XV, and I was sent to act as M.O. in fort XV. From the outside Fort XV looked like a small grass and tree covered mound. The road leading up to the fort's "back-door" was blocked at the entrance by a pair of solid steel doors, the width of the road and a good thirty feet in height. Coming up the road, this steel door was the only indication that one had of what comprised the mound beyond. Inside the steel doors was a small yard and a second set of iron grill gates which led onto a bridge. This bridge (about 30 yards long) crossed the dry moat and led into the fort proper. The entrance to the fort at the far side of the bridge was like going into a railway tunnel—a tunnel from which branching passages led to the rooms in which we lived. This meant that our rooms were well underground but they each had a window which looked out onto the moat, and across at the brick wall on the other side of the moat....

This moat was about 40 feet deep and the same across and was dry except for a small trickle of a stream in the very center. The walls of the moat were straight brick walls both on the inner and outer side. The highest

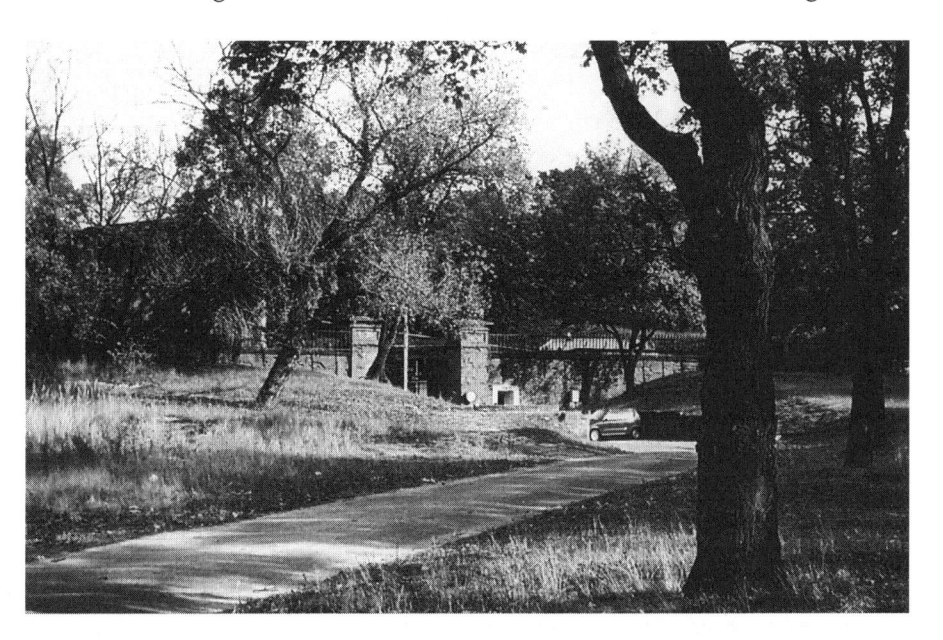

Entrance to Fort XV. *Courtesy of Jenny Feltham Setchell.*

level of the fort was the undulating path ... from which the grassy ground sloped steeply outwards towards the inner edge of the moat and inwards [toward] the sunken "platz" ... on each side. The "platz" was about [the] size of a tennis court and was well down (about 50 feet) below the level of the path. During the day we had free access to the top of the fort, reached by inside tunnels which emerged through steel doors.... From outside the whole thing looked like [an] undulating grassy mound, plentifully covered with trees and of course the moat was quite invisible to outside observers unless they came right up to the wire....

It was early evening when I was turned loose on this side of the bridge by a Goon soldier. I plodded across to the tunnel entrance on the far side carrying my worldly possessions in a kit bag, very much unheralded and unannounced. Just inside the fort I met a corporal of the R.A.M.C. who took me to the second room on the right ... occupied by the M.O. He was an Australian by the name of Meyer (known to all as "Quag"myer). He was very pleased to see me as he was feeling lonely. Being the only officer in the fort he had spent a lot of time on his own, and besides had just finished six weeks "stuben" arrest for calling a bunch of Jerries a lot of "murdering bastards." He told me all about the fort—it was for "non-arbeiters," in other words, N.C.O.s who had refused to work for the Germans. Well, we settled down for the night with the prospect of some pleasantly quiet days together in this room, which really was quite comfortable except that it had only two beds and a table with two chairs as extra furniture. But next morning in came the Germans with orders for Meyer to move and in an hour he was gone.

I was left as M.O. and the only officer in the fort with about 400 N.C.O.s to take care of. There was very little work to do and plenty of time to fill in, as I soon found; but the men in Fort XV had been there for four years and more and were adept at passing the time. The temptation for them to volunteer for work in the fields, just to relieve the awful monotony, must have been pretty strong, but with very few exceptions they had flatly refused work of any kind and took a pride in their attitude. Having sampled a little of that boredom myself I have every admiration for those fellows—how they stuck it out for so long I don't know. They even made little badges out of tin-foil—a laurel wreath surrounding a shovel with a broken handle, and underneath the words "NIX ARBEIT." They wore these "medals" which infuriated the Germans, but of course they could do nothing about it.

My first taste of this "new life" came the following morning. I was sitting reading one of the few medical books available when a sergeant major of the guards came briskly into the room, saluted smartly and handed me two pages of writing … "Times, Sir[,]" [he said]. Then with a request to burn the pages when I had finished he went out, leaving me with a summary of the B.B.C. news of the night before. After the careful and secretive way in which news had been passed round the Oflag I was startled by this casual way the "non-arbeiters" handled their news service.

Later it was pointed out to me that there was only one way the Germans could enter the fort (i.e. over the bridge)—a fact which gave them plenty of time to destroy any evidence of this nature. In fact internal "security" in the fort for this reason was excellent although to my mind the men ran too many unnecessary risks.

The next evening the same sergeant [major] returned and asked me to go with him if I wished to hear the news. We went down to the ground floor and along to one of the end rooms where, to my surprise, were a group of men sitting around a table on which was a slap-up five valve wireless (even to the polished cabinet) and they were listening to Tommy Handley! One man was posted at the window carefully watching the bridge, but the rest were enjoying every minute of the broadcast. The wireless ("canary") was kept under the floor of the bathhouse, next door to the room in which the news was received. It was certainly a great morale-raiser to hear the good old B.B.C. after so many months of nothing. How this and other wireless sets came to get into the fort would take too long to tell and perhaps is best left unsaid till I see you.

At the time I arrived at Thorn there were five wireless sets working in Fort XV as well as one set not working. This latter was kept hidden in an "obvious" place so that if the Germans did carry out a search they would find this set and go away satisfied. This very thing happened after I had been at the fort no more than about three weeks and here is what happened. Johnnie Fulton…, one of the M.O.'s in the district, was ill, and I had to go to Fort XIII to do his sick parades each morning. One day I was coming "home" complete with German guards, with two eggs in my pocket (a gift from the padre—but where he had acquired them I don't know) and I was struck by a strange "Je ne sais quoi" about the entrance to the fort. The outside steel doors were shut—a rare event except at night. I looked at the guard and he shrugged his shoulders and said "Gestapo." Bidding a fond farewell to the eggs I left them in a ditch and marched into the fort. What a sight was there! Four hundred Gestapo police had been let loose in the place for three hours and had turned the place upside down. My first thoughts were of the wireless and I didn't hold out much hope that it had survived. I was taken to my room which was in a shambles. A nasty looking goon shouted at me to undress for searching and I refused, saying that I was "protected personnel" and produced my identity card ... which has "Nicht Kriegsgefangen" printed across it (i.e. "not a prisoner of war"). The Goon saw red, and grabbing the lapel of my battle-dress tried to rip it off. I am sure I would have hit the blighter then and there if Maxwell (the medical orderly) had not grabbed my arm and pulled me back. The German security officer of the area, a much more reasonable man, explained to me in English that I would *have* to undergo a search sooner or later so I stripped and was searched, not without some muttering on my part about the doubtful parentage of that Gestapo hound.

An hour or two later the b__ds departed with their booty which included the non-working wireless set. As soon as the coast was clear and the last German had crossed the bridge the Corporal O.C. Wireless came and told me what had happened. For some reason or other the wireless had been out on the table in his room instead of under the floor in the bath house. The bugle blew for the daily rollcall, and he was going to leave the wireless on the table till after the roll-call. Before leaving his room he happened to glance out of the window and was horrified to see the column of police doubling across the bridge into the fort. He put the canary to rest in record time and had just got back to his room when the Gestapo arrived at his door.

Four police to each room, they searched everything. Bedding was pulled to pieces, clothing torn, every scrap of paper saved for further scrutiny. Here and there pieces of wall were pulled down and all the ground on top of the fort was gone over with detectors. Then they came into the bath-house. The Corporal O.C. Wireless was officially O.C. bathing and was required by the Gestapo to stand in the room while it was being searched. He stood there and sweated blood while by his side (and this is gospel truth) stood the O.C. Gestapo—a civilian—little knowing that he was standing right over a five-valve wireless separated from it by about 1 inch of floor boards. They emptied the tanks and boilers, they tore down the furnace and chimney and they found nothing.

The Gestapo chief gave the signal to depart and as he was about to follow his men from the room he took a pace forward and stamped hard to test the resonance. If he had stamped before taking a pace forward it would have been a different story for the corporal, but his fairy was watching over him....

I quickly settled down to life in Fort XV—a life of boredom punctuated by interesting episodes. We rarely saw the Germans inside the fort, a fact which made life much easier and more pleasant. Now I remember only the amusing things that happened and forget those lonely hours when

27. POW of the Germans

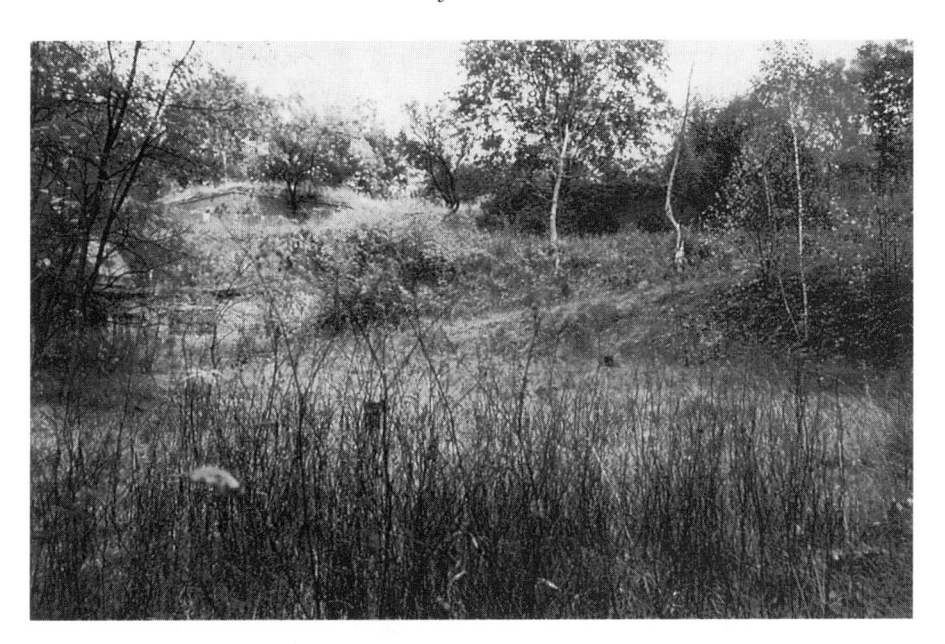

Fort XV, almost covered with earth. *Courtesy of Jenny Feltham Setchell.*

I sat alone in my room with very little to do and less moral energy to do it. Every meal for several weeks I had to eat alone, a sort of sop to custom and an endeavor to keep away from the men as much as possible in the interests of discipline. The men were very cheerful and friendly, always courteous and polite and during my stay in XV not one incident of unruly behavior occurred—due entirely to the sense of discipline and high morale of the inhabitants of the Fort.

One day two very meager-looking men in civilian clothes were thrust into the Fort. The Sergeant Maj. was suspicious of the pair and asked me to question them. I called them into my room and asked for their story—it was a curious one. They said that in 1941 they had been occupied in some commando-cum secret work in Tunisia where they had been captured by the Vichy French and interned. There they stayed in a jail in Tunis until the 8th Army crossed the Mareth Line—then they were released but were picked up by the Germans and flown to Germany. Then they were taken to Berlin where they were court[-]martialed and sentenced to death. (Such a sentence in Germany had to be followed by three months "grace" while the British Government was informed). Awaiting sentence to be carried out they spent the time in solitary confinement in Berlin prisons. The three months passed and turned into six. At the end of 12 months solitary confinement they were told that their case had been reconsidered and that they were recognized as British soldiers—hence their appearance in the fort.

Well, it sounded fishy to me, but they spoke good English and certainly looked the part—a pair of physical and mental wrecks. I thought that if their story was true they must have had a hell of a time and needed all the help we could give them. On the other hand they might be "Stoolpigeons" put in by the Jerries to get information. They had no proof of their identity and we could not accept them as "one of us" for security reasons. So I gave them red-cross food and ordered everyone to be careful not to discuss anything except the most ordinary everyday matters in front of the two newcomers. It must have been pretty hellish for those chaps—I discovered later, on return to England, that they were genuine enough.

I had pointed out to them that under the circumstances we couldn't take them into our confidence, and they certainly saw our point of view. They had done a very dangerous job, had lived within earshot of a firing-squad for 12 months expecting every day to be their last, and then having gained the comparative safety of a prison camp and the company of their fellow countrymen they were denied the comradeship which would have meant so much to them. Yet they didn't grumble and even thanked me for the trouble I took to make them as happy and comfortable as I could under the circumstances. They were just two examples of the fine type of Englishman I met in the "bag." It is interesting to know that when war broke out one was a traveling salesman and the other a "counter jumper" in a drapery shop in Liverpool....

After about two months of my semi-hermit existence Fort XV was suddenly closed down. My friends were shifted to one camp and I was sent to Fort XIII. Fort XIII was an exact replica of Fort XV but it housed the ordinary Tommies who were sent out on working parties each day. In this fort the officers' room was in the same position relatively as it had been in fort XV, but here I had some companions....

The day after I arrived at Fort XIII Johnnie Fullton [Capt., R.A.M.C.] became sick and went off to hospital (Fort XIV) leaving me all the work, which in this instance was heavy. It included two large sick parades each day and the care of patients in three wards. Of course there was a good deal of malingering but I didn't mind that as long as the men were honest with ME. I encouraged the men to get out of working for the Germans if they could put on a convincing "act"—a highly unethical state of affairs but very amusing on occasions. Once a week the German M.O. held a sick parade to check over my list of men on "light work" and "excuod [sic] duty" and it was a long and tedious day when that occurred.

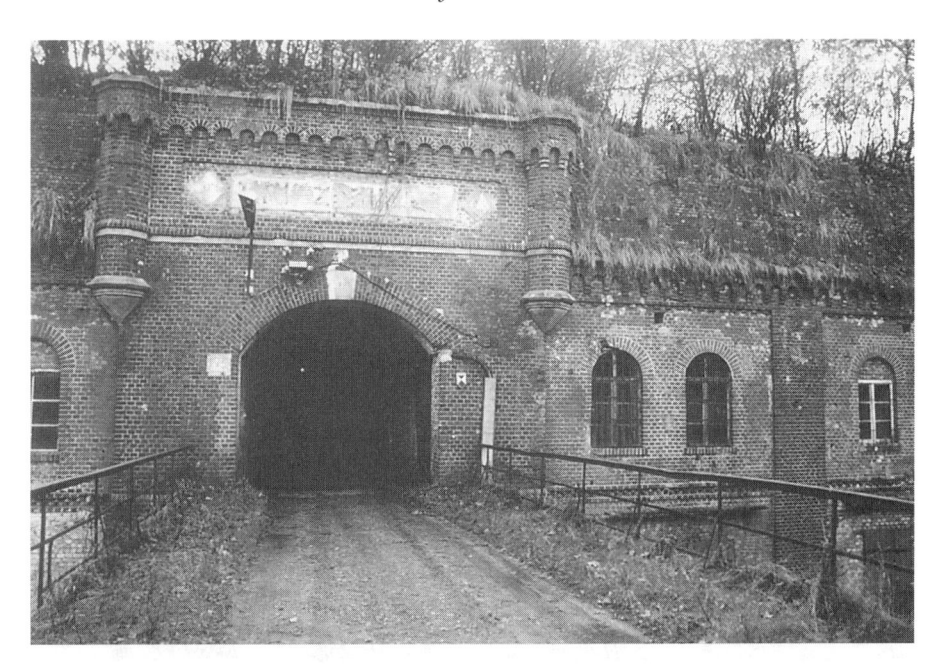

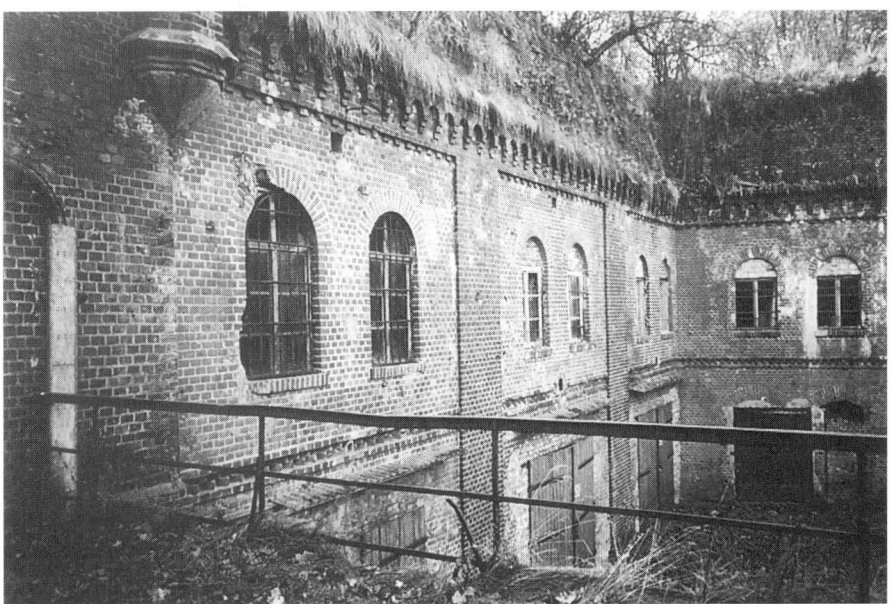

Top: Entering the tunnel at Fort XIII; *bottom:* Outside Fort XIII. *Both photographs courtesy of Jenny Feltham Setchell.*

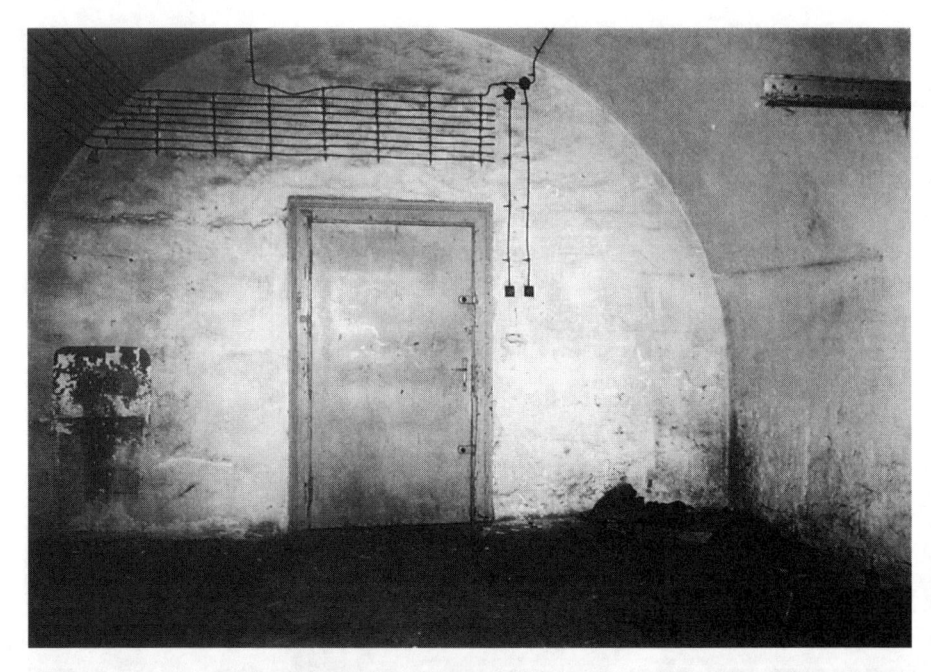

Top: Dr. Feltham's cell at Fort XIII; *bottom:* View of windows in Dr. Feltham's cell at Fort XIII. *Both photographs courtesy of Jenny Feltham Setchell.*

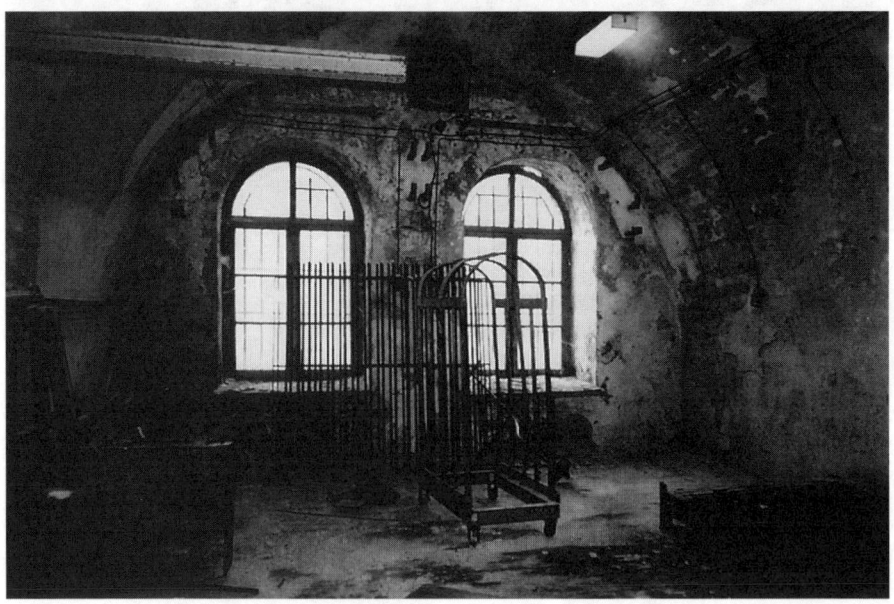

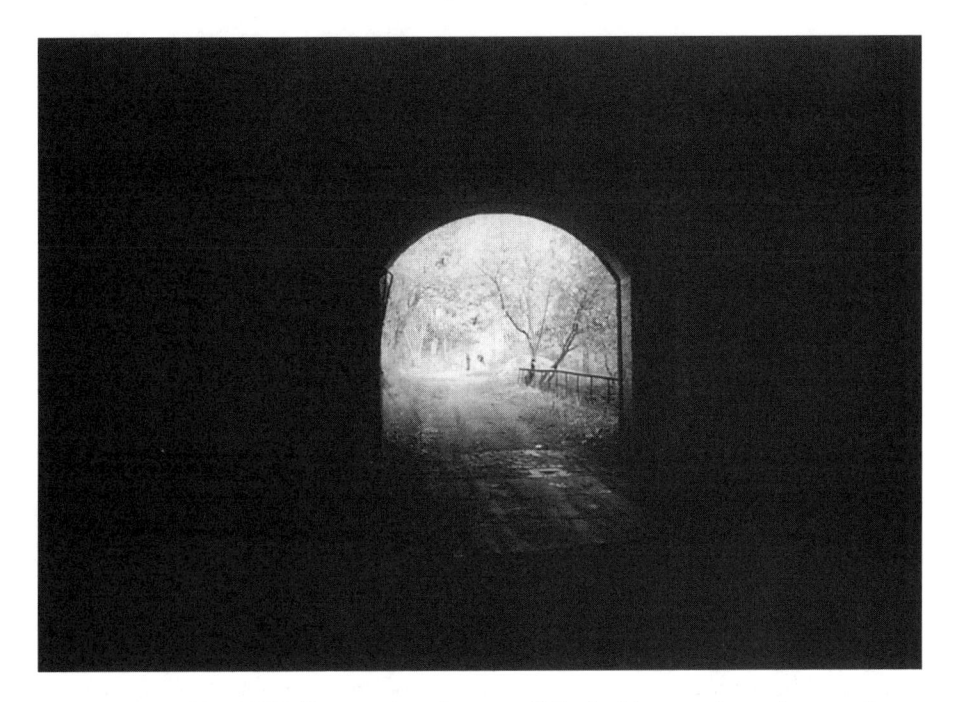

Entrance to Fort XIII (from within the tunnel) "...looking out from the tunnel towards the wall and down the road—from the darkness into the light ... how many of them longed for freedom down that road."—Jenny Feltham Setchell. *Courtesy of Jenny Feltham Setchell.*

But the sight of some "wag" coming into such a parade doubled up with "lumbago," his face the picture of misery, was somehow very funny when perhaps I had seen him a few minutes before kicking a football around on the Platz.

The first few weeks passed and I had more or less settled down to the routine when one day after doing some exercise on the Platz I had a severe pain in my back—the same pain I had as a schoolboy. Next morning my legs gave way while I was coming back from the bathhouse and I had to finish the distance on my hands and knees. After a rest I went slowly to the R.A.P, to start the sick parade but the pain was excruciating and was really getting me down. I stopped the sick parade on one occasion and felt a little better after vomiting into a bucket, but I doubt whether I've ever felt as miserable as I did that morning. But everything has its lighter side. After the sick parade I was sitting hardly daring to move and thinking what a bloody existence it was, when the door opened and in came two Tommies supporting between them an Aussie Corporal whose plight was exactly the same as mine. We just stared at one another for about 30 seconds and then burst out laughing—both stopping short when the laughter caused more bouts of pain. So we sat and giggled, almost becoming hysterical in the end. It all sounds so silly now, but such happenings as these were all that made one day different from the next, when anything was a welcome change from daily routine.

I stayed in Fort XIII until halfway through the summer of 1944 when quite suddenly we were ordered to move and the entire camp was shifted about 2 miles to what was commonly known as "Einheit III." "Einheit III" (pronounced "eyenheit dry") was just an ordinary camp consisting of a few rows of wooden huts on the sandy plain and surrounded by barbed wire, sentry boxes, machine gun posts etc. (See the film *Captive Heart* and you've seen this and many other camps like it in Germany). The officers were given a room at the end of one of the huts and we set about making our new home as comfortable as possible.

These huts were prefabricated frail wooden affairs raised about 18 inches off the ground on wooden piles and as draughty as they come. However, we didn't care. It was summer and the war would be over long before Christmas—I'd heard that same statement before the two preceding Christmases but still believed it. We were all very soon well settled in and life once again took on its monotonous routine—but this time with a difference. I think everybody's temper was getting a little short. We were all impatient for the war to end and most of us not a little disappointed as the months dragged on towards Christmas and the end of the war seemed no nearer.

The five of us began to have little quarrels—we had been living together for too long and constantly got on one another's nerves. Annoying little habits became more noticeable and tempers were lost over trifles. One lost the desire to read although there were plenty of books at this time. Outside there was nothing to see. The country round about was almost dead flat and my god how dreary—and every view was framed in a meshwork of that damned barbed wire. We all had our fits of depression, mail seemed to be coming in less regularly and one found it increasingly difficult to see the funny side of things. Then the winter came.

How bitterly cold it was. Clothes hung outside to dry even on the finest day became frozen to the line and could only be got off by softening them with warm water. Fuel supplies became low and we began to run out of stocks of Red Cross parcels. Even the sanitary arrangements were deplorable. The lavatories consisted of a shed, some 150 yards from our hut, built over a long concrete pit covered with concrete and pierced at intervals with holes about one foot square. At one end of the hut the pit was open to that piercing cold wind which swept across the Northern

Polish plains, so that when we used the lavatories the icy wind whistling up through the holes made the cold almost unbearable.

Even in the sickroom conditions were not much better. Half an hour before I started sick parade a fire was lit in the grate and the entire day's ration of coal for that fire place was burned in an attempt to warm the room. Every day for the week before Christmas, dressed in battledress, greatcoat, scarves, balaclava and mittens, I began the sick parade with the temperature inside the room between five and ten degrees below zero. Water in bottles was frozen and everyone was miserable. The coal ration per room was one shovelful per day.

Christmas that year came as a welcome relief from the monotony. Somehow we felt that this must be the last Christmas behind the wire, and we looked forward to the New Year with much more hope than we had done previously.

A few days after Christmas I was transferred to work in the hospital which had been shifted from Fort 13 to a camp similar to the one we were in and known as the "Russian hager" or "Copernicus harger." This was a very large camp cut up into blocks of about a dozen huts, one block being the hospital for the British and French POWs in the area.

If Einheit III had been dull and dreary this place was a thousand times worse. What a depressing outlook! One side of our compound was bounded by a road but the other three sides had just huts and yet more and more barbed wire. The neighboring blocks housed Russian prisoners in every stage of decay. Men with bilateral amputation above the knee shuffled round in the snow with the stumps of their legs wrapped up in dirty bits of sacking. Their wounds were healed but the Germans had made no effort to ease their lot by giving them any sort of artificial stumps. Their clothes were indescribably tattered and filthy, and all were in a state of severe malnutrition. During the course of the war some thousands of Russian prisoners had died in this camp and were buried in a common grave only a few hundred yards outside the main gate. Every day a sort of tumbrel cart rattled past out the entrance to the camp with its load of naked bodies which were tipped unceremoniously into a hole—and that was that.

So desperate were the Russians for food that if one of their number died during the night his body was propped up on his bed till after roll call so that others might have his meager food ration. As often as we could we smuggled tins of Red Cross food to their hospital, and occasionally they would come through the wire for more at night—many of them being caught in the act and ... shot by the sentries, ... no questions asked.

There were two things which made Copernicus bearable for me—one was lots of work, and the other was the presence of David Wild. David Wild, a tall thin Englishman, a Master at Eton before the war and back there now, had a fund of stories and sense of humor which was infectious. He had the happy knack of making us forget our plight and could stimulate a discussion which enlivened an otherwise dreary evening....

I had hardly become used to work in this hospital when things really began to happen. One day we were jogging along as we had done for the best part of three years, and a couple of days later we were involved in the most exciting and anxious time I've ever known. One moment we were prisoners with no immediate prospect of a break in the inevitable boredom, and yet three days later we were free!...

It began for us on the 17th of January when our canary informed us that Warsaw had fallen. This to us was really significant. Our camp was four or five miles to the East of Thorn ... but on the road running from Thorn to Warsaw. We were about 180 kilometers from Warsaw and also we knew that Thorn was the next German strong point after Warsaw on that line. Thorn was well fortified and was completely ringed by two huge anti-tank ditches—the importance of this was that we were between these two anti-tank ditches and also on the road along which the Russians were advancing. We talked things over that night and decided that we had better be prepared for any eventuality—but considered that in all probability the Germans would move us out of the battle zone before the fun began.

Next day the Germans made no announcement and we had to carry on as if nothing had happened, but inside the huts we organized the men into little groups, told them to get prepared to move out, to throw away any unnecessary kit and to carry only food. All that day down the road at the side of our camp came columns of the retreating German armies, pouring back into the stronghold of Thorn. The sentries were obviously becoming scared. Still no word from the Germans. Rumors came into camp of hurried evacuation of German civilians from Thorn and the wireless that night reported rapid advances west of Warsaw. The position was getting tense. Snow still lay thick on the ground and the days were bitterly cold.

At 3 a.m. next morning January 19th we were awakened by the German Camp Commandant stamping into our room with shouts of "Raus! Alles Aus!" He said that we had to be prepared to move within half an hour when transport would be arriving. Hurried preparations were made. My bed cases (12 in number) were transferred to stretchers and in half an hour all was set for the move. Nothing happened. At 6 a.m. the Germans returned, told us there was no transport and that we would be moving shortly on foot. We protested that such a move was impossible, we just couldn't carry the men who were too sick to walk and demanded to be left as we were. After a lot of argument the Germans agreed to let the sick men and a skeleton staff remain, and left the choice of staff to us.

We were faced with a difficult decision. Would it be better to encourage the men to remain behind or would they have a better chance in the open countryside on the march? We expected the Germans to put up a fierce fight for Thorn. We knew the position of local fortifications and that there were plenty of guns and troops in the town. If Thorn was defended then the area of our camp would be the center of the battlefield. On the other hand the weather was bad, the nights were intensely cold and this was the biggest factor against going on the march. But the weather was just beginning to improve and on the whole most of us considered that the open countryside was preferable to the possibility of being mixed up in a battle. We decided to present both sides of the argument to the men—tell them it would probably be better to get out while the going was good, but to leave the final choice to them.

Numbers of them wisely decided to go. They moved out of Camp with German guards shortly after 8 a.m. and we watched them go with rather mixed feelings. Capt. Allen went on the march. Lake, David Wild and I remained in camp. We three sat down and tried to think out what sort of precautions we could take for the safety of the patients. There were not nearly enough slit trenches for every one to take shelter, and the ground was frozen hard, making it impossible to dig more. Under the cookhouse there were some cellars, and we were considering giving orders for all patients to be moved up there, when our deliberations were interrupted by a heavy air-raid on Thorn and a low-flying machine-gun attack by squads of fighters on some nearby railway yards.

During the "shemozzle" a group of our men from Einheit III who were marching past our gates were pushed into our camp and their guards left them with us. They included Cookie (Capt. Cook) and old padre Gallaher. This brought our total strength up to 150 or thereabouts. It was decided that we could all squeeze into the cookhouse cellars and so as quickly as possible we had everyone shifted in to their new quarters. By midday the shift was complete and we sat awaiting events. The cellars were none too roomy and damp. I had 12 stretcher cases to care for—three of them with pneumonia, one case of T.B. peritonitis and one poor fellow a schizophrenic, a raving maniac. What a picnic! Poor old ... I had to keep him strapped to a stretcher with two orderlies constantly in attendance. Luckily I had managed to grab two boxes of German Evipan and most of the time had to keep him quiet with intramuscular injections. The day passed and evening brought no change in the situation. Late that night we heard the sound of track-vehicles in the distance and several bursts of machine gun bullets passed across the camp close to the cookhouse.

Next day, January 20, things seemed a little more quiet. There were a few air raids but nothing ... [much]. At dusk we saw what we took to be a German patrol sneaking up the road, and a little later, excitement ran high when our pickets reported what they took to be a Russian patrol passing in the opposite direction! At about 10 p.m. some Russian artillery, from somewhere in the woods to the East of the camp, sent a few shells whistling over our heads into Thorn. The anxiety of waiting for something to happen was making us all a little nervous and jumpy. At midnight things settled down, but we expected the dawn to bring some unpleasant surprises.

...At first light, German patrol troops were seen moving back down the road to Thorn. An hour later we were thrilled by the sight of a Russian patrol, in white cloaks, moving carefully over the snow. At this stage we could still see the Germans about a mile down the road towards Thorn behind the second anti-tank ditch. What a tense situation. It is not a pleasant sensation to be hiding in no-mans land, able to see troops of the opposing armies and expecting any minute to have a battle around our ears. We had persuaded a Russian prisoner to act as interpreter for us, and he sneaked out to the wire and tried to contact the Russian patrol—but without much success. Thereafter, we could only sit in our cellars and hope for the best.

The day passed quietly enough. No more patrols were seen and we just sat, and waited. Just after dark the Russian artillery began shelling again and soon the sky over Thorn was a deep red from some fire which had broken out. A terrific explosion right over the cookhouse made us all jump, keyed up as we were after so many hours of waiting. The whole building shook and dirt poured in through the air-vents at the side of the cellars. A quick inspection showed a hole blown in the roof of the cookhouse at one end. It was thought to be an air-burst ranging shot from the German artillery in Thorn, and had gone off right above our cookhouse. Unable to do anything about it we just sat there silent and miserable waiting for the worst to happen. Five minutes, ten, thirty then an hour passed and no further shots came. We expected that. The first light of dawn was the time we feared most—that is when most attacks begin. So we went on waiting. Nobody could sleep. Nobody talked. We just sat and waited. The hours slowly dragged on and as dawn approached so also, down in the cellars, the tension increased. Ever so slowly the sky began to lighten, but still nothing happened. With daylight our spirits rose. Somehow we felt comforted by the light—at least we could see what was happening.

We began to hope that the Germans had evacuated Thorn. We could see no sign of the Germans down the road but then neither could we see any Russians. At about 8 a.m. a small group of Russians came down the side of the road by the wire. One of them came through the wire and we waited eagerly to hear what he had to say. Through our interpreter he told us that they knew who we were, that the Russians were expecting the Germans to counter attack in this sector at any moment and that we were given ten minutes to get out of the camp. We were told to get behind the Russian lines just as quickly as we could. Believe me, we lost no time. But first we had to cut holes through two sets of wire large enough for stretchers to be passed through, and we had no wire cutters. Cookie found a spade and with all his 14 stones [196 pounds] behind it started hacking away at the first obstacle. It seemed to take an age but finally it was cut and then there was the second fence. This too seemed painfully slow but at last we were out and on the road. Slowly, dreadfully slowly it seemed, we got the stretcher cases onto the road and then began one of the most strenuous days of my life. Up that road we went, taking turns at carrying the stretchers, slipping and sliding on the icy ground and hoping like hell that the Germans would delay their attack just a little bit. It was an uphill grade and the road was ice-covered and slippery. Russian, French and British prisoners jostled up the road in their hundreds. Soon we gained the comparative shelter of the woods but nobody thought of stopping for a rest.

Advance groups of the Red Army passed—first a few members of a patrol in their long white cloaks, then odd groups of infantrymen. A Cossack officer rode past, a drawn saber in his hand, and then a small cart with the body of a dead German soldier overtook us. Occasional shots rang out from somewhere in the woods and we passed more groups of Russian infantry as we slipped and struggled with the heavy stretchers.

And so it went on. No thought of what had happened—I don't think any of us appreciated the fact that we were free at last, we were too intent on putting the miles between us and Thorn. When we had covered about five kilometers we were ordered to halt and to sort ourselves into nationalities. We lined our men up and took a rollcall; nobody was missing. I think most of us were a bit dazed by the happenings of the last two hours after those days of tense waiting in the cellars.

Regular groups ... [of] stretcher bearers were organized and in a few minutes we set off again. This time we marched in orderly columns,

British in front. We settled down to a marching pace (slow, on account of the stretchers) and, resting from my turn at stretcher-carrying, I began to take an interest in my surroundings. Although cold, it was a beautifully still and "crystal clear" morning and the snow covered trees were pretty to see. It was wonderful to be walking along without German guards. I wasn't a bit tired but felt happy and glad to be alive. Then suddenly I found myself thinking—"My God, I'm free. I'm out! I'm really free. I'm on my way home! All those days and nights of loneliness and longing are over. I'm really free. I'm on my way home! Soon I'll be seeing Bobs and Christopher. Gosh, isn't it great. Maybe a few weeks will see me back in Raetihi. I wonder what Mother and Dad are doing now? How soon will they [K]now what has happened to us? No more barbed-wire thank God."

Realization of freedom came to me suddenly, just like that. One reads in novels of people shedding tears of happiness. Well, it certainly happened to me. I found that I was crying, with tears just pouring down my cheeks, but I didn't care. It was great to be alive. When I had recovered I looked around. Nobody was talking. Everyone was quietly plodding along obviously absorbed in his thoughts, and several faces were wet. I'm sure that in those few minutes of "reaction" we all thought of home, and how wonderful it was to be "on our way" at last.

On and on we plodded, with no time for a rest. We began to pass bigger units of Red Army troops and what a disorderly rabble they looked. At first there were groups of infantry—very Mongoloid types—and all their transport was horse drawn. Then a small group of cavalry, followed perhaps by a single tank—a few trucks would slither by, then more infantry. A Russian officer drove past in a gig with his girlfriend on the seat beside him. The roads became more congested; Cossack infantry, tanks, artillery, more infantry and horsedrawn vehicles surged down the road—terrible congestion and utter chaos. A Russian interpreter at the head of our column kept telling the oncoming traffic who we were—and as the trucks passed we were received with shouts of "Anglecani," "Angleski," and "Amerikanski."

Reaction began to set in. The initial stage of excitement was wearing off and I began to feel the effects of the anxiety and tension of the past few days. We began to stumble and slip on the road, longed to put the stretchers down for a few minutes. Arms and legs began to ache and collar bones were becoming tender from the pressure of the laden stretchers (we were carrying them at shoulder height). Wouldn't we ever stop for a rest? Then, after covering about 12 kilometers in all, we were directed off the road to a small farmhouse. Gratefully we lowered the stretchers to the ground and sat about resting our weary limbs. Where were we? What were we going to do? Nobody seemed to know—or care, for that matter. After about an hour we were told that fit members of the party would have to continue on foot to a place called Alexandrovo and that the stretchers would be sent by transport as it became available. Padre Gallaher was showing signs of exhaustion so we made him stay behind with the unfit and soon we were on our way once more....

We moved along more quickly now, anxious to reach this town before dark. However, time and again we were held up by the congestion on the roads and darkness saw us still with five or six kilometers to go. We left the road and cut across the snow-covered fields, just a long line of hungry refugees plodding wearily in the footsteps of those in front. I think it was "Cookie" who gave a short summary of the situation with the words: "Consider yourself nothing more or less than a bloody refugee now, Horace!" At least, it was after midnight, we straggled into Alexandrovo. It was snowing, the streets were deserted and there wasn't a glimmer of light from anywhere. I don't know who was leading the column (or rather "mob") but somehow they found billets for us in the school—a large barracks of a place that had been a Gestapo police school the day before. There was no light inside or out and confusion is hardly strong enough to describe the state of affairs. French, Russian and British POWs stumbled about in the dark but finally got settled down for the night. When things had calmed down a little I went with a guide to the local hospital where our sick had been sent. It was a small hospital run by some nuns and they had made our fellows very comfortable. We had a meal at the hospital and I was persuaded (without much resistance on my part) to spend the night on a comfortable hospital bed. Next morning I went back to the School and found things much more shipshape. Polish volunteers were cooking soup for the hungry hundreds and everyone was happy. A Russian officer arrived, said he was the direct representative of the Soviet Government and that he would look after our welfare. He told us that transport would arrive in a day or two and that we would not have to walk another step.

Later that morning I went back to the hospital to see how the fellows were getting on and found the place very changed. Hordes of Russian wounded had arrived and the place was filled to overflowing. On the floor, all along the corridor lay wounded waiting their turn for treatment; there were no Russian doctors about, all the work being done by the Polish staff of the hospital, and offers to help from us were turned down flat. During my whole eight weeks as a guest of the U.S.S.R. I saw absolutely nothing (or almost) in the way of medical organization. What little we saw on the trip to Odessa was futile and very inefficient.

Before leaving the hospital that morning, while upstairs talking to the Padre, I was attracted by a commotion outside. I went to the window and saw a stretcher containing a wounded German officer being carried down the steps of the hospital. As I looked, a young Cossack officer hurried after the stretcher, drew his revolver, and shot the German through the head. It was a ghastly exhibition, but even more nauseating was the sight some few minutes later, of Polish children stripping the body of its clothes as it lay in the street. Two days later we were given orders to move and without delay set out for a town some nine miles away (Needless to say on foot!). This was Ciechocinek ("check-o-chee-neck")—known to the Germans as Hermans Bad. (Herman's Spa—named after none other than H. Goering himself). We were billeted in the Pension Home (postcard enclosed)—and were reasonably comfortable. It had recently been a German military hospital and there were tons of beds with thick springy mattresses—but no blankets. We found a large dump of coal and as there was a fireplace in every room we soon had that building really hot. Any day we expected to move on, and every day brought various Russian officers—all with the same story—transport will be here, tomorrow or the next day. Most of us wanted to push on to Warsaw on foot but were persuaded to wait, and wait we did. Five weeks we waited there and they seemed like years to a bunch of ex–POWs eager to go home. The Russian food was poor (no fats, sugar or anything to go with the bread) although we did get some extras from the Poles. One day I was asked to go and see a Polish kiddie with pneumonia. I had some M & B and in 48 hours or so the parents were all over me with presents of food saying that I had worked a miracle. In about two days I had a practice worthy of the name—the village insisting on paying me with food. Besides all this I had our own sick to care for (they had arrived by horse drawn cart a day or so after us) and my time was pretty well filled.

At times it was embarrassing to be plied with Polish politics while we were technically the guests of the Red Army. The Poles hate the Russians and lost no time in saying so. All the villagers I spoke to were in a high-pitched state of apprehension for the future and the reason was obvious. The Russian Armies were swooping through their country; rape, pillage and murder were rife. There was very little difference between this and the German occupation, and many Poles tried to get us to take them in as one of us so that they could escape to England. I know that this Russo-Polish antagonism is an old, old, story and I know a lot of the blame rests with the Poles, but neither side seemed to be trying to meet the difficult situation in any way, and I am sorry for the Poles....

Five weeks we stayed at Herman's Bad, and just about every day the

Russians promised us transport within 48 hours. They would not let us send a nominal roll to the British Embassy in Moscow—instead they made lists of their own in Russian phonetics! When they read the list out to us the only way we could tell who it was supposed to be was by following the procedure on our own lists and calling out the names after they did. Yes, it was a muddle, and the red tape far outdid anything I had experienced anywhere before. The whole town was plastered with crude and rather childish placards of propaganda—the only thing they seemed to do at all efficiently.... Then one afternoon quite as much a surprise to the Russians as to us, fifty American trucks arrived and by midnight we were on the road. Snow fell as we started off and it [was] the coldest journey I can remember. However midday next day saw us at a place called Brischen(?) where we were to entrain for Odessa. The following day we were marched to the train and our almost "unbelievable" journey to Odessa began.

We were in cattle trucks—60 per truck and our journey took ten days. It was as haphazard as the rest of the Russian arrangements. The train was exactly one kilometer long and the engine driver was the rankest amateur. When we started off the first time we were all thrown in a heap in one half of the truck by the jolt. We soon learned to listen for the crash-crash-crash-crash of the couplings whenever starting or stopping—then we would grab the nearest piece of solid truck and hold on for dear life. We stopped and started so much during those ten days that holding on was almost a conditioned reflex by the time we reached the journey's end. We passed Warsaw at night so didn't see much of it.

Almost all the way to Odessa the country was dead flat, snow covered and indescribably dreary. Our train just plodded on and on sometimes stopping at a siding for ten minutes and sometime stopping apparently nowhere for 12 or 15 hours. Rations (bread and bullybeef) was given out daily and we were also supplied with cakes of dried Russian tea. At the first stop one of our number disappeared for a few minutes and then returned with a bucket. At the next stop he jumped out with the bucket and raced along to the front of the train. There by a sign language all his own, he managed to indicate to the driver what was wanted, held the bucket under the engine, and had it filled with boiling water—it made very good tea!

There were no latrine arrangements anywhere on the trip and we just had to wait till the train stopped, then jump out onto the rails. There was no room for false modesty as all our stops were at some sort of village or other, and the arrival of the train was the signal for the villagers to turn out to see what it was all about. The country was dead flat and consequently there was no cover. On one occasion I jumped out to "faire mes besoins," and while squatting in the snow at the side of the train heard a voice apparently addressing me. I was a bit confused to find a woman from the nearby village standing in front of me, quite unconcerned, doing her best to start a conversation!

On this trip we passed through several well known places—Warsaw, Brest-Litovsk and Kovel to mention some—and without exception they were reduced to heaps of rubble. The countryside has not suffered much but the towns just don't exist any more except in name. In such a way we traveled for ten days—sometimes bumping along at a good pace and sometimes the train would stop miles from anywhere. It was impossible to go far from the train at any of these stops as we never knew how long the stop was for, and when the driver was ready to start he just started. At Brest-Litovsk we were parked for some hours by a train containing German POWs on their way to Siberia—it was difficult not to feel sorry for the blighters.

A train similar to ours, but running about six days behind us, experienced a little Russian rough justice at one of their stops. They had stopped at one town and for some reason the train was being shunted—but with a difference. They shunted it with an engine on each end of the train. The train was broken in half for some reason and when the two halves were brought together again the impact was so great that two trucks were telescoped and three of our fellows killed. The Russian Officer in Charge of the train decided that the local station master was to blame and without further ado, shot him! (Any officer of the Red Army may summarily shoot anyone under him). This train load joined us six days after we arrived in Odessa....

While we waited in Odessa we were not allowed outside the building until after very strong representation on the part of the Military Mission. The men were taken for route marches and officers were allowed out walking, in pairs only! Cookie and I took immediate advantage of this order and made hasty tracks for the harbor. The sea was a beautiful blue, my first glimpse of it since August 1942, but even more beautiful to our eyes was the sight of two big steamers [sailing] slowly into harbor—and yes, both of them were flying the good old British ensign. We literally jumped for joy, then hurried back to spread the good news. Excitement ran high that night and we spent the time arguing how long it would take to reach England from Odessa.

Next morning we were dashed to the ground by a message from the captain of one of the ships, who said that he had to go to Alexandria and was sorry he couldn't take us this trip! However, the intelligence officer got busy with messages to the Admiralty and the result was that two days later we were marching down to the docks and at last, on our way.

What a lovely ship she looked. It was the *Duchess of Richmond* (22,000 tons). The captain and crew certainly gave us a great welcome and the food was almost too good to be true. We all found that we couldn't eat very much. I think most of us, after stuffing ourselves at that first meal of eggs, bacon, toast with butter and jam, went straight up to the bathroom and were sick. After that we took things more slowly, but it is hard to describe what a pleasure it can be to sit down to a slap up meal and really enjoy eating for the first time for three years. I put on a stone [14 pounds] in weight during the trip to England.

We embarked in the evening and the ship pulled out almost at once. Next day we arrived at Istanbul. The next interesting place we passed was the Dardanelles—we saw the Gallipoli memorials.

Naples was the next port of call. We stayed five days there and unfortunately were not allowed on shore. I tried to send a cable home but the war was still on and security forbade it. Butt Adams came an [*sic*] board one evening and it was grand to see him.

At Naples hundreds of troops were embarked and accommodation on board became pretty crowded. Among the new arrivals were several colonels and majors who objected to the dormitory sleeping arrangements and gave orders through the military administration staff of the ship that we were to be moved out of the cabins to make room for officers of higher rank. The ship's captain here turned up trumps by giving a counter order that on no account were we to be moved. A real gent! The rest of the journey was fairly uneventful, except for the sinking of an enemy submarine 24 hours out from Scotland.

Sailing past Ailsa Craig and up the Clyde was a terrific thrill. The hills looked so green and peaceful it was hard to believe that we were practically in England (sorry Scotland). All day batches of ex–POWs were disembarked. Our turn came at 3 p.m. and almost before we realized it, there we were with two feet planted on good old British soil. A train was waiting in the Station, with daily papers on all the seats, and Scots girls on the station were giving out cakes and tea. It was a welcome change to be able to read all the advertisements and to understand everything anyone said without having to scream for an interpreter. As the train steamed along we all leaned out the windows and shouted and waved to anyone nearby. It was dark by the time we arrived in Edinburgh so all we saw there was the name of the station—but even that was a thrill.

Thereafter things happened so quickly it was all a little confusing. Ten in the morning saw us arriving at Kings Cross—there a lorry arrived and took us through London to Victoria Station. The Strand, Trafalgar Square, the Mall, Buckingham Palace and lots of other places were pointed out as we hurried by—I would have like[d] to have stopped and had a good look but we had to catch a train for Margate where the New Zealand reception camp was stationed....

Now a little more than a year after my arrival in England, I am beginning to feel more or less a normal citizen. I am beginning to forget the worst side of the prison life and remember most clearly the funny bits which helped to make life a little more pleasant.

I miss the comradeship that one finds among men in such a predicament, and still feel a little resentment on some occasions. For example, there are plenty of young doctors in London who have held good jobs in hospitals throughout the war, and some of them openly boast of how they kept out of the army. I feel a little bitter on this subject but am beginning to get such thoughts out of my system. Such people are really not worth bothering about, and I feel that although I may be a long way behind them in medical matters [a] little hard work will soon put that right—and on the other hand I have had experiences which in some ways are beyond value. I've made friends with men all over the world, and I've had unique opportunities to really get to know men from all walks of life. Friendships made under conditions of privation and danger seem to mean so much more than ordinary friendships.

I didn't enjoy being a prisoner of war, but I've come out of it with a wealth of experience and knowledge which compensates in some measure for the hardships entailed in gaining it.

Love to you all at home
Dick

PS: I dedicate this "effort" to my dear wife whose constant bickering and nagging drove me to completing it.

Chapter Twenty-Eight

The CBI Theater

THOMAS J. MCKENNA, M.D.

> *"The Hump" was the name the GIs gave the world's highest mountains, the Himalayas, some of which were 26,000 feet high and, of course, Mt. Everest [is] at 28,000 feet. This was tricky for aircraft that could only get up to 12,000 feet when fully loaded such as our C-47s ... [which] had to dodge through passes with wild air currents and peaks towering thousands of feet beyond each wingtip. Planes hauling necessary supplies from India to China had to fly over "The Hump." One thousand airplanes and most of their crews were lost [in the Himalayas] during the war and today no one remembers. It is so sad.*
> —Dr. Thomas McKenna

Dr. McKenna served in the China, Burma, India (CBI) Theater of War. He was 28 years old at the time and Flight Surgeon with the Fourth Combat Cargo Squadron, First Combat Cargo Group.

Plane Crashes at Likiang

The First Combat Cargo Group with its one hundred C-47s was ordered over the Hump from India to China in December 1944. I was Flight Surgeon with the Fourth Squadron and the Fourth was stationed at Chengkung, which is a long rickshaw ride from Kunming.

Our squadron commander was Lt. Col. Loyal Penn, out of American Airlines, and if you would ask any man in the old Fourth he would say: "He's the best damn C.O. in the whole frickin U.S. Army Air Force." I would have to agree.

One day around the middle of January 1945, Colonel Penn called me into his office and said, "Doc, we've had a plane crash at a tiny, little airstrip up near the border of Tibet at a place called Likiang. The plane, a C-47, is a total wreck but it didn't burn, thank God, but they have an injured man aboard. I want you to go to Likiang, do what you can for the man and get him back here as soon as possible for probable hospitalization."

I said, "Colonel, why in the world did we have a plane up on the border of Tibet?"

He said, "We have a small radar station there, maybe five or six men, to help guide planes over the Hump. Our plane that crashed was taking in gasoline for their generator. Harold Beason, our Operations officer, will be your pilot, and Second Lieutenant Dewey Lowe will be copilot. You better leave as soon as you can." Colonel Penn had already told Beason and Lowe, so all I had to do was get my medical flight service chest, get on the plane, and take off.

We took off and headed northwest, and in an hour or so we saw huge, snow-covered peaks in the distance that towered ten or 12 thousand feet above our airplane, and most of them weren't even on our map. Eventually we saw Likiang below with a tremendous, snow-covered mountain towering 21,000 feet on its northwest side, and southeast of the town was a grassy field that served as a landing strip. And there lying off to one side of the landing strip was our wrecked C-47.

Beason came around for a landing, and I was standing in the worst possible place, back between pilot and copilot. We came in well on our approach until we got above the end of the runway. We were then hit by a tremendous crosswind boiling down from that 21,000 foot peak. Beason fought for control of the airplane, and I didn't think he was going to win for a while, but he gave her more power and eased back on the stick and finally regained control.

He then came around for another approach. The crew-chief came up and said "Wow." Beason said, "Yeh, I'd rather turn around and go home right now, but they have an injured man down there and my orders are to get him out."

We came in for another attempt at landing, and just as we got to the same spot that hurricane wind hit us again. Beason got the wheels down on the grass this time, but I looked out and saw that we had used up almost all the runway and hadn't slowed down one bit. As we approached the end of the runway Beason yelled, "We're f——d!" I was thrown back and forth from one side of the companionway to the other as Beason ground-looped the plane to the right.

The plane spun around, the right gear collapsed, the right wing-tip dug into the ground, and the right prop flew off through the air. We came to a stop off the runway to the right, with the plane facing at right angles to the direction we were heading. After we had stopped I looked at the air speed indicator, and it was registering 70 miles an hour. If he had ground-looped the plane to the left, the left prop would have flown through the fuselage right where I was standing.

The Likiang radar crew had been watching from the side of the landing strip, and as soon as we came to a stop they came out in their jeep to get us. They took us back to their small, bleak quarters and shared their C ration with us. I examined the injured man and found that his injuries were not serious and that I could take care of him out of the medical flight service chest.

We radioed back to Chengkung immediately and reported that a second plane had crashed at Likiang. I had roomed in the Basha with Colonel Penn for two months at Dohazari, and I could just hear him now. "Those damn, kid, army pilots; I'm going to have to go and do the job myself."

Sure enough, at first light next morning we heard a plane coming over the mountains. We got in the Jeep immediately and rushed down to the airstrip. We had a "drop-chute" with us that we tied together so it wouldn't balloon out in the terrible crosswind. A man from the radar crew climbed to the top of a dead tree and tied the strings of the drop-chute to the tree. The trussed-up chute pointed straight out from the tree like a long, white finger pointing at right angles to the airstrip.

I don't know whether Colonel Penn saw the chute or not, but he came straight in for a landing. He got just above the head of the runway when the hurricane-force crosswind hit him. We could see him fighting desperately for control of the plane, and he eventually gained altitude; he had won that fight. He didn't try it again. The last we saw of him was the small silhouette of a plane flying back over the mountains on the way home.

The next day the terrible wind continued so we went into town. Likiang was the cleanest, prettiest, little town I had seen in all of China. There was a river winding through it with ducks on the water. And in a place so remote we saw a woman sewing on an old foot-treadle Singer sewing machine. We also saw a caravan of Tibetans coming through on the old Silk Road. One of our GIs threw an empty beer can down, and one of the Tibetans ran out and picked it up. Dewey Lowe laughed and said, "They never waste anything. He'll make a drinking cup out of that."

There was the ubiquitous missionary in town, a Scotch Presbyterian with an American wife from Cleveland. He was delighted to have someone different to talk to and invited us to his home for dinner. We had a delicious meal and conversation that was just as welcome. He said it would take us six weeks to go out by horseback. I was all for doing that until he said, "The mountains are full of bandits who will kill you for your shoes." That snuffed out all my enthusiasm for adventure.

After we finished eating he asked us if we'd sign his book. We were very happy to do so, of course. I took the book and started to look through it. The first two names in the book were Kermit Roosevelt and Theodore Roosevelt, Jr. The date was 1920, and they had been through there looking for Giant Panda. Also in the book was the name Col. Robert L. Scott, author of *God Is My Co-Pilot*. I was truly amazed and gladly added my name to this illustrious list.

About two days later we woke up and the wind had stopped; just stopped. We got on the radio in a hurry and reported it back to Chengkung. A couple of hours later we heard the roar of a plane as it came in and landed with no difficulty. We all got on in a hurry and took off before the wind started up again. As we circled above the airstrip I looked through that little rubber ring in the center of the C-47 window and saw those two, derelict, C-47s lying there off the dirt runway, dead and abandoned.

We'll Shut Off Your Water

In the summer of '45, the war in China had been sorely fought when the First Combat Cargo Group was ordered to occupy the old abandoned airbase at Luichow that had been completely destroyed by the Americans in November '44 to deny its use to the Japanese. The old base had been burned, blasted, and bulldozed until nothing was left except the airstrip.

As we erected pyramidal tents and dug latrines, we encountered two new enemies we hadn't had to face elsewhere—Chinese cholera and amoebic dysentery. Chinese cholera ravaged the surrounding countryside killing hundreds of Chinese, and thousands more suffered the terrible complications of amoebic dysentery. Both diseases were carried by contaminated water.

On all the other bases where we had been stationed the drinking water in the Lister bags was made safe by simple chlorination because cholera and amoebic dysentery were not endemic in those areas. The bacteria that cause cholera, and the amoeba that cause Amoebiasis, however, are not killed by chlorine, and the drinking water must be boiled. Word came down fast through medical channels: "Boil all drinking water for one half hour; allow to cool; chlorinate before putting water in Lister bags."

Now this was not an easy job—to boil drinking water for over a thousand men under the very primitive field conditions that existed in rural China in 1945. First we had to "liberate" some heaters from the mess, and to liberate heaters from our mess sergeant—Sergeant Goldberg—was certainly no easy task. Then we had to liberate some aluminum, 55-gallon drums that were used, along with steel drums, to carry gasoline over the Hump. This wasn't easy either because aluminum 55-gallon drums were scarce and were guarded like gold.

The next step was to set up a team of men to keep the water boiling, which we did. We had just boiled the first 55-gallon drum of water, allowed it to cool, chlorinated it and put it in the Lister bag when Major Rosebrook, our group surgeon, drove up. He said, "Tom, it seems to be going real well." I agreed that it had gone well. We were standing about 30 feet away admiring our work when suddenly a dirty, Chinese coolie ran over, put the Lister bag faucet in his mouth, and drank deeply.

"My God!" Major Rosebrook screamed. "Did you see that; he has contaminated the entire Lister bag of drinking water." It was obvious that he *had* contaminated the entire Lister bag of drinking water.

Major Rosebrook said "We'll have to put a man on to guard the Lister bags or the entire group will be infected," so we put a guard on. There were many Chinese who tried to use the Lister bags now, and the guard tried to be nice at first. He couldn't speak Chinese, but he would motion for them to leave, take them by the shoulder, talk to them (in English), and do everything to try to dissuade them from using the Lister bags, all to no avail. When being nice didn't work, the guard screamed at them, pushed them away, and finally in desperation aimed a kick at their backside. It still didn't stop the Chinese from using the Lister bags.

It was about this time that our squadron engineering officer and my friend and tentmate, Captain Tex Enloe, from Kilgore, Texas, came along.

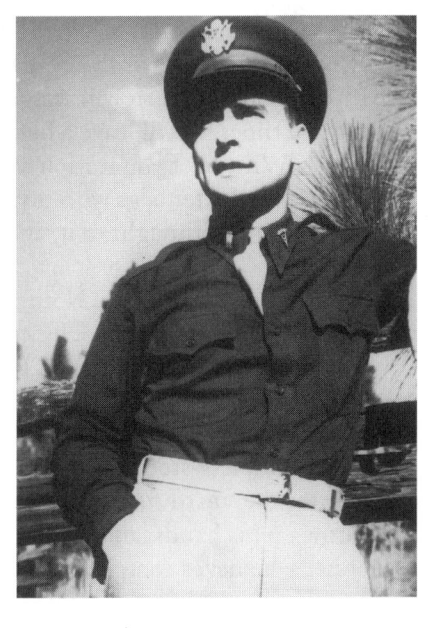

Dr. Thomas J. McKenna. *Courtesy of Dr. Thomas J. McKenna.*

He saw immediately what the trouble was. He said, "Doc, I have the answer to that. I have an air pistol that shoots BBs, and there's no sound. If you pump it once, it will sting like Hell through the clothes; if you pump it three times, it will leave a big, red welt on the skin and won't feel good, either. Why don't you station a man in our tent over there and have him protect the Lister bags with my silent air pistol." He stopped and seemed to give a lot of thought to it, and then said, "I'd just pump the pistol once though."

We were desperate. Nothing else had worked, even the guard kicking them hadn't kept the Chinese away, and we were worried that cholera would break out in the group. I said, "OK, Tex, get your pistol." Our tent was about 40 feet away with the sides rolled up. The guard sat on a cot inside the tent and wasn't easily seen, and the pistol was silent. Every time a Chinese stooped over to put the faucet from the Lister bag in his mouth, the guard fired the air pistol at his backside. He would scream, throw up his hands, and run. It didn't seem to be hard work for the guard either—he never complained.

War is a mean and ugly thing, and many people are hurt, and a very great many are killed, but this was the first time, to my knowledge, that lives were saved by the simple expedient of shooting someone in the ass with a BB gun.

Chapter Twenty-Nine

H.M.N.Z.H.S. *Maunganui*
HERBERT MATTHEW ROBSON
AND GRACE ROBSON

Bert's rank on the Maunganui was officially corporal, but in rank he was actually sergeant when he went on the ship. They could only have a set number of sergeants, so he became a corporal. However, he was a "ward master" and was in charge of a ward, and they worked long hours when they had patients, which was often on the outward and homeward journeys. The last 12 months the ship was attached to the British Pacific Fleet, and they had some pretty scary times there.
—Grace Robson

Herbert (Bert) Robson served for six years on the New Zealand Hospital Ship Maunganui. *He kept a diary of all the trips, recording the many incidents that occurred. The following are excerpts from that diary, contributed by Robson's wife, Grace.*

Grace Robson was a V.A.D. [Voluntary Aid Detachment] Nurse on her way to Egypt onboard the Maunganui *when she met Bert Robson. She, too, shares her story here.*

Herbert Matthew Robson's Story

VOYAGE VIII

Nov. 17th, 1942: At 10 A.M. a Catalina signaled us to go to aid of a Dutch tanker which had been torpedoed 500 miles south of Cocos Is. The tanker had been attacked by two raiders, one of which she had sunk complete with two aircraft. The second raider had put 2 torpedoes into her side,

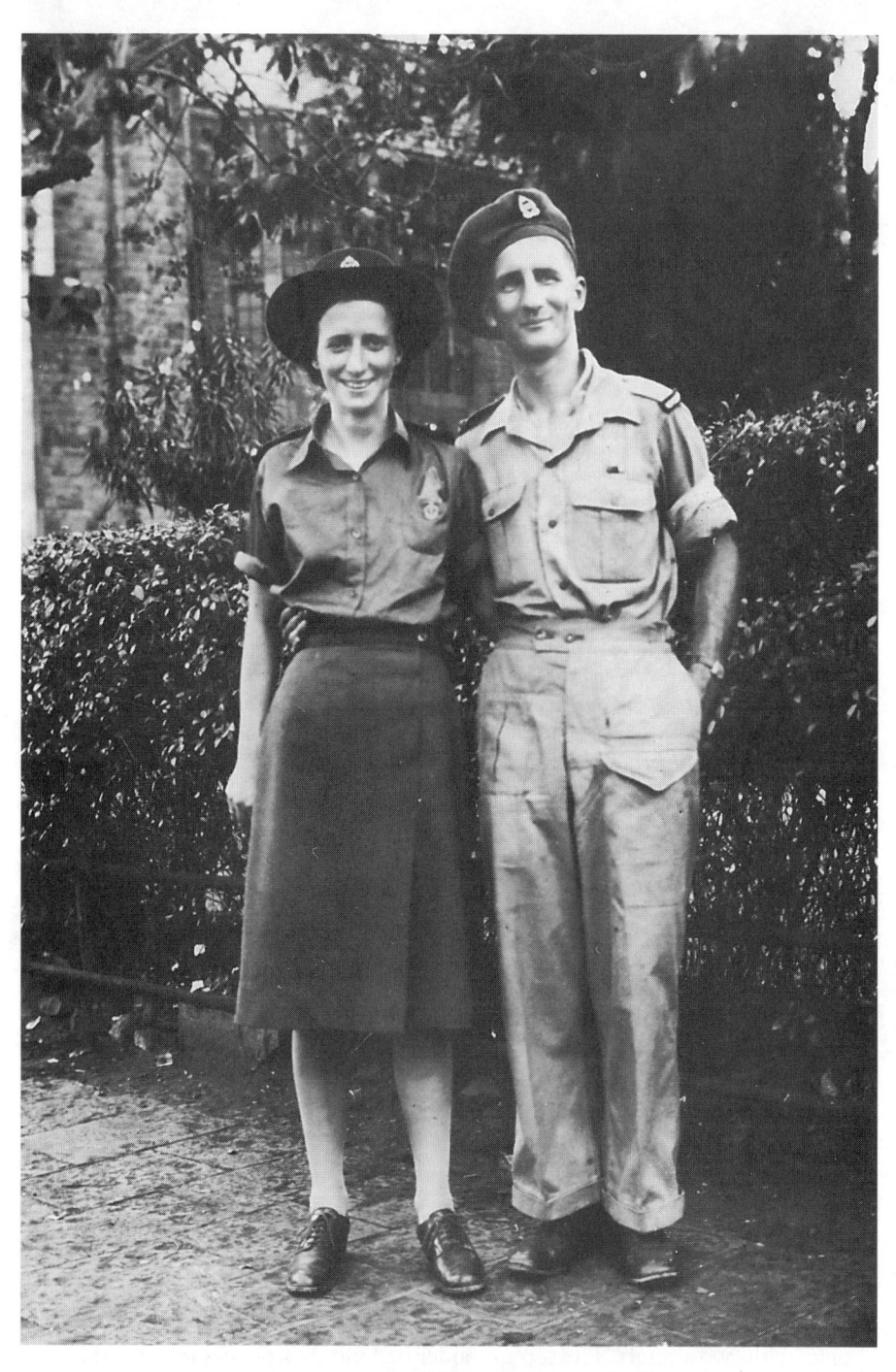

Grace Smith Robson and Herbert Matthew Robson in Bombay, January 1945, on a voyage to the Middle East. *Courtesy of Grace Robson.*

but the crew who had abandoned ship were able to reboard it and proceed to where we found them. The skipper and 1st Engineer had been killed when their life boats were machine gunned. Over 70 bullet holes were found in the life boat. After fixing some of the wounded we proceeded.

Nov. 1942: Arrived at Colombo [Sri Lanka] about midday. Leave from 1:30 P.M. to 11 P.M. Melvin, Neil and I met two Scotties who showed us round. We had an excellent day and were fortunate to have such good guides. I was fortunate in meeting Ken Robinson who was based on the island. He heard I was on the ship and spent most the day trying to find me. We arrived back at the ship with about 300 bananas on one stalk.

Dec.: Arrived Aden [Yemen]. Saw my first camel.

Dec.: Arrived at Tewfik [Egypt]. Neville went to Cairo, so Smithy and I went to Suez, said goodbye to boys in reinforcements. Spent evening in Tewfik. Grocer's store stocked all sorts of spirits and liquors. Suez: Long-eared donkeys and scraggy ponies. Filthy streets—dirty Wags and dilapidated clothes.

Dec.: Embarked 360 patients. Train 3 hours late because it ran out of coal about 2 miles down the line. Left Tewfik at 1200 hrs. Started work in Pantry.

Dec. 1942: Picked up 3 German sailors from a small dinghy. They had been interned in the Portuguese settlement of Goa on the west coast of India. They had escaped from Goa and put to sea in a small dinghy ... in the hope of reaching a Japanese island. They were without food and had little water left when we found them. About a dozen sharks were following the boat, as well as a school of porpoises and some exquisitely beautiful fish...

This incident of the three German castaways was recorded in a British newspaper.

The Maunganui returned to Wellington, New Zealand, before starting on another voyage.

Voyage IX

Feb. [1943]: Nothing of importance occurred until we reached Fremantle [Australia], where we saw again the Dutch tanker which we had helped last trip.

Feb. 5th: In the harbour when we arrived were several warships as well as some American submarines...

Feb. 28th: Arrival at Tewfik. Spent a good day looking around the bazaars at Suez.

Mar. 1st: We embarked patients who consisted of Sth. Africans, British, Greeks, Poles, Yugo. Slavs.

Mar. 3rd: Called at Port Sudan, which seems to have very modern port installations, with excellent deep water for large ships, and great cranes and derricks. The town is quite small and the natives as black as is possible.

Mar. 10th: Arrived Mombasa. Did a little shopping but most goods very dear and of shoddy quality. The following ships were in port: *Revenge, Resolution, Ramilles, Warspite, Mauritius* (all battleships), and 7 destroyers.

Mon., 3rd May: Arrived Fremantle. Ernie, the aft cook, and Clive … suspect of "smallpox," also two others taken off ship. Shorty Russell went to help the hospital. No leave. Left Fremantle 9:30 P.M.

ANOTHER VOYAGE

Sat., Oct. 16th [1943]: Land on Port side. Near Derna. Convoy sighted. Wireless broadcasts our position every four hours.

Sun., Oct. 17th: Mishap to crankshaft during early hours of morning. Compelled to cut down speed. We passed an Italian hospital ship. Arrived Tripoli 7:30 P.M.

Tripoli: Three ships sunk at entrance to harbour and several others inside. The wharf where we tied up was the hull of a ship on its side. Planking at each end made it level, and an excellent wharf it proved to be. Evidently Tripoli was a fine modern town built on Italian…, but it had been badly damaged. No. 3. NZGH was located here for several months, but when we arrived was all ready to go elsewhere. Very few shops were open and very little could be bought. The curfew for civilians is 8 P.M. Many servicemen have been knifed or shot. Many of our crew brought aboard shell cases of Italian and German origin. On the top of the granary lie the bodies of a German gun crew. No one can get them down because of the condition of the building which stands alone amid piles of wreckage and debris.

Mon., Oct. 18th: The trouble was diagnosed as a broken crankshaft so will now have to await further orders. Repairs may be affected at Malta or Alexandria. Leave from 2 P.M. till 11 P.M. Looking at the harbour in daylight I was able to count 21 ships which were either badly damaged or partially sunk. One of these was an Italian hospital ship, which I was told, hit a mine. It was piled up against the breakwater. No. 7. H.S. *Amarapoora* in port.

Tues., Oct. 19th: Embarked Tommies, Basutos, Germans, & Italians.

29. H.M.N.Z.H.S. Maunganui

Wed., Oct. 20th: Left Tripoli 0700 hrs. using one screw.

Sat., Nov. 6th: Went for a swim ashore. The boys marched past Admiral Cunningham "without noticing" him and were called back. When we arrived back we were told that we were to go to 1 GH. [General Hospital] and 2 GH. while the ship returned to NZ to be repaired.

Sun., Nov. 7th: Collected my gear together to go to 2 GH.

Mon., Nov. 8th: Left ship by launch at 1 P.M. then took a truck to Kantara where we arrived at 7:30 P.M. The staff of the clothing store invited me over for supper which consisted of omelets. We spent the night in the Gymnasium.

Tues., Nov. 9th: We dug the sand from our tent space and put up two tents, made our bed on petrol cases and adjusted our mosquito nets. After a good shower and tea, Melvin and I and about 10 others went down to the Bengal Club where a weekly cabaret is held. It turned out to be a beautiful evening. We sat on the verandah overlooking the canal, and listened to and danced to a first class orchestra.

Mon., Nov. 15th: …The ship is still at Tewfik. There has been a fire in the mattress-store. It seems probable the ship will go to Alexandria now to be fitted. We are all on 4 hours' call.

Wed., Nov. 24th: Left Kantara 7:30 A.M. to rejoin ship at Suez.

Thurs., Nov. 25th: Began night duty

Fri., Nov. 26th: Embarked patients for England. The second train was due at 1030 hrs. but did not arrive until 1530. Ward K.L. had 40 Psychiatric patients, several of whom were epileptics and two of suicidal tendencies.

Sat., Nov. 27th: Left Suez to go up canal. We stopped for the night in the lake at Ismailia, where King Farouk's yacht is moored and where two Italian battleships lie at anchor.

Sun., Nov. 28th: Continued our trip up the canal, and reached Port Said at 1330 hrs. where we remained overnight. H.S. *Vita* No.14 in port.

Mon., Nov. 29th: Left Port Said at 1500 hrs. We were late because there had been a hold-up over maps of English waters. We were making about 11 knots on one screw.

2nd to 4th Dec.: In sight of land several times each day. Patrol vessels, convoys, hospital ships and large numbers of landing craft seen.

4th Dec.: Off Cap Bon the H.S. *Vasna* No.4 was waiting to go through the channel with us. Three minesweepers swept a passage for us while we followed in line…

Sun., 5th Dec.: Large convoy passed with good "air cover." The big three "Roosevelt, Churchill, & Stalin" concluded conference in Teheran.

6th Dec., Mon.: Arrived Algiers 1030. Leave for a short time at night.

Enormous quantities of stores stacked all the way down the main streets. Very good facilities for shipping. Large numbers of ships in port including H.S. *Vasna* and H.S. *St. Andrew.*

7th Dec., Tues.: Left Algiers at 1230 hrs. H.S. *Amarapoora* No.7 arrived....

8th Dec., Wed.: Sighted Spanish coast. Spanish and German aircraft seen.

9th Dec., Thur.: Arrived Gibraltar 8 A.M. Collected orders and were on the way out within about half an hour. Convoy had just arrived. Great number of destroyers, frigates, and corvettes on patrol.

There is a discreapancy of dates beginning here.

14th Dec., Sat.: Sighted lighthouse on Irish coast 0230 A.M. At 0730 we passed a fleet of fishing vessels. It was not light until 8:30 A.M. Every few miles on the port side lighthouses could be seen flashing and twinkling.

15th Dec., Sun.: Passed Isle of Man. Temp. on deck 35 degrees. Portholes blacked out in preparation for sailing up the Clyde tonight.

16th Dec., Mon.: ...Left our anchorage near Greenock at 9 A.M. and arrived at Glasgow about 1400 hrs. It was cold, bleak, misty weather, with the temperature very near zero. The Union ship *Aorangi* was tied up immediately in front of us. About a quarter of our patients were disembarked. On guard for two hours during the night, complete with great coat, battledress, balaclava, jersey and gloves. Even then it was—cold.

17th Dec., Tues.: Leave in Great Britain for 28 days announced. Remainder of patients were disembarked. On guard from 8 P.M. till 11P.M.

18th Dec., Wed.: Finished cleaning ward, then prepared for leave. Received 20 pounds pay, and issued with the following:
1. Ships leave pass.
2. Dock pass.
3. Authority to travel.
4. Rail warrant.
5. Permit to buy sweets & Tobacco (NAAFI). [Navy, Army, Air Force Institute; the equivalent of an American PX].
6. 2 Ration food cards.

[The discrepancy in dates is resolved after this point.]

Sun., Dec. 19: ...During the night bombs fell about a mile away, but I did not even hear the "alert."

Mon., Dec. 20: We saw planes returning from Germany, mainly Lancasters and Halifaxes, one group numbered 36...

Tues., Dec. 21: ...Went to "News" theatre at 1 P.M. and then to Madame Tussauds, where we spent the remainder of the afternoon. Spent the evening at NZ Club. Caught out in street in "air-raid." Heavy gunfire grew louder, then suddenly several searchlights intersected at the one spot. A great shower of "flak" went up as the bomber commenced to dive. However it was soon shut out by clouds, and we were unable to see the result. "Alert" lasted from 6:30 P.M. until 7:30 P.M.

Sat., Dec.25: Xmas dinner at NZ Club. Four sittings. Mr. Jordan present and Brig. Hargest. Dance in afternoon. Went to R.A.F. Xmas tea and party at 101 Warwick St. Three U.S. officers present. Missed tube and had to walk the five miles into town finally arriving at 2 A.M.

Sun., 16th Jan. [1944]: Met Garnet Fairfar at 2:30 P.M. and went to see film *Sahara*, then had tea in Piccadilly. It was extremely foggy and all bus services stopped, with the result that I had to go to Whitfords from tube station at Latimer Road. Did not arrive there until 11 P.M. instead of 8 P.M.

Mon., 17th Jan.: Left London at 10 A.M. and arrived at Glasgow at 8:45 P.M.

Fri., 21st Jan.: We went by motor ambulances to our new temporary home at Turnberry, with the 74th G. Hospital.

Sat., 22nd Jan.: Commenced night-duty. Under me were two general duties orderlies, Rogerson and Hayfield.

Fri., 18th Feb.: Worst fire raid on London since 1940–41.

Sat., 19th Feb.: Received first mail from NZ

Sun., 20th Feb.: Worse air-raid on London than the one on Friday night.

Mon., 21st Feb.: Said goodbye to all our new-found friends at Turnberry ... to report back to the ship....

Wed., 1st March: Snowed hard from early hours of morning until 4 P.M. 3 or 4 inches of snow on the wharf and "A" Deck. A "battle royal" ensued when our boys arrived back from town. All those on board pounded them with huge snowballs.

Fri., 10th March: The Italian ship near us has a new name inscribed on her bow *Empire Clyde*. We left the wharf at 2:30 P.M., remained stuck on a sandbank for a time, then set sail up the river. We passed the *Queen Mary* about 5 P.M. then arrived at Greenock at 8 P.M.

Thurs., 16th March: Arrived Gibraltar 7 P.M. and stayed the night. Depth charges could be heard and felt every few minutes, keeping us awake most of the night. The harbour was a mass of twinkling lights, searchlights from "the rock" lit up the runway for the Batalona flying-boats.

Fri., 17th March: Left Gibraltar 7 P.M. for Bizerta.

Sun., 19th March: Arrived Bizerta at 10 A.M. The skipper wanted to take on water but he was refused permission to do so. At 5 P.M. we left Bizerta, having remained off-shore for seven hours. U.S. Hosp. Ship *Chateau Thierry* left just before us.

Tues., 21st March: Arrived Taranto 10 A.M. Lay alongside the French destroyer *Le Fantasque* which had just returned from a successful sortie with Germans in the Adriatic. Embarked 150 NZ patients and some Sth. Africans. Left at 5 P.M.

Sat., 25th March: Passed through Port Said, then down the canal to Suez, where we berthed in our usual place about 5:30 P.M.

Sun.-Mon.-Tues.: Remained in Suez. Patients were to have been embarked on Tuesday but a sandstorm covered over the railway line between Cairo and Suez so train was unable to get through.

Wed., 29th March: 120 patients were embarked from 5 N.Z.G.H. They had been in the hospital-train since Monday night due to the sandstorm. NZ troops at Cassino are having a bad time and the fighting is pretty severe.

Mon., 3rd April: We put on the "radio show," "Shorty's 21st," which I had written specially for patients. It included Harold Wheeler, Doug. Fyffe, Claud Burrell, Doug Russell, Bill Hinds and myself.

Sun., 9th April: Arrived at Colombo at 9:30 A.M. Ship remained in port over night. I was a "special" for the night, looking after a cerebral case, on whom Maj. McKenzie had operated that morning. Depth charges were dropped at the harbour entrance continuously during the night.

Wed., 19th April: Arrived Fremantle. Leave granted from 10 A.M. to 3:30 P.M. We left at 5 P.M.

Sat., 22nd April: 3rd anniversary of H.S. *Maunganui*'s first voyage as a hospital ship. During her 3 years' service she has steamed more than 250,000 miles, and carried over 5,600 patients.

Sat., 29th April: Arrived Wellington. [New Zealand] Leave granted from 2nd to 17th May.

Wed., 24th May: Lt. Colonel Reid to be our new O.C. Left Wellington 10 A.M.

Mon., 5th June: Rome fell to the Allies.

Tues., 6th June: ALLIED INVASION OF FRANCE

The Invasion of Europe began today, with landings on the coast of Normandy, and intense aircraft activity. Submarine sighted and alarm sounded. Its identity is still unknown.

Doug ... taken to hospital with T.B. Staff shifted into Ward D. for rest of voyage, under Maj. Caughey's instruction.

Tues., 13th June: Arrived Colombo. Made ship ready for 100 patients...

Tues., 4th July: Passed through Port Said on way through canal to Suez. Arrived Suez 7:30 P.M. and remained in stream until the morning.

Thurs., 6th July: We made up our full quota of patients by embarking a further 140, quite a number of whom were Australian and NZ repats. Left Suez at 4:30 P.M.

Fri., 7th July: Heat is becoming more intense. Temp. in ward 92 degrees F. Sat., 8th July: Temp. in ward 96 degrees F.

Sun., 9th July: Water consumption reached an all-time high today when the total used in 24 hrs. amounted to 170 tons. Temp. today 108 degrees F.

Mon. 10th July: Passed out of the Red Sea at 3:30 A.M. Much cooler and there is a slight breeze. Water will be severely rationed until we reach our next port...

Sat., 15th July: Weather is much cooler now, but heavy seas have been running for several days.

Thurs., 3rd Aug.: W.N. [War News] Turkey has broken off diplomatic relations with Germany.

Sat., 5th Aug.: Arrived Wellington.

Sun., 6th Aug.: Left Wellington at 5 P.M. for Lyttelton.

Mon., 7th Aug.: Arrived Lyttelton 8 A.M. and reached home just in time for lunch. Leave granted till Sun., 20th Aug.

Wed., 23rd Aug.: Embarked 19 sisters [Registered Nurses] and 28 V.A.s. Left Wellington at 7 A.M. Paris is said to have been captured by French partisans. News came that the German troops in Paris had broken their truce and fighting was still going on.

Aug., 26th Sat.: Allied troops have now captured Paris. General De Gaulle was attacked by snipers outside Notre Dame Cathedral.

Fri., 1st Sept.: W.N. Russian troops in Rumania have captured the Ploesti oil fields. We arrived at Fremantle today. I went ashore with Doug Russell, Doug Tooby and three of the V.A.s. Leave until 2359 hrs.

Sat., 9th Sept.: ...War news: British troops are now thrusting towards the Dutch border after capturing Brussells. American troops are fighting in Luxemburg.

Mon., 11th Sept.: Arrived Colombo. 110 patients were aboard at 3:30 P.M. but the staff off duty were granted leave from 1 P.M. until 11 P.M. I was treated to afternoon-tea by a Sth. African Colonel and two captains. They were dressed in jungle uniform, technically known as "cellular bottle-green battledress."

Tues., 12th Sept.: Beautiful calm sea, and plenty of time for sunbathing.

WAR NEWS: The Americans are fighting on German soil 5 miles from the border. British and U.S. airforces have secured big victories against Jap. shipping...

Thurs., 14th Sept.: At 0230 hrs. we hit a 413 ton dhow [an Arabian vessel] and cut it clean in two. We were awakened by the warning whistles ... amidships. At the moment of impact the *Maunganui* was in reverse, but our momentum carried her right through the wooden dhow, which was only built in 1941 and cost 23,000 Rs. (About 2,300 pounds)

The work of taking off the survivors was not an easy one, owing to the non-existence of a strong spot-light. There was a floodlight on the bridge, but it was of little use in the inky blackness.

After the first survivors were aboard, the dhow had disappeared in the dark, and it was some time before it was rediscovered. 19 of the crew of 21 were saved. It is thought likely that the two missing were killed when the collision occurred. One of [those] rescued had a fractured femur, another suffered lacerations to the face.

Fri., 15th Sept.: Arrived Bombay 9 A.M. and disembarked all the Indian patients including two lepers. Leave from 1 P.M. till 10 P.M. I bought some brassware, pyjamas, etc., then six of us went out to see the Hanging Gardens but were stopped by a[n] M.P., so the taxi driver took us round the city for a trip. ... We learned later that Ghandi and Mr. Jhinna [Jinnah] were holding talks near the Gardens and that was the reason we were prevented from going there.

Wed., 27th Sept.: Arrived Port Tewfik 10 A.M., then proceeded to far side of harbour to oil.

Tues., 2nd Oct.: Arrived at Taranto. The H.S. *Dranje* and the H.S. *Toscanh* were in port. The *Dranje* left at 2 P.M. for England. We were due to leave at 4 P.M. but a bearing broke on the forward winch so the anchor could not be weighed. It was soon fixed, however, and we sailed out of the harbour at 5:30 P.M.

Tues., 10th Oct.: Embarked 50 patients at 10 A.M. Left Tewfik 6 P.M.

War News: Mr. Churchill is in Moscow to discuss the final assault on Germany.

Sun., 15th Oct.: WN.: Allied H.Q. in New Guinea states that in raids this week on Formosa 150 ships and 520 planes have been destroyed.

Mon., 16th Oct.: The German town of Aachen is under intense artillery fire and bombing after the rejection of the American ultimatum to surrender.

The Greek towns of Athens and Piraeus have been occupied by British troops.

After the destruction of the German towns of Kleve and Emmerich, the R.A.F. have now wiped out Duisburg, the greatest European inland port, with 4,500 tons of bombs dropped by 1000 bombers in 25 minutes. 1200 American bombers attacked Cologne, on the Rhine, directly ahead of the Allied Armies closing in on Aachen.

Tues., 7th Oct.: Hungary has asked for an armistice. Duisburg has been attacked again with 2,000 bombers of the R.A.F....

Sat., 4th Nov.: ...Display of articles made by patients in the new Occupational Therapy Dept. under Nurse Cullen...

Wed., 6th Dec.: Left Wellington. Travelling personnel included 61 V.A.D.s and 27 sisters for passage to M.G.

Fri., 15th Dec.: Arrived Fremantle. A shipping strike was in progress so the staff had to load the supplies. I was on the first shift which worked from 1–4 P.M. Allan Gilkison did a great job at the winch, but was unfortunate in losing four bags of flour which fell off one of the slings into the hold. The evening was spent with Grace, Ann and Len Paulsen, at the film *True to Life*.

Sat., 23rd Dec.: GRAND FANCY DRESS BALL

Grace was dressed as a sheik, while I wore Jenny Thompson's sunsuit as a pair of rompers.

Grace and I decided to have our engagement announced on Xmas Day.

Sun., 24th Dec.: Christmas Carols on "A" deck.

Mon., 25th Dec.: Grace and I went to Church in the morning then I told Col. Bennett of our proposed engagement. He suggested that it be announced at the Christmas Day celebration in the afternoon.

At Xmas Dinner the O/Rs were waited upon by the officers, each of whom had on white pyjama-suits and a card bearing his Christian name.... In the afternoon gifts were distributed by George Scandrett, from the Xmas Tree. ... Grace & I were called up by Colonel Bennett and presented with a couple of huge pink bows and an enormous ring and silver bell.

Patriotic parcels were distributed.

Tues., 26th Dec.: Arrived at Colombo. Grace & I went ashore with Noel and Ann. We had afternoon tea and then a swim out at Mt. Lavinia, ending up with a walk along the waterfront before returning to the ship. About 130 patients were embarked, mostly T.B. cases.

Sat., 30th Dec.: Arrived at Bombay. I was on guard from 6 A.M. till 3 P.M. The travelling V.A.s & sisters, however, were not able to get passes for shore leave until 7:30 P.M. Nevertheless Grace & I had a most enjoyable night looking around Bombay.

Sun., 31st Dec.: New Year's Eve. The R.S.M. gave me permission to leave the ship by the 2:30 P.M. launch as there was no other until 5 P.M. so Grace and I went with Ken Wright and Rea Glass on a sightseeing expedition. For 15 Rupees we went to the Hanging Gardens on Malabar Hill, the Tower of Silence and Beach Candy, then to the Hindu crematorium after getting special passes from the city. We were fortunate enough to see an actual cremation take place. Huge pieces of wood were piled up, then smaller pieces, then the body was taken from the litter that it had been carried on, and placed on top of the pile of wood, then more wood was laid on top of the body. The priest sprinkled holy water about the pyre before setting fire to the twigs at the bottom.

We arrived back at the ship shortly before midnight. At 12 A.M. all the ships in port started sounding their sirens and whistles, making a terrific noise which lasted until after 1 A.M.

Mon., 1st Jan., 1945: We went into the wharf at Ballard Pier (Berth 18) but there was no leave until after lunch. Ken, Rea, Grace & I went to Juhu Beach for the afternoon. It was quite a lot of fun getting there as we had to first get to Victoria Station. There the girls bought a huge basketful of fruit. We then caught a train for Bandra, then another to Santa Cruz, where we went by bus to Juhu. After a stroll along the beach we all went for a swim, ate some of our fruit, then found our way back home again.

Tues., 2nd Jan.: Grace & I paid a visit to the Crawford Market, where we bought a silver tea set for 32 rupees. In the afternoon we went by bus to Beach Candy, and in the evening to the Town Hall to a dance.

Wed., 3rd Jan.: We embarked 120 patients, including 12 Italians and a German off a U-boat. Travelling personnel had leave from 9:30 A.M. to mid-day. We left Bombay at 1500 hrs.

Fri., 12th Jan.: Arrived at Suez. All patients were disembarked, including Italians and the lad in the iron lung. The V.A.s & sisters remained on board for the night so Grace & I spent the evening in Tewfik.

Sat., 13th Jan.: 10 V.A.D.s including Grace, and 10 sisters disembarked at 2 P.M. to go to Helwan. The remainder of the travelling personnel and a few of the staff went into Cairo for the day. 10 more sisters and 10 more V.A.D.s were embarked.

Sun., 14th Jan.: 14 W.A.S.A. (South African girls) and 200 Yugo Slavs were embarked....

Wed., 24th Jan.: Arrived Port Said at 6 A.M., and remained there until 1 P.M. Nse. Leonard's brother paid her a surprise visit...

Thurs., 25th Jan.: Went in to the wharf at 8 A.M. Sister Farland's brother arrived on board to see her, all the way from Gaza. At 10 A.M. Grace arrived so I changed over to "divided" shift, and spent the rest of the time until 3 P.M. with her, when she had to return to Helwan. We embarked about 35 patients including a Palestinian A.T.S. and Wren married to New Zealanders, a couple of Wrens married to Australians, and an English nurse married to a New Zealander. At 4 P.M. we pulled out into the stream and waited for some new laundry machinery to arrive from Cairo. It arrived at 10 P.M. and the ship got under way immediately...

Tues., 6th Feb.: Arrived Colombo at 9 A.M. 3 Woolworth escort carriers were in port. ... As we left Colombo, planes could be seen taking off and landing on two carriers some miles away.

Wed., 7th Feb.: A flying fish landed on one of the patients as he lay asleep. After breakfast the Matron and two M.O.s came down to see it but I had already tossed it overboard.

Sat., 17th Feb.: Arrived Fremantle at 1 P.M. Leave from 3–7 P.M. for patients, 3–11 P.M. for staff. No beer available in the hotels so the patients were very quiet getting back to the ship.

Sat., 17th March: Left Wellington at 0700 hrs.

Thurs., 22nd Mar.: Received Radio Signal to return to Melbourne. We picked up pilot at 7:30 P.M. and went up the Yarra River, dropping anchor about 12 P.M.

Fri., 23rd Mar.: Tied up at Port Melbourne at 9 A.M. when we were told we were now under orders from the Admiralty. Our new address was given as: R.N.Z.H.S. *Maunganui* c/ British Pacific Fleet.

All traveling personnel were disembarked and went to a camp handy to central Melbourne. Our cargo for Middle East was also unloaded but no indication of our future was given. We surmise going to the Philippines where we understand the B.P.F. is making an advanced base.

Sat., 24th Mar.: We went out to the Zoo in the afternoon, ... During our absence the carpenters had been at work making deadlights for all the port-holes.

Thurs., 29th Mar.: Arrived Sydney at 7 A.M. Anchored just inside the boom and stayed there until 4 P.M. when we left without the four signallers who were supposed to come aboard. Several dozen swing cots were brought aboard for use in an emergency.

The entire staff was called together by the Colonel during the evening. He told us we were bound for the Admiralty Is. and in all probability would go thence to the Philippines, probably Leyte, where we would act as either a base hospital or run a ferry service between Leyte and Sydney.

We were introduced to C.P.O. Lawrence, R.N.DS.M. who will act as liaison officer and supply all information, re., navy routine.

The colonel impressed upon everyone the necessity for very great care with water as it was extremely short in the Philippines. C.P.O. Lawrence said that monotony would be our greatest problem and gave some suggestions in regard to entertainments. We were told it might be six or eight months before we would be relieved. It was stated that nine hospital ships were required in the north, but we were only the second on the way there.

Tues., 3rd April: All portholes were covered with blue paper.

Thurs., 5th April: Arrived at Manus, Admiralty Is., an advance base of the B.P.F. The weather was peculiar. Heavy showers were experienced all day.

Tues., 10th April: ...The following notice was placed on all of the notice boards:

"Fresh water time table while at Leyte"

Fresh water showers between 1630 & 1830 hrs.

All heads of departments are to ensure that a "brown-out" is observed until 2300, after which a strict blackout must be maintained.

Wed., 11th April: Arrived at Leyte. A huge fleet of merchant vessels were in harbour. A fleet of mtbs. left as we came in. Planes of many types flew around the harbour all day—B25 Mitchells, Venturas, Marauders, P40 Lightnings and Black Widows.

Fri., 13th April: Embarked 45 mumps patients (N.Z.S. *Gambia*) from H.S. *Oxfordshire* (No. 6.). We will be acting as a base hospital ship and will probably be here for about two months.

Sat., 14th April: President Roosevelt died this morning (13th April). American troops within 40 miles of Berlin. The Stars & Stripes flown at half-mast for the day. The NZ merchant flag to be flown for the next 28 days.

Two American naval men & their landing craft were attached to the ship, also two R.N. signallers. No mail has reached us since we left Melbourne.

Wed., 18th April: The *Illustrious* arrived today having had her steering-gear damaged in the present action of the fleet.

Fri., 20th April: We went for a trip in the launch, past the *Tjitjalengka*, along the shore bordering the adjacent landing strip, past several LSTs, over to the beach, a distance of about 7 miles, had a swim then returned to the ship. The beach is called Tolosa, and we had to take off our shirts as the place is reserved for "officers only."

Sun., 22nd April: All the mumps patients came out of quarantine today. A trip in the LVP was arranged for both patients and staff to the main harbour about 15 miles away.

We followed the beach past the second airfield which had about a hundred planes on it, also dozens of damaged planes had just been run off the landing strip straight into the sea. Many more ships were found when we rounded the headland towards Tacloban. We saw for the first time the latest American night-fighter "The Black Widow," which bears a close resemblance to the P-38 "Lightning."

We had a couple of hours in the township of Tacloean, but it was dreadfully hot and the usual native smells were a little too abundant, and money meant nothing as regards buying anything. You could get more for a packet of cigarettes than you could for a couple of "pesos" ($1). Clothing is very scarce and terrific prices could be got for anything in the way of clothes. I managed to get some of the Japanese occupation money, (a 10 peso note).

On the way home we trailed our feet in the water and everyone got thoroughly wet as a slight swell was running and the flatfront of the LVP threw up showers of spray over us all. It was most enjoyable, and even though we arrived back late for tea, and dripping wet, everyone wore a happy grin and soon made short work of all that was left on the tea-table.

Mon., 23rd April: 4 cruisers including the HMNZS *Gambia* arrived here this morning. 1200 hrs.: A number of destroyers arrived. 1230 hrs.: Battleships *King George V* and *Howe* arrived, also aircraft carriers, *Victorious*, *Formidable*, *Indefatigable*, & *Illustrious*, also more cruisers and destroyers...

Tues., 24th April: We disembarked 30 patients to the *Gambia*. 13 more mumps cases came on board, also a few battle casualties, as well as a number of Americans and other navy personnel. The dentist has been kept busy fixing teeth for some Americans off some of the U.S. destroyers.

Wed., 25th April: Anzac Day Service...

Thurs., 26th April: 1st Party from the *Maunganui* went over the Aircraft Carrier *Victorious*, which carries 48 aircraft, (Corsair fighters and Avengers) and 2 walrus amphibians...

Tues., 1st May: The fleet left on another operation.

Thurs., 3rd May:
1) Berlin has been taken by the Red Army.
2) Italy has signed another armistice with the Allies and virtually all fighting in Italy has ceased.
3) Australian troops have landed in Tarakan, Borneo.
4) Hitler is dead.

Sat., 5th May: Rangoon has been captured by the 14th Army. Denmark & Holland are to be occupied by the Allies under a treaty signed with the Germans in that area...

Tues., 8th May: Celebrated by BPF as VE day. The official announcement of Germany's capitulation in both Germany & Norway was flashed to us from RAFT (Rear Admiral Fleet Train) (HMS *Lothian*).

Today is to be the End of the European War as far as the Brit. Empire is concerned. Station WVTK (Voice of Leyte), however, gave what is evidently the American official opinion "that although the capitals of most European countries were celebrating VE Day on Tues., May 8th America would await an official statement from President Truman. The patients were all granted an extra issue of beer today.

SERVICE OF THANKSGIVING ON B. DECK AT 9:15 A.M.

May 8th, Tues.: VE day Word was received of the *Formidable* having been hit. 37 casualties arrived on the HMS *Striker*, an auxiliary carrier, and were embarked on the *Maunganui* at 7:15 P.M. They were casualties from a bomb which landed at the base of *Formidable*'s "Monkey Island"; the *Formidable* is still in action. 3 LVPs carried the casualties from the *Striker* to INZHS. When the carrier arrived, it signalled "How soon can you take off casualties?"

Our reply was "As soon as you drop anchor." One amusing sidelight was in connection with the speed of our embarkation. The P.M.O. came over to watch the embarkation of patients, but arrived just as the last LVP began to unload its patients. It was just 57 minutes from the moment *Striker*'s anchor went down till the last patient came aboard. Most of the patients were badly injured, keeping the Theatre staff going until 5 A.M. in the morning.

"Shorty" Russell came back to bed just as the rest of us were getting up at 6 A.M.

10 P.M. VE Day: Mr. Truman was rebroadcast over the Leyte Radio, telling the World of the German capitulation. Up on "A" deck we could hear also at the same time the loudspeakers on the Striker tuned in to Mr. Churchill on the B.B.C.

Wed., May 9th: America has stated that the war to date has cost the U.S. $275,703,000,000. We embarked 60 patients from H.S. *Tjitjalengka* this morning. We "spliced the main brace" at 9 P.M. Patients at 8 P.M.

Wed., 16th May: 8 Reinforcements arrived on the transport *Maidstone*.

Sun., 20th May: Gave a farewell supper to the two Americans who had manned L.V.P. 15.

Mon., 21st May: Left Leyte at 1400 hrs. for Manus in the Admiralties...

Sun., 27th May: Arrived Manus 9 A.M. Many units of fleet train had already arrived. Radio WVTD. The Jungle Network.

Mon., 28th May: Despatched 1st batch of 20 patients by air to Sydney. Remainder of fleet train arrived.

Tues., 29th May: The new aircraft carrier HMS *Implacable* has just arrived from Sydney. Also the H.S. *Oxfordshire*.

Wed., 30th May: Fleet arrived at Manus. The only major units missing are the HMS *K.G.V.* and the cruiser *Black Prince* which are taking part in the bombardment of the Sakashimas.

Thurs., 31st May: Patients still being sent to Sydney by air at the rate of twenty each day. The task force left during the forenoon leaving the *Howe*, a couple of cruisers and a few destroyers behind. The *Implacable* went with the task force.

Fri., 1st June: Left Manus at 9 A.M. to pass the *Tjitjalengka* at its boom. We are bound for Sydney. During the afternoon a huge waterspout was observed a few miles away. The questions being asked are:
1. Will we go home to NZ?
2. Will the Div. In Egypt come home?

Sun., 3rd June: Picked up a patient from a U.S. Liberty ship. He was brought over by launch. Some difficulty was experienced in getting him aboard due to the considerable swell. The skipper was mad about the delay as he had hoped to get through the treacherous reefs before dark. This interruption put us about an hour behind schedule.

Thurs., 7th June: Arrived Sydney 5 P.M. Arriving at Sydney Heads we found that a major part of the fleet had already arrived, the *Howe* being conspicuous along with several of the carriers. The NZ ships *Gambia*, *Achilles* and *Arbutus* were all in port.

The walking patients were all disembarked immediately after tea…

Fri., 8th June: …5 P.M.: News came through that we were to leave Sydney tomorrow at 3 P.M. for NZ. Rumour has it that this is the last trip…

Sat., 9th June: Left Sydney 3 P.M. for NZ. Meeting of staff called. We were told that the ship was to remain part of the fleet train. Also that there would be fourteen days leave on arrival in NZ. We are due back at Manus by the 7th July.

Sat., 7th July: Arrived at Manus at 1030 hrs. The *Tjitjalengka* has gone to Borneo and the *Oxfordshire* to Leyte.

Wed., 11th July: …Air Raid Alarm 9 P.M.

Sat., 14th July: Went by launch to Piti Velu, the navy recreation area, where facilities are provided for all sorts of sports, hockey, cricket, football and basketball. There is a canteen on the island and a marvellous spot for swimming. Hundreds of men from the various ships in the roadstead go to this island every day.

A reef runs the length of the island leaving a huge natural swimming pool between the island and the reef. The vast variety of marine growth and tropical fish is amazing, while coral of every colour is to be found on the sea-bed.

Sun., 15th July: Sgt. Greer, Gwen Leonard and I went out for a sail in the dinghy after church. In the afternoon I was to have visited the *Pioneer*, a Carrier-Repair ship of the same class as the *Unicorn*, but was notified of a new patient arriving, so had to remain on board.

Tues., 17th July: Went to the RNZAF staff at Los Negros, where we were shown over the aerodrome, where C47 [sic] transports were taking off for the Philippines, NZ and Australia. Three units operate from this NZ aerodrome, the CAU (Corsair assembly unit), the fighter patrols and the bomber squadron. Planes on the tarmac included Corsairs, C[-]47s, Venturas and Liberators.

Wed., 18th July: Air-raid alarm 9:20 P.M. Mr. McTaggett placed on Dangerously Ill list.

Fri. [sic], 24th July: British Election Results. Sweeping victory for Labour. Mr. Attlee new premier. British–U.S. carrier forces still striking hard at the Japanese mainland.

Fri., 27th July: ...Hospital Ship *Gerusalemme* arrived.

Sun., 29th July: ...U.S. Hospital Ship *Bountiful* arrived.

Sun., 5th Aug.: Battleship *Duke of York* arrived from Sydney.

Tues., 7th Aug.: Went over to Los Negros to play the RNZAF at cricket...

Wed., 8th Aug.: Allied planes dropped the first ATOMIC bomb on Japan. The naval base of Hiroshima was completely annihilated and the ... inhabitants killed instantly. (8:15 A.M. August 6th)

Thurs., 9th Aug.: Russia declared war on Japan at 5 P.M. today...

Fri., 10th Aug.: ...It was announced that Japan had asked for Armistice under the Potsdam declaration terms with the exception that they wished the Emperor's prerogative as sovereign ruler to continue.

Sat., 11th Aug.: James F. Byrnes (Secretary of State for U.S.) after consultation with other Allied leaders made a declaration to Max Grassls, Charge D'Affairs [sic] of the Swiss Legation, to the effect that the United Nations would accept no conditions from Japan short of total surrender.

Mon., 13th Aug.: The world is still awaiting Japan's answer to the Allied declaration.

Wed., 15th Aug.: At 10:30 A.M. the sirens ashore began to shriek—a U.S. corvette let go a few ack-ack shells—Station WVTD announced that the war was definitely over as Japan had agreed to surrender "unconditionally."

29. H.M.N.Z.H.S. Maunganui

V.J. Day 1945 ...At 7 P.M. the shore was a mass of coloured flares and lights of green, yellow and red. At 7:30 P.M. the official signals were sent from the flagship *Montecalm* [*sic*].

Immediately we let go a ship's rocket, then the whole harbour was lit up like day, as searchlights of forty-odd ships flashed to & fro amid exploding rockets and parachute flares.

The H.M.S. *Tyne* pointed her two huge searchlights skyward to form a gigantic "V." Ships flashed the V sign to one another (···–) and periodically sent up flares of all colours.

By this time the Yanks had a tremendous bonfire going ashore. As far as the eye could see, the fifteen miles of coastline was just a maze of colours and fires as GIs and gobs celebrated the end of World War II.

The only hitch to the day's enjoyment was the inability of the officers to secure rum for the "splicing of the mainbrace."

At 8 P.M. we commenced a dance, Harry Miller picking the records while I acted as MC. Shortly after 10 P.M. we went down to Ward J. where the patients were trying to sing themselves hoarse. The accordian helped things along until 11 P.M.

Thurs., 16th Aug.: Special Thanksgiving Service held on A. Deck at 10 A.M. Lessons read by O.C. Troops and Capt. Prosser.

Beer and soft drinks dispensed to staff, crew and patients in lieu of rum...

Fri., 17th Aug.: ... On returning from Pityilu we discovered that all our patients were to be transferred to the *Gerusalemme* tomorrow and that we will be leaving for the Philippines on Sunday, for the purpose of "carrying back refugees and prisoners of war."

The rum arrived today. We "spliced the main brace" at 9 P.M.

Sat., 18th Aug.: In charge of Isolation ward until Bob Strang is fit to carry on again. Sister Farland is helping me.

Much amusement was caused by a signal sent to the fleet train requisitioning the following: Babies' bottles, teats, baby foods and napkins. It looks as though we are in for an interesting time.

During the morning the *Gerusalemme* drew up a quarter of a mile away for us to transfer our patients.

Part of the fleet arrived this morning, The *Implacable*, *Victorious* and *Formidable*, the *Achilles* and *Argonaut* and six destroyers.

Sun., 19th Aug.: The cruisers *Uranian* and *Swift-Sure* arrived this morning along with two carriers, the *Indefatigable* and *Indomitable*.

The *Formidable*, *Implacable* and *Victorious* left in that order at 1:15 P.M. escorted by destroyers, for the South.

Fri., 24th Aug.: Arrived in Leyte Gulf. An official count of ships in harbour was 842. We anchored in a maze of shipping well up towards Tacloban, but during the afternoon we were shifted near our old position near the British warships, *Bermuda* and *Argonaut*.

Sat., 25th Aug.: A tanker came alongside with oil. A U.S. seaman was brought aboard from the tanker with Cerebro-Spinal-Meningitis. He was very irrational causing us quite a lot of concern. Lt. Moore did a Lumbar puncture while Bryan Thompson & I held the patient still.

The U.S. authorities sent for the seaman at midday so our worries are over for a little while...

Mon., 27th Aug.: We received instructions to leave at 10 A.M. All boats were hauled aboard and the hatches battened down. At 9 A.M. instructions to leave were cancelled. At 9 P.M. a landing craft came alongside with vital stores. It then transpired that the stores we were supposed to load yesterday were cancelled because the Americans had wiped out "lease-lend [*sic*]." The Admiral on the Bermuda paid for our vital stores with hard-won golden sovereigns. Censorship of mail ceases today.

Tues., 28th Aug.: At 6 A.M. SOS was to be seen taking the mail down the gangway to the ship's launch, for transit to the *Argonaut*. A sure sign that we are moving soon.

At 7:30 A.M., as we sat down to breakfast, we left our anchorage. Giving the land a wide berth we sailed up the east coast of Samar, en route for Hong Kong via Subic Bay in the Philippines.

As we left the gulf, 45 LSTs came in a double line and grouped in fifteens.

The aircraft carrier (fleet class) *Colossus*, was lying off the entrance to the gulf, along with some 50 ships of all classes.

WVTK announced that the first airborne troops had landed at Atsugi airport to prepare for the main forces on Thursday.

SAN BERNADINO STRAITS—SUBIC BAY

Wed., 29th Aug.: An American transport signalled us that they would lead us through San Bernadino Strait. A mistake was made, however, from the wrong signals of a bouy with the result that both ships nearly ran aground on a sand spit. The mistake was soon rectified by the radar & asdic apparatus on the transport, enabling us to proceed.

The trip through the straits was most interesting for all of us. Islands dotted the seascape, while every here and there could be seen small native villages hidden away amid the almost tropical foliage that covered the hills almost to the seashore.

Thurs., 30th Aug.: Arrived at Subic Bay 7:30 A.M. The only other

British ship in harbour was the Australian minesweeper *Red Rose*, although there were countless American ships of all types including two cruisers and some twenty destroyers. During the morning nine submarines left the port, and in the afternoon eleven others returned.

We saw Martin-Marriner flying boats heavily laden with supplies taking off with the aid of rocket propulsion. They were able to clear the water in about a hundred yards but made hard work of their ascent once the rockets slung beneath the wings were exhausted.

Nobody here knows anything about us: either where we are to go or when we are to leave. A wireless message has been sent to the fleet asking for further instructions. A reply is expected tonight.

Fri., 31st Aug.: We sailed from Subic Bay at 10 A.M. for Hong Kong.

Sat., 1st Sept.: A typhoon hit Subic Bay during the night so it seems we got out just in time. B.B.C. news at 9 P.M. said that British forces had seized the docks at Hong Kong. We are due in Hong Kong tomorrow at 10 A.M. I wonder what awaits us. Preparations are in hand for handling more patients than we have ever handled before.

At 6:30 A.M. we are to be met and escorted through the minefields, which according to the maps on board are several miles deep.

Sun., 2nd Sept.: We arrived off Hong Kong at 6:30 A.M. to be met by an escort-carrier and a destroyer. They gave us instructions by lamp while everybody kept a life-jacket handy in case we struck a mine.

After negotiating the minefield we entered the harbour and berthed a few hundred yards from the *Anson*. Also near at hand were the *Indomitable*, the *Swiftsure* and the *Oxfordshire*.

During the morning we bartered with the Chinese who had come out in their sampans. Vast quantities of valueless Japanese occupation currency were offered for anything in the way of food.

At night the warships were all lighted from bow to stern, and their searchlights played about the hill above Hong Kong and the streets of Kowloon where British Marines and Japanese occupation troops were rounding up Chinese looters. All day dozens of planes kept up a constant patrol over Hong Kong and Kowloon.

During the afternoon 3 destroyers arrived at Kowloon with Japanese prisoners.

The crew of the Oxfordshire were granted leave last night but no more will be granted until the looting diminishes.

Mon., 3rd Sept.: It is six years today since we declared war on Germany.

Hong Kong Radio stated that there are still about 4000 Japs to be rounded up in Hong Kong. The *Empress of Australia* is due tomorrow, having been held up by the typhoons. Owing to an outbreak of dysentery and enteric fever very special precautions are being taken with the city's water supply.

Colonel Bennett went to Camp Stanley to see the POWs and to arrange for their evacuation. Of the 22 New Zealanders in camp only two or three wish to leave Hong Kong. The remainder want to see whether they can resume their various business connections in the city.

The *Oxfordshire* left during the afternoon.

Tues., 4th Sept.: We went alongside the wharf at Kowloon. The Canadian armed merchant cruiser was also at the wharf loading refugees. (*Prince Robert.*) The *Empress of Australia* disembarked 3000 RAF personnel for the purpose of aiding the marines in their job of policing the trouble areas.

Wed., 5th Sept.: Leave from 10:30–12:30 A.M. in Kowloon. Squads of Jap guards are still doing picket duty, preventing looting and preserving law and order. We saw battalions of Japanese being marched into the barracks to be disarmed. Inside the barracks we saw huge piles of Japanese equipment including thousands of the traditional officers' swords.

Points of particular interest: The streets are gaily decorated with Chinese and British flags—the Chinese are celebrating their release from tyranny by letting off fire crackers—looting is going on at an astonishing and unprecedented rate as gangs of toughs try to get goods that have been off the market for years—the Chinese are to be seen punishing collaborators (we saw them stoning some women who had been living with Japanese officers)—everywhere, British marines and Jap soldiers are rushing to prevent the unruly elements over running the town and stealing much needed foodstuffs.—Currency is upside down—the British supply of "Freedom" money has not yet arrived—food is worth thousands of pounds—tins of meat are worth many pounds sterling.

Thurs., 6th Sept.: Leave to Hong Kong. Three parties were organised; one in the morning, two in the afternoon. 100 internees were embarked. I took over Ward H. temporarily, with L/Cpl Chudleigh and L/Cpl Bendall. In the ward we had 27 men from Stanley Camp. Most of them were between 45 and 70. Among them were most of the top-line civil servants of the colony including the District Superintendent of Police, the Assistant Secretary, the Colonial Treasurer and the Superintendent of Works.

Two naval ratings from the *Swiftsure* were in an explosion at a Jap ammunition magazine. They died during the night owing to the very extensive burns which they had both sustained.

Fri., 7th Sept.: Left Hong Kong 7:30 A.M. Owing to two firemen being missing we were one and a half hours late leaving, still minus the firemen.

We are being escorted all the way by a corvette HMS *Helford*, which will sweep a passage for us through the minefields to the port of Kiirun in Formosa.

Sun., 9th Sept.: Arrived Kiirun at 10 A.M. About 100 patients were embarked during the afternoon, most of them seriously ill with dysentery and in terribly undernourished condition. KL took only eighteen patients but they were the worst to come aboard.

I asked the Sgt. Major for extra staff and received another Sister and two orderlies.

We were still unable to catch up on the work to be done. The doctor, Sister Keyes and I worked through till near midnight before we had all the injections and infusion sets functioning properly. The Sgt. Major dispensed with the telephone orderly and put him into KL to help the night orderly...

Mon., 10th & Tues., 11th: As a typhoon passed just outside the harbour entrance we were not allowed to leave. We took on twelve men from a U.S. Liberator brought down during the typhoon en route from Okinawa to Manila. Only 12 survivors out of 20 were picked up by the HMS *Ursa* which put out to sea especially for the rescue.

Just across the wharf from us flew a Japanese flag, while on an adjacent building flew the Stars and Stripes.

The Japs brought presents to the Admiral in the way of fruits, etc. The Admiral refused this but said that it would be given to the Hospital Ship.

A Japanese officer came aboard with a great pile of post-cards and silly childish toys which he said was a present from the Japs of Kiirun. Colonel Bennett said he would not accept these on account of the treatment meted out to our patients while they were POWs.

Wed., 12th Sept.: Left Kiirun at 4 P.M. in fair weather for Manila where we anticipate taking on Aussies.

Sat., 15th Sept.: Arrived Manila. The *Empress of Australia* is also here. We are going to embark 170 patients on Monday. Odds are being laid by the patients as to which of the two ships, the *Empress* or the *Maunganui*, will reach Sydney first. Some of the patients have wives or husbands aboard the *Empress*.

Sun., 16th Sept.: Padre Ball conducted a special Thanksgiving Service.

Tues., 18th Sept.: The *Empress* is not now going to Aussie as she has insufficient blankets for the voyage south. The new arrangement is for her to go direct to England via Suez and Singapore.

Wed., 19th Sept.: Embarked 160 patients, which with the previous number of 217 makes 377, about 13 more than usual.

We went alongside a water boat during the afternoon and took on water during the night.

Thurs., 20th Sept.: In the morning the waterboat was replaced by a tanker. Later LSTs brought out supplies. At 5 P.M. we left Manila, en route for Sydney via Manus.

Thurs., 27th Sept.: Arrived Manus 8 P.M. Several bags of precious mail arrived today, but there is a lot missing.

The O.C. gave a talk tonight over the P.A. system. He told the staff and patients that we were going direct to NZ, where the patients were to be the guests of the NZ Government until they were fit enough to travel on to England.

Mon., 8th Oct.: Arrived Wellington. The cot cases were disembarked to Lwo. [Lower] Hutt, Palmerston North and Wellington Hospital. The Australian patients went aboard the *Tjitjalengka* which sailed immediately for Australia. Left for Lyttelton at 5 P.M.

Tues, 9th Oct.: Disembarked 180 patients to Burnham Camp and the Cashmere Sanatorium. Left the ship at 11 A.M. for a week's leave.

The *Maunganui* made two further trips for the NZ Government, both to England:
1st   taking the English POWs home.
2nd   taking the Victory Contingent to Gt. Britain.

After this the *Maunganui* was overhauled and sold to Greece, still capable of riding the roughest seas and cruising along at 12 to 14 knots with an occasional boost up to 16 knots, which is not bad for an old lady who has ploughed the seas for over 35 years.

Grace Robson's Story

V.A.D. stands for "Voluntary Aid Detachment," and as we were Voluntary Nursing Aids the term was used in general for us nurses. We did our own training and sat exams set by the Red Cross such as "First Aid," "Home Nursing," "Hygiene & Sanitation," and then we did 60 hours unpaid voluntary work at our local general hospital. When all that was completed we were officially classed as VAs or Voluntary Aids. Then we could apply for army service if we were over 21.

We were issued with uniforms when we were accepted for army service: khaki serge in winter and drill for summer. Underclothes were not supplied but we received a small allowance for this. Basic pay was ³/₆ per day (about 70¢).

I served in Helwan, which is a few miles out of Cairo. We had our No. 5 General Hospital there. I also served in Alexandria where we had a convalescent hospital at Sidi Bish along the coast about four miles. This was very enjoyable as we were right on the coast where swimming was the order of the day.

Service in Helwan was quite tough. We would have one qualified nursing sister, two VAs like me, and mostly one medical, male orderly and sometimes two. We worked 11-hour duties, six days a week, and had up to 150 patients mostly confined to bed. Materials in 1945 were in short supply, and we washed and boiled things such as bandages and then rerolled them for further use. Food supplies such as sugar, butter, eggs, and fruit were carefully rationed and were kept under lock and key in the ward kitchen, or they were pilfered by the Egyptian servants who did the rough cleaning. I might mention that Maadi camp where our New Zealand forces were based had an "Ice Cream" unit, and we were supplied with ice cream once a week from there. It was a great treat and was made from New Zealand dried milk, and it tasted just like our own ice cream from home.

Life in Egypt was not very easy. You could not just go out and about, and we always went in groups with boys from our own unit or from English and Scottish units nearby. There were also South African units, and those men were very good to us, too, and very gentlemanly. Sometimes we went into church at St. Andrew's in Cairo, and we were given a warm welcome there. The male personnel from whatever units were very protective of us girls and would always make up a group to go sightseeing to such places as the Pyramids, the Zoo, the Museum, Mosques.

We lived in houses close to the hospital which was originally a three-storied hotel, and we had an armed guard on every gate, and at night we had a roving armed guard who escorted us between places. It was forbidden to walk unguarded.

Then life apparently became too dangerous for us to remain in Egypt so we packed up, closed the hospital, and in three days we left for Bari in southern Italy. It was just as dangerous there, and we always went in large groups.

Later on I had leave in Florence, and that was most enjoyable as it was not dangerous on the street, but we went in large groups as that was what we were used to. Florence was largely in ruins. The Germans bombed the bridges and a lot of places as they retreated. There was no public transport, so we walked miles to see anything that was gradually being brought out of hiding. The people in Florence were very poor and also friendly, so chocolate, sweets, soap, and half-worn-out clothes were very good for barter, as were cigarettes. When driving through Italy we were amazed to see children clothed in pants and dresses contrived from grey and khaki army blankets.

We were quartered in a hotel right in the center of Florence which was staffed by Italians, and we were well served. If someone wanted laundry done, the room maid took it to do, but the customer had to supply the soap—enough for the job. If the maid had any over, that was her perk. Italy was the place where I learned to eat spaghetti à la Italien. To this day I can't stand spaghetti out of a tin.

I had two weeks' leave in Palestine, and that was also a strange place to be. We visited Jerusalem, Bethlehem, and some of the tourist attractions such as "The Church of All Nations"—which is a rather modern but beautiful edifice—the Garden of Gethsemane, Jericho, and the Dead Sea, where we actually had a swim. We were supposed to make a trip to Damascus, but at the last minute that city was put out of bounds, so we went to the ancient Roman ruins of Baalbek instead. We camped near Tel Aviv, but were warned not to attempt to go there as it was also very dangerous. It is not much better today, is it?...

I met my husband on H.N.Z.H.S. *Maunganui*. It was just one of those chance encounters, and we had an instant attraction which lasted all our married life of 42½ years. We were best friends.

We were married in April 1946 soon after I returned home, and we had two daughters.

Chapter Thirty

The U.S. Army Nurse Corps
Lee Threlkeld

Lee Threlkeld Jansak served with the 65th General Hospital, affiliated with Duke University.

As I look back and reminisce about my army days, I have a deep sense of appreciation for all who served in the armed forces. It was an honor and experience that I would not exchange anything for … yet I would not like to repeat it. It never seemed special at the time, for everyone around me was also serving.

Growing up on a farm in the Piedmont section of South Carolina during the Depression years, I graduated from high school in 1937. My father died when I was 16 with a massive heart attack, leaving my mother with four children to raise and educate. I was aided in school by President Roosevelt's National Recovery Act, specifically the National Youth Administration. In exchange for this aid, I was required to perform light tasks at my high school. College was never an option; funds were not available. My grandmother, whom I loved and adored, was a midwife, so it just seemed my calling to be a nurse.

I entered nurse's training in January 1938. Books were furnished and tuition was at no charge. We were given $10 per month during the first and second year; $12 for the third year. My class consisted of ten trainees. We lived in nurses' quarters and experienced strict discipline. Our meals were served in the hospital dining room where absolute decorum was always required. The first six months we were on "probation," and our classes were taught by staff doctors and nurses.

It was a three-year diploma program, which I completed in February

1941. I prepared for the state boards that June, and after learning I had passed, I joined the Red Cross. Almost immediately, I received a letter from the Army Nurse Corps saying "we need you"—very similar to that received by potential service inductees. So without much thought, I volunteered for the corps and reported for duty at Fort Bragg, North Carolina, on August 2, 1941.

I was assigned hospital duty and also received indoctrination into the army way of life. I learned how to salute, whom and when, marching in formation, bivouacking, pitching pup tents, eating out of mess kits, and drinking from canteens. All of this was in preparation for overseas duty. It might be of interest that our salary was $70 per month, which was better than the $50 average for civilian duty! The army furnished our blue dress uniforms and white hospital duty uniforms. We lived in barracks, which by today's standards were rather crude; however, the rooms were private. Bottled cokes at break time were five cents.

I was fortunate and honored to be asked to join the 65th General Hospital unit, affiliated with Duke University. The unit was activated at Durham, North Carolina, and staged at Fort Bragg, North Carolina, for initial duty training. The unit consisted of 1,000 enlisted men, 50 doctors, 120 nurses, three Red Cross personnel, three physical therapists, three dietitians, and six administrative army officers. Our commanding officer was a World War I veteran, and a full colonel with 27 years of military service.

In order to officially join the unit, it was necessary for me to receive permission from the chief nurse—a captain with 26 years of army service. She was not enthusiastic about the idea because I would be joining a unit composed of career army nurses with no army background myself. She ultimately relented, and gave her assent. I was to learn later how fortunate I was to be assigned to a general hospital rather than an evacuation unit.

We departed Fort Bragg in *winter* uniforms in August 1943 by unair-conditioned troop train. The train was three days en route to our destination—Camp Shanks, just out of New York City. There we changed uniforms from navy blue to olive drab. An overall uniform shortage caused a delay of our departure for overseas, and we were sent to Fort Devons, Massachusetts, until we could be resupplied. We had further training there, including ship evacuation procedures and negotiating obstacle courses. Our gear consisted of a helmet, gas mask, mess kit, and canteen.

In October 1943, we sailed aboard the *Queen Elizabeth* from New York to Scotland. As we marched up the ship's plank, the band was playing "Pistol Packin' Mama"; suddenly, they stopped and started playing "I

Want to Marry a Girl, Just Like the Girl That Married Dear Old Dad." We were to learn later that a World War I army nurse, a sister to then Secretary of War Henry L. Stimson, was an official greeter for the nurses boarding the ship. She approached the band leader, saying the music was very inappropriate for a group of nurses boarding a ship for overseas duty in time of war. Thereupon, he abandoned "Pistol Packin' Mama" for the latter selection.

We zigzagged across the Atlantic Ocean in a record-breaking three days, dodging enemy submarines the whole way. At the time the *Queen Elizabeth* was the fastest ocean liner on the seas. The ship was designed as a luxury liner, but that role was interrupted by the war and she was converted to a troop carrier. Only two ports in the world could accommodate the ship: New York City and Southampton, England. The ship docked in the Firth of Clyde off Glasgow and the Scottish coast. Troops were ferried to land and boarded troop trains. However, before anyone was allowed to leave the ship, the British air commodore came aboard to address us over the loudspeaker system. After welcoming us to British soil, he issued the announcement that although there was class distinction in his country, there was no color distinction, and that we would remember at all times!

After boarding the troop train early that evening for an overnight ride through Scotland, we were pleased to see people throughout the countryside lining the railroad tracks and displaying the "V" (victory) sign. The gesture, which was initiated by Winston Churchill, was a great morale builder.

Our maiden duty assignment was in the Great Malvern area, near Worcestershire, England. This was a mountainous resort with lovely hotels requiring the best of dress. Many wealthy Londoners, the elderly, and

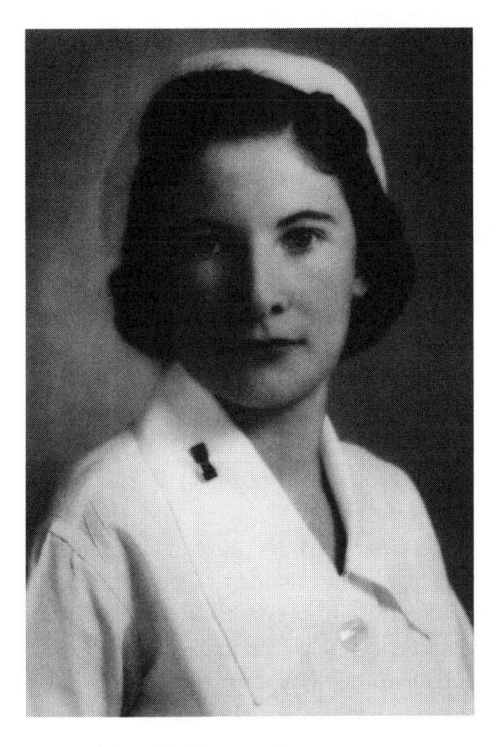

Lee Threlkeld Jansak. *Courtesy of Lee Threlkeld Jansak.*

children were evacuated there to escape the blitz. There I had my first experience owning and riding a bicycle, as this was the most common form of transportation.

The English were great hosts and freely shared their homes for afternoon tea and occasional evening meals. I particularly remember a family that invited four of us for dinner and were very proud of their son, a member of the Royal Air Force. The son had been seeing an American girl, and the parents were anxious for their daughter to meet an American soldier. Our foursome included a prospect who was a staunch Republican and heir to large textile mills in North Carolina. As we gathered around the fire after dinner, he offered a negative opinion about President Roosevelt. Our host then practically ushered us out of the house, signaling an abrupt end to the soldier's future with the daughter! I would also like to give honorable mention to Peter and Don, child refugees from London, who often ate their meals with the unit.

We established a general hospital at Great Malvern, receiving casualties from North Africa, Sicily, and Italy. The majority of our patients were rehabilitated and returned to their units in preparation for D-Day. In March of 1944 the air corps was suffering heavy casualties, and their nearest medical facility was a station hospital with minimum staff and surgical expertise. The 65th was requested to replace the station hospital, and I was selected for the advance cadre of hospital personnel.

Our hospital was formed at Bottesdale in Suffolk, England, and it served Eighth Air Force casualties and thousands of others. My first patient on the neurosurgical ward was a young lieutenant, a fighter pilot, who had overestimated the airfield on returning from a mission, crash-landed, and lost a portion of his frontal skull. He was awake during the surgery while bone fragments were removed from his skull. After the surgery his head and face were bandaged including his eyes, with his nose and mouth as the only openings. The patient was warned that he should not cough or sneeze and should lie perfectly still, for fear of spinal cord rupture. He remained under our care for six months, made good progress, and was sent to England Hospital in New York, where he received a silver plate in his skull. The silver plate accompanied him to the States, as it was crafted by a silversmith in London, located by the unit's neurosurgeon. This was considered quite revolutionary at the time. After the war I enjoyed a visit with this patient, whose surgical scars were barely visible. He often commented during those months of recovery that he pictured me in his mind's eye. Upon removal of the bandages, he remarked that I looked exactly as he had imagined!

Our unit experienced numerous air raids, and we were required to don our helmets, take a gas mask, and return to our duty station in complete darkness with only a flashlight to guide our way. On one occasion during the buzz bomb scare, a bomb fell just outside our compound, leaving a large crater in the ground. Also, when the war was winding down and blackout conditions were less observed, the village where our hospital was located was strafed by German aircraft mistaking it for an air corps runway. Two of our enlisted men were injured during the episode and given Purple Hearts—even though they were actually in a pub at the time!

At the close of the war in Europe, a point system based upon length of service was used to determine who could return first to the States. Due to my longevity, I soon boarded the *Queen Elizabeth* for what proved to be its last voyage from the Firth of Clyde in Scotland. Afterward, the ship returned to its home port of Southampton to be converted into a luxury cruise liner.

The army plan for me was to return home, enjoy 30 days' leave with family, and be redeployed to the Pacific. However, the atomic bombs dropped on Hiroshima and Nagasaki caused the army to no longer need my services. Following my leave I reported to Fort Seibert, Alabama, which has long since been deactivated. The Alabama post provided a temporary home for 6,000 nurses awaiting return to civilian life. Since I was in the Reserve, I received a discharge.

Bringing matters to the present day, I attended a reunion of the 65th General Hospital in May 1999. These reunions have been an annual tradition since the end of the war. The 1999 event was held back at Duke University. Regrettably, only two of the unit's physicians were still living, and they both attended the reunion. A total of 70 persons were present, including ten nurses.

Although our numbers thin with each passing year, we still have a great spirit of unity and enjoy reliving many of our World War II experiences. This was a period of great adventure and a remarkably character-building influence in our lives. I shall always be grateful for that opportunity to serve my country and to work alongside some of the finest personnel the medical community had to offer. Thank you for allowing me this opportunity to share those days with you.

Chapter Thirty-One

Physical Therapy in the South Pacific

FORREST WALKER

...I was 21 when I enlisted in the navy. I had just graduated from Pasadena Junior College in February and had stayed on to take three emergency wartime postgraduate courses. In doing this I was able to be included in the June graduation services which were held at one end of the Rose Bowl. That was the only time I "played" in the Rose Bowl. At the time of Pearl Harbor I was working at Lockheed Aircraft Company in the final assembly line, manufacturing P-38 Lightnings. I worked on the graveyard shift so that I could finish at PJC.
—Forrest Walker

Boot Camp, San Diego Naval Training Station

Given ten days to get things in order, I reported to San Diego Naval Training Station on July 8, 1942. We were formed into companies of 150 recruits each, our hair was shorn, and we were issued our allotment of clothes, ditty bag, blankets, hammock, mattress and a sea bag. Then started the indoctrination which, of course, is one of many facets of any military training program.

In new issue "whites" we reported to sick bay for our first round of shots, the bane of all recruits. They shot us in both arms at the same time, and I was surprised that it didn't bother me. I recall an instance where the third man in line ahead of me got his shot okay, but as the corpsman tried to pull the needle out it separated from the syringe and stuck in the recruit's arm. The man standing in line in front of me passed out cold.

On another occasion a recruit didn't move smartly in the line, and he got shot twice, just like that. Oops! About three weeks later, we went through all this again with the additional discomfort of being very sunburned.

Selecting a Service Training School

About the fourth week we were given the opportunity to select a service school or career direction. We were told to report to an assembly hall where we filled out classification papers which were to assist the officers in charge to arrive at a decision as to which school, if any, one would be sent to. This was the most important moment in our tour of service, and it came up without much fanfare or notice; few had even thought about it before. The event caught men unprepared and, for many, the three choices available were the same as no choice. The limited choice may have been intentional as the navy always needed many able bodied seamen who could be assigned wherever the command needed men the most. There were three schools available at the time.

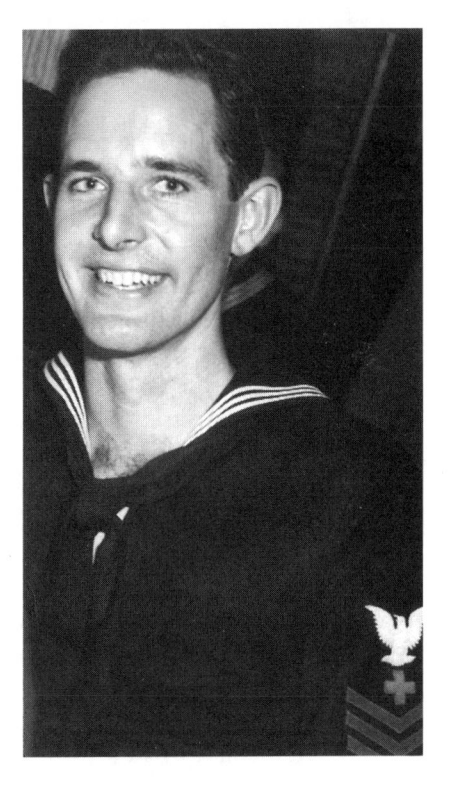

Forrest Walker in San Diego upon return to the United States. He lost 25 pounds while overseas due to heat, hard work, long hours, and diet. *Courtesy of Forrest Walker.*

Hospital Corps School was the school I signed up for, and my thinking was thus. I would most certainly get married after the war and probably have children. Any training or education I received would come in handy in raising a family. It was almost as simple as that. The other reason actually had to do with my basic faith beliefs. I would really rather help people than kill people. This value system came from my family and the church teachings. Dad and Mom were basically pacifist, but not activist in their beliefs; however, never once did they not do their utmost to support the war effort, and service men in particular. My earlier go at the Naval Air Service must have been an aberration, probably only the good Lord really knows.

Hospital Corps School, Balboa Park

After five weeks in boot camp, I was transferred to the Naval Hospital Corps School at San Diego. We were housed in the Balboa Park exhibition buildings where we formally inducted into the Hospital Corps for training as hospital apprentices. Most of the six-week training program was in a classroom setting, and we studied from the Hospital Corps Handbook primarily. Topics covered included materia medica, nursing practices, tropical diseases, food sanitation and cross-infections control in hospital settings, to name a few. I can't go on without saying a little more about the Balboa Park building experience. These buildings were the coldest, draftiest places in which to house men; they were heated with large heater-blower combinations that were meant to be used in factories or warehouses. After spending several fitful nights, I found that I could keep fairly warm by using a couple of pieces of newspaper slipped in between my two, regular navy blankets. It was very noisy but effective, and soon many of the men were using those "paper blankets."

There were five corpsmen by the name of Walker, but I can only remember one... I remember him because of an event which occurred between us. I had a top bunk and Walker was across an aisle from me. A bully type of guy was on the lower bunk and boosted me out of my bunk several times. I had just finished a double shift so I was sort of pooped out and needed to get some sleep. Walker was a Golden Gloves champion and could have beaten me to a pulp with one hand tied behind him. He wanted to get in on the fun and pulled the blankets off my bunk for starters. In a moment of rash carelessness I propelled myself over the foot of my bunk and, with a loud screaming yell, planted one foot on his chest and the other on the side of his head, surprising him more than stunning him. I immediately changed my demeanor to one of cowardly defense. I reacted as though I had temporarily lost my sanity, so that he and quite a few others bought it. I'll have to admit that I enjoyed not being approached in a hostile manner by anyone for some months after that event, my only Golden Gloves "fight."

Ward Assignment

My first work assignment was to ward 134 down the hill from the main buildings. In these buildings were sailors and marines who, for the most part, were from scattered operational activities from all over the west. Within a week we became deluged with casualties from such places as Tulagi, Tanamboga, Gavutu, Guadalcanal, and other islands and the seas of the Southwest Pacific. The flood became greater as the Matson liner *Lurline* came into port and discharged a full load of patients, some ambulatory, but many in stretchers. I use the term "in" advisedly because we used a stokes stretcher most of the time. It is metal-framed, basket-like, and about six and a half feet long, and for safety's sake the patient was strapped into it and transported thus up the stairways or to other ships at sea. In a cruise ship there are stairs, but in navy ships they're called ladders.

It took us about 14 hours to get everybody off-loaded and over to the hospital. I made four trips or five, and it was amazing to see how the conversion to wartime use had changed the interior of the ship. I particularly remember carrying a stretcher case out of the emptied swimming pool where many of the patients had been stacked four tiers high. All this was not a problem for most of the patients as they were glad just to be back stateside. One could still see beautiful paintings, murals, and chandeliers that were still hanging, along with other signs of its former opulence.

I passed the test to hospital corpsman second class in a few months and soon advanced to first class. I learned early on that one had to study as much as possible to be eligible to "strike" for the next higher rank. In the meantime I had sent in a request for assignment to a physical therapy training program. I didn't know much about it, but it seemed like a good idea at the time.

Vernie Rice (Cajun)

I guess everyone on a station assignment has a best friend, and I suppose the nearest to that for me was a fellow corpsman by the name of Vernie Rice, from near Lake Charles, Louisiana. He claimed to be a Cajun and could tell stories until there seemed no end to them. Most of the stories were "funny as a crutch" so it was a real pleasure to hang around with him. At times he would keep three or four of us in stitches for hours. He was one who would blow most of his pay on one night on the town by way of busses, streetcars, and ferry boats. We hitchhiked up to Los Angeles two or three times as I knew my way around there, and he soon learned how to stretch his funds. He shipped out to the Pacific with a mobile hospital, and that was the last I heard of him until the summer of 1994.

I need to insert this bit of more recent history as it is quite special. In 1994, my wife Helen and I drove across the southern part of the country for the first time. One night we stopped overnight in Lake Charles, Louisiana. While at the motel I looked in the phone book and found the name "Vernie Rice" listed with the number. I dialed the number, and a lady answered. I identified myself quickly and began to tell her about having known Vernie. She stopped me and told me that he had died in 1976 in a V.A. Hospital. Then she relayed this story to me.

Vernie had been assigned to a mobile hospital which was sent to Saipan. They had set up everything and were reasonably comfortable. Shortly after that he was transferred to Okinawa where he was to help set up another hospital that was to receive patients from the expected invasion of the Japanese mainland. After he arrived in Okinawa he and a buddy were in tent quarters, and they got word of a typhoon which was predicted to sweep through the area where they were quartered. (It swept through that island, coincidentally, just before the A bombs were dropped.) He and his friend didn't get to a safe area, and Vernie was struck down by some flying debris which paralyzed him from the neck down. After returning to the States he was started on physical therapy and regained most of the use of his arms, but that was all. During his hospital stays he became the favorite of many of the nurses, and one of them married him after a long courtship. This was the lady I was talking to. I asked her why she still had the phone in his name, and she said just so people like me would call to say hello or ask for him. She never remarried, and said she never would, and that their life together, some 17 years, was the greatest blessing anyone would want.

Assigned to Physical Therapy Training Program

I had gotten quite comfortable at my job at the commissary, and while there I made pharmacist mate third class. I kept studying and pushing for another step up and soon made it to pharmacist mate second class. I figured that this was about as far as I could go without some sea duty or an assignment overseas. But out of the blue I received notice that I had been accepted for a three-month training program in physical therapy. I had completely forgotten about signing up for the course back in the fall of 1942. This was a new ballgame, and it did mean I had at least three more months of stateside duty. The program was very intense as they needed many men trained in this specialty. We were given a lot of material to read as well as the beginning of hands-on training where we learned about various methods of massage, rudiments of the use of diathermy for back pains and other muscle spasms, and galvanic currents to aid in treatment of certain damaged nerves and even scars. Most of this type of treatment was designed to overcome certain conditions of the body and limbs left paralyzed from wounds, but of course some of it was for sprains and strains.

We were always under the supervision of a navy medical doctor. The two senior physical therapists were inducted directly into the Hospital Corps as pharmacist mate second class since they were already chiropractors in the state of California. The most experienced one's last name was Shuth; next was Craig Crockard who was from my home town and had lived about a mile from me. There were only ten of us in the class, and some were transferred out almost immediately after our three months' training was over. I learned about several types of hydrotherapy treatments: hot and cold contrast soaks, Hubbard full-body tank, smaller hydro tanks for arms or legs, and hot-towel compresses.

I was happy to hear I had been selected to stay on staff at San Diego as a "physio" pharmacist mate. Another corpsman by the name of Carl Palange was also selected to stay on, and his claim to fame was that he had already sung with the San Francisco Opera Company. He was following in his father's footsteps who was an accomplished opera singer, having sung at the La Scala Opera House in Italy before the war.

Drs. Brillig and Rosenberg: "Tendon Stretchers"

Carl and I were assigned to monitor and guide hundreds of marines and a few navy men to see that they did some prescribed exercises intended to loosen the hamstring tendon and generally improve their mobility. This, in turn, was to cure some of the back problems, knee pains, and the pains caused by flatfeet. Carl was a little larger than I was, and as a team we would not take any guff from the patients, some of whom would rather stay in the hospital than go back to duty. The two medical doctors in charge of this particular program were a Dr. Brillig and a Dr. Rosenberg.

We had 700 patients under this program, and after three months all but about 30 had gone back to duty including about 15 for limited duty. Many men stopped complaining of pain and chose to go back to duty rather than do the painful exercises. Some of the girlfriends or wives, many working in war industries, started doing some of the same exercises to prevent or lessen their menstrual cramps. That was the last straw for many of the men.

This experimental treatment program had about run its course when my name appeared on a list notifying me that I was to report to Camp

Shoemaker near Pleasanton, California. There were over 3,000 enlisted men at the hospital, and by this time I was number five on the enlisted men's pay line (seniority). The orders only stated that I would be there FFT (for further transfer).

Camp Shoemaker and Dispensary Duty

I had about three days to get stuff in order, and I was on my way by train to Shoemaker. We went up over the Tehachapi Pass and through the San Joaquin Valley, then toward the bay area and over the Altamont Pass to the camp which would be my home until I left for overseas. We were traveling for 27 hours and were handed a sandwich and a beverage about three times during the trip. Men would be at Shoemaker for a few days, weeks, or sometimes months prior to leaving for their particular theater of operations, so I guess it could best be called a holding and reassignment area. The second day I was there the person in charge of the barracks called me out after the regular muster and said that the doctor at the dispensary wanted to see me at 9 A.M. The doctor asked me to report for duty at 1 P.M. that day and said that he would have the necessary paperwork at hand to make it official.

All was in order as I reported to Tony Beerbaum, pharmacist mate third class, and was informed that I was to be in charge of any physical therapy treatments that would be referred by the medical officer. Tony was from Wisconsin and had worked in a drugstore when he was recruited into the navy. He told me up front that he had referred to the Corpsman Handbook, but had no training at all in physio, and said he was really glad to have me aboard and wished me well. Since I was just "passing through" and he was on permanent assignment, he was in charge. Tony was about 35 years old, so for me it was like having a much older brother around.

On the second day I heard a patient yell out in pain, and as I was on a break, I was at the far end of the unit. In a few minutes I heard another yell and went to investigate. A corpsman was trying to treat a new patient with diathermy. I lifted up the well-padded coil from the man's leg and noticed a long scar. I asked the patient if he had ever had a broken leg, and he responded affirmatively. I then said, "They put in a metal plate, didn't they?" He said yes, and of course I knew what was going on. It would be like getting cooked inside the leg with a microwave. Of course, treatment was changed posthaste.

It was slow for the first week, but then things started to pick up. I surmised the M.D. thought things were going well as he sent us more cases. About this time most of the men I knew in San Diego were sent on over to Treasure Island FFT so that left me kind of alone, but such was navy life.

My Last Trip Home Before Overseas

I went on liberty while stationed at Shoemaker, but not with the gusto that I had while in San Diego. On the 29th day of March, 1944, I made arrangements for coverage to visit my folks in Baldwin Park.

I visited some friends not yet relocated by service, occupational, or marital changes, and helped a little with some things that needed doing at the ranch. Frances and Mom fixed a holiday dinner with all the trimmings, and as we were enjoying the meal, the phone rang and a voice said, "This is Tony up at Shoemaker, and I'm calling to let you know that your name was just posted, so you better get your tail back up here posthaste." I responded with, "O.K., sure, and I also know this is April Fool's Day." But he said, "Yes, that's true, but you're really on the list for the Southwest Pacific Command. We'll answer muster for you in the morning, but you better be here by 2:00 P.M. at the latest." So that was that.

Life in the Southwest Pacific

We'll pick up just as we clear the continental shelf off San Francisco. The water goes from a green tone of blue to an almost iridescent indigo. We saw a few dolphin and flying fish, but no birds for the first few days. We were headed almost due south, and as I reckoned, there was no chance of our going by way of the Hawaiian Islands. About five days later we picked up an albatross that escorted us to our first landfall almost two weeks later. The green of those islands was really a relief after seeing nothing but blue for that extended period of time.

There were two reports of submarine contacts that reached our ears, so we were aware of the possibilities. We picked up a New Zealand destroyer escort vessel, and he stayed with us for only a couple of days. In the evenings we observed the beautiful traces left by the phosphorescent plankton which we disturbed on our way through their home waters. During the day we watched or played pinochle and poker intermittently all the way across the Pacific, and if we took a break from that, it was probably spent in reading, or sharing tales of home and girlfriends.

The New Hebrides

After being at sea for 31 days we pulled into a harbor on a "real live" tropical isle. It looked great, but even a dry desert isle would have looked good after that much time at sea; after all, most of us were landlubbers. As we pulled along side a dock large enough for only one ship at a time, we found that we were in the New Hebrides on the island of Espiritu Santo. We noticed a navy seagoing floating drydock, so we knew it was a fair sized base. We went ashore and were walked several hundred yards to the receiving station where we would be quartered until we were sent "north," which meant up the Solomon Island chain toward some of "the action that was going on" at the time.

The marines had already moved up into parts of Bougainville as well as captured New Georgia, Rendova, and the Treasury Islands. The Solomon Islands continued some 600 miles to the north, and we had no idea when or how we would go that way. This was the only time during my stint in the navy that I really had time on my hands. I found myself tracing girls' pictures which I would pick at random from magazines or newspapers—talk about weird. Letter writing was without a doubt a better way to pass the time, and I did send dozens of V-mail letters to home and friends.

The best way of spending time was to hitch a ride out to a beach area that was actually part of a bay; I got in a lot of swimming. I was on the island about a week, and I started having low back pains, so I found my way to the base carpenter shop and talked the head person into giving me a two by three foot piece of thin plywood. I placed it under my navy mattress, and in a couple of days I began to feel much better. I spent all that time in physical therapy training, so why not put some of that knowledge into practice.

I got out to an airstrip where "Pappy" Greg Boyington had his squadron headquartered for several months and found that there were still many F4Us active there. I used to go out quite often just to watch the aviation activity that was always going on. Many DC-3s, a few Catalinas, and some army B-25s made flights through there at different times. I was shown the site where the *President Coolidge* sank as a result of hitting one of our own mines and some poor ship piloting. Only one or two lives were lost, and everyone that saw it firsthand said the low casualty rate was a miracle.

Nearby, there was a large crane mounted on a barge made up of many of the five by five steel "Magic Boxes," one of the simplest but most useful (nonkilling) products to come out of the war. It was said the crane was large enough to lift a P.T. boat or the smaller auxiliary craft. There was also the large, floating drydock which was large enough to handle a destroyer. A short distance beyond the pier area was a large, steel girder bridge which had been built some years before the war and was an important link in the road system.

Food Poisoning

Now comes a tale of something which had a lasting effect on my life — an illness commonly known as food poisoning. (The area of public health, in which I was to serve a lifetime after the war, was very actively engaged in preventing the occurrence of such illnesses). About 1,200 men were being fed out of the particular mess hall where I was billeted. I had eaten lunch and headed to my favorite swimming spot at the northern part of the island. After a 20-minute truck ride I arrived at the beach, got into my swimsuit, and walked out into the very gently sloping beach swimming area.

After five minutes or so I began to feel a little weak and turned back towards the beach, which suddenly appeared to be twice as far away as it had been a few minutes before. I looked to my right, and two other swimmers were choking and sort of staggering out of the water, too. I dressed and reached the roadway where I hailed a truck for a ride back to the base. Others climbed aboard at the same time, and some started throwing up as we traveled along. They took turns heaving out of the back end of the truck, and I wasn't feeling too well myself by that time.

I hung on until we reached the base where I jumped off the truck, and then as my feet hit the ground, I upchucked violently. I went towards the "12-hole" head which was so crowded I couldn't get in, so I looked for an open space between the coconut trees, dropped my pants, and let fly. I quickly upchucked again, and in two or three minutes let go the other way once more. I was beginning to feel like a spinning pinwheel, and it got worse as I crawled some distance away from the mess, dodging the places where others had done likewise before me. In five or ten minutes someone came along and announced that everyone feeling ill was to report to the hospital (Mob [Mobile Hospital] 6, I think) on the trucks that would be available in a few minutes. Several days later the service paper called the *Scuttlebutt* reported 600 men were checked into the hospital, and most were released after a couple of hours.

Four of us, however, were held overnight because of complications or extreme dehydration, and I vividly remember the following sequence of events. I told someone I was a corpsman, and I had no business being sick. A nurse asked me to remove my shoes as I was going to be here for a while. I sat on the edge of the bed and leaned forward to take off the first shoe and fell forward off the bed. I barely recall some people helping me onto the bed and getting me into hospital attire, and I must have faded away again.

Sometime later I heard the nurse say something about "Doctor, can you check this man?" The next thing I knew, someone was raising my eyelids one at a time and saying, "Yes, um! uh huh," and I remember thinking, "Oh, boy, this is serious; I may be at the end of the road." They gave me two one-liter bottles of saline solution and watched me for a while, then discharged me the next day. We were told later that someone had not put some creamed peas, the causative food, into the refrigerator the night before, so that a typical case of food poisoning had developed.

While in the islands one of the things that kept my spirits up was receiving copies of the L.A. *Daily News* through the mail. I would read the papers from cover to cover and pass them along to others in our area and would take some over to the hospital. Dad would send a few magazines along which also kept me connected with home and, of course, these made the rounds, too, even if they weren't the "girly" type.

After three or four weeks 50 of us found our names posted on a shipping-out list, or draft, as it was called. We were to board a ship the next morning and go up to the Russell Islands, which were northwest of Guadalcanal, and report for duty at Mob 10 Naval Hospital. As we were sailing north in a navy freighter of the Liberty ship class, we learned over the radio that the Normandy landings were under way in Europe.

Mob 10 Naval Hospital: Russell Islands

We pulled into the Guadalcanal anchorage, and dropped off some personnel, mail, and some equipment. We stayed there overnight, and the next day set out for the Russell Islands, which are only 15 miles off the north end of Guadalcanal. In the morning we heard the engine begin to rumble again and the sounds of casting off. We proceeded northwesterly, up the Slot, and cleared Cape Esperance while an officer explained a little of recent local history about the war through this part of the Solomons between August and December of 1942.

At about 1300 hours we pulled into the outer anchorage of Renard Sound on the Island of Banika, and an announcement was made: All hands assigned to Mobile Hospital Number 10 were to debark with their gear immediately. We dropped over the side by the way of a cargo net into a landing craft and were taken to the beach. The landing craft dropped us off in an absolutely deserted place. Nothing was there except a landing area where we could see a small navy barge making trips across this inlet. We could look across the water several hundred yards away and see a large freighter tied up to a dock and a lot of activity going on.

I was one of five second-class pharmacist mates and also the youngest. The rest of the men were either third-class pharmacist mates or hospital corpsmen. After observing all the activity across the harbor, I said I would go over to the other side and see what the holdup was. No one else stepped forward, so I went on alone with comments like "You're going to get in trouble" following in my wake. I learned from the bosun's mate that we had been put ashore on Red beach, and he would escort me to Blue beach.

I saw a control tower with the words "BEACH MASTER" clearly visible, and when I finally got his attention for a moment, I told him our plight. He summoned a rating who took me to a phone where I called the hospital. I was transferred to a Chief Joiner who was, I learned later, the personnel officer. The first question he asked was "Who has the orders?" I told him that no one had been given a copy of any orders, but there were 50 men waiting over at Red beach. He asked my name and rating and told me to have everyone get on the next ferryboat and form up with our gear at my phone location on his orders, and wait for transportation.

I went back and told everyone what I had found out. Some, including a couple of the older pharmacist mates second class, didn't want to go over on my say-so, but we finally got them to agree to stay with us. After getting a ride on the barge to Blue beach, we still had to wait another hour for the trucks, but at least there was a single drinking fountain which satisfied our greatest need at the time. Again the same guys were developing really nasty dispositions and were blaming me for screwing things up for everybody.

Finally, three trucks pulled up led by a jeep. Chief Joiner jumped out yelling, "Where's Walker?" "Here, Sir," said I. He then asked a few more questions of all of us in general and told us to get our gear together and board the trucks. The barracks to which we were assigned had 50 cots and lockers set up, and we were milling around when the chief came in and said, "Attention, men. Walker will be the rating in charge of this barracks until everyone has permanent details and quarters. Walker, your bunk is at the far end, starboard corner of the building. Everyone else is to take bunks in alphabetical order, starting at this end of the building, clockwise, ending here. Walker, see that this is done; here's a clipboard and duty belt; you're in charge. I want a temporary, alphabetically arranged roster with last name, initials, and current rating of every man ASAP." With that he told us a special chow would be served in the mess hall in a few minutes, and he departed.

Later in the day he came by to see how everything was going and to give us a little pep talk. He announced that evening, "It has come to my attention that several men were senior to Walker in time-in rate, but he was placed in charge because he took the responsibility to see that you all didn't spend the night on the beach with the coconut crabs, and by the way, don't believe everything you hear about never volunteering."

Things started moving first thing in the morning. A detail office yeoman had a typed copy of the roster we provided; he called roll, and then we had to check the information for accuracy and add to it our serial numbers. As an added incentive he said if the list was not correct, we might not get paid or receive mail for quite a while. We had the rest of the morning to get our stuff squared away, and after chow the chief came over and had a list of 20 men who were assigned to pick and shovel work repairing the coral paths between various buildings. Everyone else was to stay close in and police the barracks and area outside. This kind of stuff went on for a week or two, but gradually all hands were sent on to a permanent work and bunking assignment except me. Chief Joiner came over, and we talked for a few minutes. He asked what my training and work history was. When I got to the physical therapy part he said, "Hold it; I think I have a spot for you."

Sydney S. Sideman, M.D.

A little later Joiner told me to report to a Dr. Sideman in the plaster cast room next to the x-ray room at 1600 hrs. Sydney S. Sideman, M.D., from Chicago, was an orthopedic surgeon about 45 years of age and was to be a father figure and teacher during the time I was on Banika. After talking for a while, the doctor said he'd like me to take charge of the plaster cast room. I would be making all of the plaster of Paris bandages which would be made from scratch with the materials he had already procured. He commented that regular plaster bandages from the States were not working out as they were not impregnated with enough plaster to suit him or this humid tropical environment. He went on to say that cast material would be in great demand every time we received a shipload of casualties, so it was important that a plentiful supply be ready to go at all times.

31. Physical Therapy in the South Pacific

To begin with I had no experience with plaster of Paris, let alone casts. As a physio man I had seen the effects of prolonged wearing of casts and what it does to the limbs, i.e., they become atrophied, develop skin lesions, lose the sense of touch, and do not function properly. I had to keep an adequate supply of bulk plaster of Paris on hand and see that the two-, three-, four-, and six-inch-wide plaster cast bandages were kept dry. I made the bandages from fresh plaster—which came in 25-pound, well-sealed cans—and bolts of plain white crinoline. A cabinet was made which was six feet tall and had five shelves to store the cast material. A 60-watt light bulb was installed to keep the moisture to a minimum so that the plaster was always fresh.

Using this fresh plaster I could make first-class bandages to suit the preferences of either of the medical officers, as well as having sufficient supplies ready for any emergency. The real benefit of the fresh plaster bandages was that we could put on very lightweight casts to replace the ones which tradition said had to be about an inch thick because of the humidity that was ever present in the tropical latitudes. In practice, we did not find the thick casts were better for patients, or the staff that had to care for them over longer periods of time.

On the other hand, when applying emergency casts on casualties on the beach or even aboard the very busy evacuation ships, things were quite different, and allowances for moisture and haste had to be built into the quantity.

After some firsthand training from Dr. Sideman, I learned how to remove any cast that came my way with very elementary tools: a plaster cutting knife shaped like a carpet knife; a small oval shaped saw blade about two inches long; and a pair of scissors. I quickly developed a feel for the difference between cutting cast material and the stockinette that was next to the skin. Many a nervous marine asked me if I'd ever done this kind of work before, and my response was often colored by the way I sized up the man. If he was a certain type, I would answer in a way that was not too reassuring. Of course, other patients on the ward, who had already been cared for, knew what was going on,

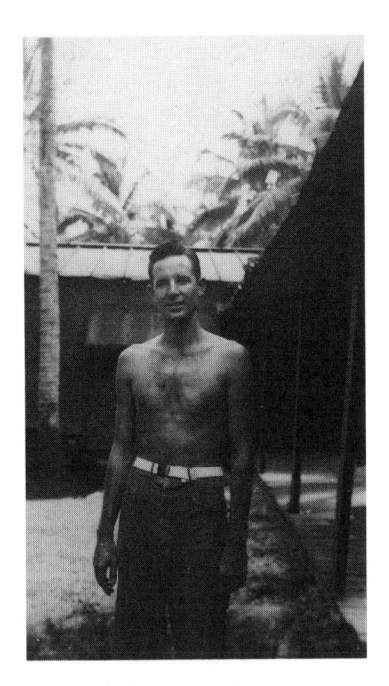

Forrest Walker outside plaster cast room on Banika. *Courtesy of Forrest Walker.*

would chime in right away, and later have a good laugh about it. About a year later we received a compound jaw plaster cutter similar to long handled pruning shears which made a lot of the work more efficient.

One of the hospital ships that brought beachhead casualties from the Marianas campaign hit a coral reef on its way to us and had to lay to for a while and then proceed slowly to our location. By the time the patients got to us, most of the beachhead casts had been in place over two weeks and were very "ripe." I had to remove 16 of the upper body/arm horizontal casts during one day's activity. The casts were made of the usual inch to inch and a half thick plaster cast material and were very difficult to cut through with the simple cutting devices we were using. Almost without exception these casts were soaked with body fluids and had a green tinge of color to them as well as the attendant odor. I remember working through lunch and just grabbing a bite of a sandwich now and then, as I cut off the casts just described. Some of the patients as well as corpsmen were aghast at my eating and working at the same time. It shows what you can do if you really feel you have to.

Although we always had local operational casualties, the real impact of the war was felt when we received patients directly off the hospital ships. Not too long after arriving here we learned that the official name of our unit had been changed to Fleet Hospital 110 to concur with other Mob Hospitals' designations. While stationed here, we were treating patients from the Northern Solomons, New Britain, New Georgia, Bougainville as well as Peleliu, Guam, Saipan, Iwo Jima, and the Okinawa campaigns. Since I was in orthopedics, most of the cases I worked with were wounds where the bullet or piece of shrapnel had hit a bone and broken it. Many of these marines were kept here for months until they were able to go back to duty. A few were sent back to the States and even fewer to New Zealand or Australia.

An Old Friend

One of the more distressing things to happen occurred at a time between campaigns. When I passed by the outpatient building, I noted a shore patrol person with a marine inpatient in tow. The marine's skin color was yellow with Atabrine poisoning, but he looked familiar to me. As I spoke to the S.P., I recognized the patient and got permission to talk with him. I remembered him as a first-class, parade-type marine who had been a guard at the main gate at the naval hospital during most of my stay in San Diego. Since coming overseas he had been on three landings and had worked with mine clearing details most of the time. I found out later he had cracked up and overdosed on Atabrine (antimalaria tablets) and was consequently suffering from Atabrine poisoning. I was glad I had taken the time to talk over old times with him while I had the chance. It brought home to me that there are many kinds of casualties in times of war, and that there is little concern shown for the alternative cases.

The highest ranking patient that I became acquainted with during my stay overseas was Brig. General Bill Rupertus, USMC, who was in command positions during several of the marine campaigns. He had a severe sprain in his ankle which required the application of a plaster cast. Dr. Sideman had me assist him with the application of the original cast and told the general to come back in seven days for a walking cast so he could be somewhat mobile. At the appointed time the general appeared at the door of the cast room and said he had come back for the walking cast. I found that Dr. Sideman was in emergency and would not be available for several hours. He told me to cut off the cast and apply a new walking type of cast myself, then wrote a short note to the general which I was to give to him. The general read it and with a big "Harrumph!" said, "Well, Son, let's get at it." I did, and everything came out O.K.

Other Events and People

Movies were a great outlet for us. We usually took our ponchos and tropic helmets with us, as there was a 50 percent chance of rain any evening. A fellow by the name of Applegate was in charge of procuring the films and selecting the music played over the sound system before the show. "Steel Guitar" seemed to be his favorite tune, as we heard it at least once every night. We had a Bob Hope, Jerry Collona, and Frances Langford USO show. Some months later Bob Crosby and his Bobcats Dance Band put on a daytime program. Later in the day Bob himself came around to the wards and even visited the plaster cast room, where I was able to share one of my private stash of 7 Up as well as talk with him for a while. When I mentioned Baldwin Park being my home town, he said he remembered going to the Al G. Barnes winter circus performance there a few years back.

A most somber experience occurred when a B-25 bomber crashed upon landing on the island. Drs. Sideman and Disbrow, a Roentgenologist, seven or eight corpsmen, and a couple of nurses worked many hours to save the lives of the five crewmen. Only two survived. Hours of effort went into trying to save the other three but the bodily trauma was too great to allow recovery. Although I had no exposure to surgical training, I did many things I had only heard about or had studied in corps school. I recall painful discussions by the doctors as to the efficacy of setting broken bones right then and casting them, bringing on more trauma, or setting and casting them at a later time.

With all the problems of "jungle rot" and plain itching misery that occurs with casts, accentuated by the heat and humidity, some experimentation with repairing fractures was done using Roger or Stater external fixation or splinting. Long screws or pins were inserted into the bones, and then they were "fixed" by rods and clamps in a way that the broken bones were held in proper position to bring about the growth of bone callous and healing. Most people shuddered when they first saw these devices, but many of the patients thought it was okay because if it itched they could get at the source, and they were not nearly as heavy as the plaster casts. About halfway through my tour of duty there, I was promoted to pharmacist mate first class.

A very unusual assignment came up while I was on duty there. A patient needed a brace for his upper ankle and lower femur area. Dr. Sideman procured a piece of canvas, a grommet tool and grommets, a hand drawn pattern, the loan of a sewing machine, and some heavy shears. He then instructed me to make the needed brace. I don't remember exactly what my response was but he said, "Go ahead; you can do it." I was really bewildered as this was so far from any experience I had had previous to this, but the doctor commented that I had worked with sheet aluminum at Lockheed, so it shouldn't be too different. I got at it and came up with a fairly reasonable looking device, and it served the desired purpose for the six weeks the patient needed it.

As the hospital was being built,

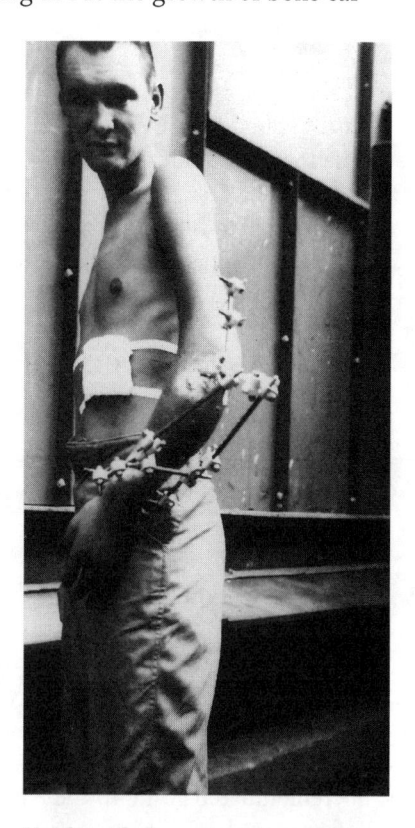

Unidentified marine wounded in the Marianas Campaign wearing Stater splintering or Roger Anderson Splints. With these splints, there was none of the itching common to plaser casts. *Courtesy of Forrest Walker.*

long before I arrived there, I was told the enlisted men and officers got along fine and were on very informal and friendly terms. But as soon as the nurses started coming on staff, barriers arose overnight, and soon there were "officers' country," an officers' club, and uniform of the day. There never was an enlisted men's club or meeting place, as the navy didn't seem to consider these types of facilities were desirable. The nurses had a barracks compound surrounded by barbed wire and rather brilliant lighting. One night a ne'er-do-well corpsman named "Charlie" had a few too many beers and decided he wanted to visit the nurses' compound, and proceeded to crawl under the fence.

About 0100 hours the general alarm went off, and everyone had to "stand to" outside their respective quarters for an hour or so. The MPs were running all over the place, checking out the fencing around the nurses' quarters, and making sure the roll calls were accurately made. It took several days to get the real story, which was as follows. Charlie had gotten in the compound but fallen asleep under one of the nurses' Quonset huts, and his snoring gave away his presence. One of the nurses reported the incident, and all hell broke loose. End of story.

To complete the circle I'll share the story of one particular flight lieutenant. It seems he and a nurse had gone to the movies and then on a

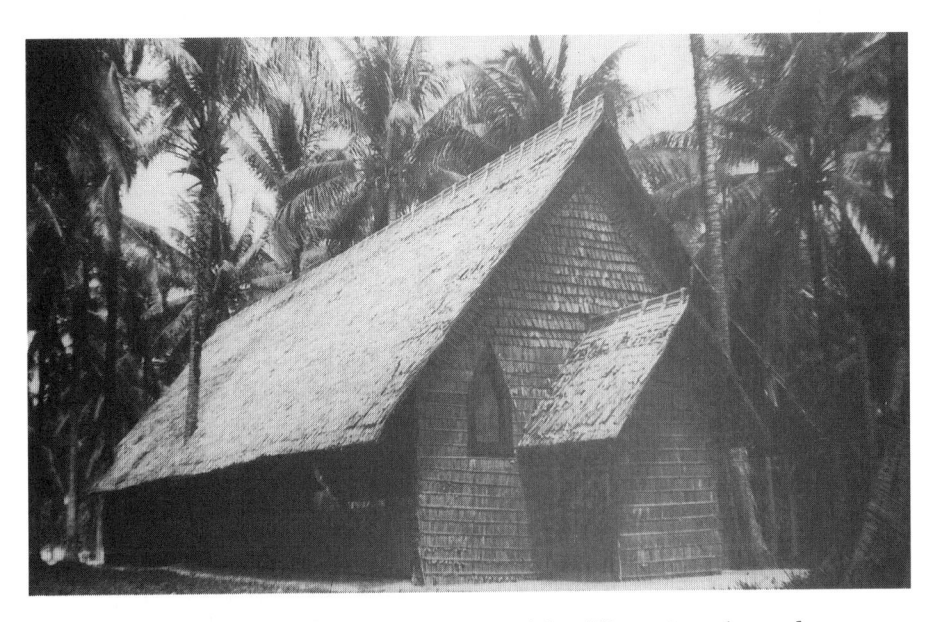

Chapel built on Banika by navy CBs and native labor. The natives observed a special Mass there on Christmas Eve 1944. "Beautiful singing of hymns was a real blessing to all who heard."—Forrest Walker. *Courtesy of Forrest Walker.*

drive to the moonlight parking spot known to many of the officers. It seems he got a little rambunctious with his lady friend, his pistol went off and blew out a good sized hole in his gluteus maximus. He couldn't lie on his back or sit for a couple of weeks. Needless to say, he was the butt of jokes for the duration of his assignment on Banika. The cover story was put out that he was shot by persons unknown as he checked the jeep for some mechanical problem.

New Station Tulagi

Quite a few family men were being rotated home on the point system, so the anticipation for movement stateside was growing. My name came up on a list, but instead of stateside the orders sent me to the island of Tulagi where I was assigned duty in the small hospital there for an indefinite time. I got my gear together and with seabag and hammock properly secured, boarded a small APC [All Purpose Craft] vessel and said goodbye to Banika and the Russell Islands. We left by the same channel that we came in on, but this time crossed north of Savo Island, and as we passed by we heard the first news that a "superbomb" had been dropped on Hiroshima and that it had destroyed much of that Japanese naval base and city.

The one amenity located at Tulagi was a refrigerated drinking fountain, and with the tropical heat there, that is something most unforgettable. It was also the fountain where I received great relief from dental pain from a dry socket that had developed after an extraction. The dispensary had two Quonset huts linked together with about 20 beds in each one, and it actually served as a small hospital. The corpsmen and pharmacy shared another Quonset hut, and another set of buildings housed the surgery and other facilities.

A road built by the Seabees circled the island a few feet above the high-water mark. I recall that I could walk around one half of the island in 25 minutes. We could explore the machine gun pits and wander most anywhere about the island, as most of the ordnance materials had been removed some time before. There was very little flat area, and what did exist had been covered with buildings, and the remainder of the island was very rugged and densely covered with typical jungle growth. Our most distinguished guest while I was assigned to ward duty was the son of a village chief. He was about 16 years old and had welts on his back where the Japanese had beaten him for some infraction after their occupation of the island almost four years before. He could speak very good

English and seemed to enjoy easy talking with any who took the time to listen.

On the second day of ward duty I watched a corpsman give an older patient a shot in the buttock and noted the loud yell from the one stuck. It didn't surprise me because the manner in which he gave the shot was, in no way, by the book. He placed the needle on the surface of the skin and just pushed it slowly in. I told the corpsman to call me when the next shot was due, and I would see if we could be a little easier on the poor patient. The patient was actually a merchant mariner who, along with his buddy, had pneumonia. I prepared and administered the shot with all the zip, zing, and flourish of an old timer, although it had been six months since I had given anyone a shot. Much to the patient's surprise, he had been given the shot while I was talking, and he didn't even feel it.

Goin' Home

About the first of November I received orders to go Stateside, which was, of course, music to my ears. Dr. Ernie had just left, and the last of the patients were accompanied by him over to Guadalcanal. That left a new warrant officer and three enlisted men to close down the dispensary operation. We were sent over to the "Canal" on an LCT along with a lot of supplies, and were put ashore for a few hours until a ship known as the AKA 159 USS *Darke* was docked. We boarded her by a gangplank, and it was our first real step back into civilization. There were four landing craft in the davits, and the larger caliber guns were still installed. Some of the really scary types said they kept all the ships "at the ready" in case the "Russkies" got some ideas.

We pulled into San Francisco Bay and stood offshore for an hour or so and moved slowly toward a long wharf to tie up and offload. When we were still a hundred yards off, I noticed a large man with hat, coat, and tie strolling out onto the open part of the pier. I was in my dungarees as were all the enlisted men in transit, and I had climbed up onto as high a spot as any of the "troops" were allowed to go. The man on the pier took his right hand in an exaggerated way and grabbed his ear. A half a minute later he did it again. So I did it right away, and he repeated it. At this time I remarked to some of the fellows nearby that the man, still a great distance away, was my dad. Of course the kidding started in and the remarks about getting a medical discharge not being necessary now, so on. But it *was* my dad. Those of us who had people waiting at dockside were told they had 30 minutes to say hello and then go by navy bus to

Treasure Island, where we would all be reunited with our seabags and stand by until released for liberty.

There were no bunks available at Treasure Island, so everyone was told to go ashore as soon as possible and return in 24 hours for further information or orders. We did this for several days until orders were posted regarding leaves or assignments. Of course, I spent that first night with the folks out at San Quentin. I stayed in town the second night and went to the El Patio Dance Hall on Market Street. This was a place which was frequented by many service personnel and some civilians. On this night, November 20, 1945, I had no idea of what was to happen to me and that it would have a most profound effect on the rest of my life.

I met a navy yeoman by the name of Helen Moses from Indianapolis, Indiana. We danced the evening away, gabbing most of the time, and for my part I tried to find out all I could about her before the evening ended. Her quarters were on Sutter Street, six or eight blocks away, so, of course, we hoofed it. After the goodnight stuff I caught a bus for San Rafael and then hitched a ride out to the prison. The folks, who both worked for the Department of Corrections, lived in a state-owned house just outside the main gate. As I came in I noticed that Mom's reading light was still on, so I stuck my head in to say hello and goodnight before hitting the sofa. Mom repeated the story many times in the following years, stating that she knew that I had met the girl I was going to marry because I had that look in my eyes and the sound in my voice that gave it away. (Mom always thought she had a little clairvoyance in her make-up.)

I had to report into Terminal Island, San Pedro, for reassignment about this time, so off I went again, fully expecting an assignment to some naval hospital at least for a few months because physio personnel were frozen, and I would have to serve a while longer.

I got into a line and soon was at the window. I was asked for my papers and asked a few questions, then told to go to "window B," which was the window for those getting out of the service. I didn't say a word, but went to that window where they stamped some things and gave me a pay envelope. Then I asked, "What's next?" He said he didn't have any idea; it was entirely up to me as I was out of the navy. I heard some chuckles as I left and went into the lounge. I sat down—collapsed would be a better description—and I remember thinking, "Wow! What now?" After a short time I went to the phone and called the folks as I knew Helen was to be there for New Year's Eve. I said "Hi" and quickly asked for Helen and said right off, "We've got a big change in plans; I'm out of the navy as of now." It was December 30, 1945. Thus closed my military career....

Chapter Thirty-Two

British Red Cross Nurse
Mona Stanton

Mona Stanton of Auckland, New Zealand, was only 20 when she joined the British Red Cross. She spent four and a half years on active service overseas.

At the outbreak of war my whole family was on holiday in Great Britain, and my father immediately joined a New Zealand battalion that formed over there and was sent to the Middle East. My mother and four younger siblings were lucky enough to get passage on a ship and were able to return to New Zealand in 1941. My younger brother joined the Air Force and was sent to Canada to train as a pilot. At the time I was working for the BBC, but resigned to join the British Red Cross to serve as a nurse for the duration of the war.

In Great Britain when someone joined the Red Cross they were posted to either the navy, army or air force. I was lucky enough to serve in the navy. Even though I served in Royal Naval Hospitals they were onshore, but we used nautical terms, so that if we left the hospital to go out for the evening it was termed "going ashore." The cabin was the small office at the end of every ward. I tried very hard to transfer on to a hospital ship, in the hopes that I may get to the Pacific and see my family from time to time, but this never happened.

Only trained nurses can be made sisters; one sister was in charge of each ward. Above them was the matron who mainly played an administrative role, but was in charge of all nursing personnel.

As a Red Cross volunteer what little training I had was as a nurse. The only registered nurses we had were the sisters, one to a ward. The nurses who were training to become registered nurses were in the civilian hospitals doing their training. Apart from the base naval hospital I was in for a few months and a few around the country, most forces hospitals were huge palatial homes which had been adapted. The hospital I served in for some years had previously been an old people's home.

All Red Cross nurses were young women who had left their own careers to nurse the masses of casualties for the duration of the war. Indeed, Britain's own Princess Royal (Princess Mary, the only daughter of King George V), was a V.A.D. in the First World War. My colleagues had come from all walks of life. They were office workers, typists, telephonists, housemaids, shop assistants, and dancers, and many of the British gentry also joined up as nurses.

I was lucky as I had learned first aid in the Girl Guides and had had a fortnight pressure-cooker course given by the Red Cross in London, and was also able to spend a fortnight on a civilian ward before I was posted to my first Royal Navy hospital. Some of my peers didn't even have that much, as we were so short, and there were so many casualties, when a ship was torpedoed for instance. Often several ships in a convoy were sunk. But for the Red Cross V.A.D., there was no one else to nurse them. Even though we did not have the theory, we became very efficient practical nurses, and did the work of nurses who had trained for many years to pass exams. We always had a sister on a ward for any advice if we needed it. All dressings and treatments were written up in the treatment book.

At first it was pretty horrific, the severe casualties we had to nurse. Often when I felt I couldn't take it any longer, the reality hit me that if I didn't do my job, it wouldn't be done. When I was nursing the first of the POWs that had been rescued from Japanese prison camps, the only thing that kept me going was the thought, "I am lucky I am the nurse and not the patient." There were very few who could not carry on and had to leave; others were given alternative jobs such as working in the library or the dispensary.

In 1996 came the publication of Four Glorious Years, *Mona Stanton's memoir of her World War II service. In that memoir she writes:*

Reporting to each nurse in turn, I found I had to watch a DCL, a patient on the Dangerous Case List, who had been given approximately only two more hours to live. The staff had been expecting the worst at any time, as he'd had a temporal operation that morning, and had not yet recovered

Opposite: **Mona Stanton.** *Courtesy of Mona Stanton.*

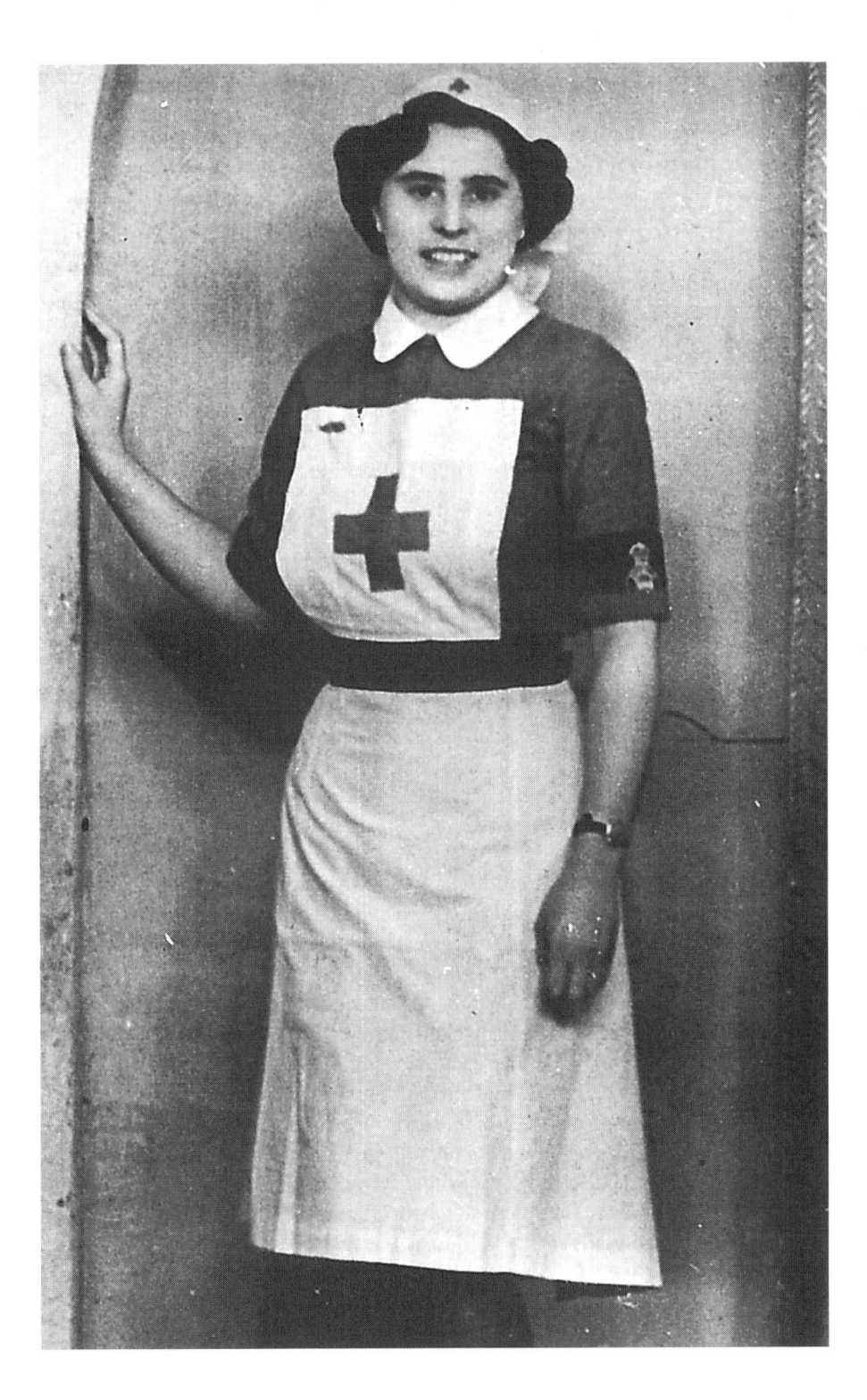

consciousness. Studying his bed-ticket in the cabin first, I then silently entered between the screens that surrounded his bed. Only 22 and not even on his own soil weighted my heart. The little I could see of all that was left visible, from a large, pure white turban of bandages and cotton-wool, gave me the impression there was a decent family or some-one, hoping and waiting for his return. Man had pitched in all his skill on this delicate op, and now no-one but God could determine his destiny. Silently praying with all the reverence at my command, I pleaded from my heart that he be allowed to at least get home. As the silence of the night gradually wore on, he still just lay there unresponsive to my taking his TPR, Temperature, Pulse and Respiration, every quarter of an hour. His expected time came and went without a movement. When my relief came for me to go to supper, I did not want to go ... [and I didn't even feel] hungry. I wanted to see this boy come round. With his temperature down to 95, and his respirations which were very hard to take dropped to 10, his pulse rate down to only 44, and midnight ... come and gone, I still did not want to leave, nor could they convince me I must have a break. The long vigil lost its tension, when at 2 A.M. he slowly opened his eyes and asked, "What's the time, Nurse?" I seemed conscious of my whole body and mind relaxing as he quietly spoke, and felt my prayers had been answered. He would at least go home to his own people.

Elsewhere in Four Glorious Years, *Mona relates what it was like tending a severe injury that took her completely by surprise.*

Before any conversation could take place with the older patient, "Nurse, would you do the arm dressing?" was asked of me. Standing alongside the dressing trolley was a tall patient, wearing a jacket over his white shirt.

"Is it your dressing I have to do?" I inquired.

"Yes, nurse, you only have to use meths and rub it well in," he told me, as he began removing his jacket sleeve.

To my horror his whole arm came off. I was speechless and could only drink in the sickening realization that this rugged young man would have to go through life with only one arm. The other was artificial.

Commandeering my self control, and suppressing the nauseating feeling that seemed to shock my whole system, I did exactly as I was asked to, and thanked my guardian angel for giving me the strength to overcome my emotional shock. As soon as the task was completed, my shock must have registered visibly, as although not fainting, I became aware of Sister asking me if I was all right. When I replied in the affirmative, she asked a nurse who ushered me to the ward galley to make me a cup of tea.

32. British Red Cross Nurse

Mona also describes what it was like nursing the returned POWs from Japanese prison camps.

Soon the Hospital Ship *Oranje* arrived in Sydney. Our wards were almost empty, and we had been having a pretty easy time. While having afternoon tea, the first POWs began to arrive. As I looked up the ramp to where they were coming down towards our ward, I had never in my life witnessed such a heart-rending horrible sight. How any human being could possibly survive in such a state of deplorable malnutrition, and sheer neglect, is beyond human comprehension. A surge of hatred rose and subsided as each emaciated individual either walked, or was helped, or was borne on a stretcher towards us. I could not believe my eyes. My God, it isn't possible that they are really still alive, stuck in my throat.

With a weeping heart, and tears burning the backs of my eyes, I silently and unnoticed slipped behind the galley door. Determinedly summoning my self-control, I was sandwiched in by my colleague, who broke down, too. Smiling at each other through our tears, we egged each other on to start work, but neither of us moved. Before we had time to reappear, Sister called us as she too peeped round the door. With misty, sad eyes, "I'm coming, too," she whispered. "In all my years of nursing, and I have had some shocking cases, I have never seen anything like this in all my life," she quietly told us. Comforted by her sincere natural understanding, we suppressed our emotional shock and began with our usual calm efficiency, which had developed over the years, to receive our pathetically wasted patients.

Tucking in one patient who just stared glassily at every move I made, I learned she had an abdominal cancer, and had suffered excruciating pain for six months, with no drugs or treatment whatsoever. Not even any proper food to give her a few moments respite. Her condition was so serious, there was no hope of optimistic speculation, and she was transferred after a rest later that same afternoon to a civilian hospital, where she died a fortnight later. Her one wish was to hang on, until she got to her own soil, and [she] was granted that wish.

Many bore the telltale marks of inhuman acts of sadism. Many broke down just to see the long forgotten comfort of white sheets, to rest their exhausted bodies between. It was impossible to comprehend how they had survived. One felt so desolate and inadequate, as for so long they had been completely deprived of relief or palliation. Into our sympathetic ears poured many tragic stories. The Red Cross emblazoned on the bib of our spotless white aprons, signifying our status, put us on a pedestal to them. Many of their eyes filled with tears. While still in captive hands most had openly wept, just to see the Union Jack hoisted again. "Oh, nurse, you are so kind and gentle" fell on most of our ears, touching our hearts very deeply, as we were only doing the job we had joined up to do.

Leaving the ward next day to collect the lunch from the main galleys, I noticed, too, that there were a lot of New Zealanders amongst them. In a passive way they wandered about, with a glassy look in their eyes, and some seemed so vacant. Some were yellow from Atabrine, and some were fat and flabby from Beri-Beri. Pity, anger, hatred and fear surged through my whole body. Pity for the unnecessary, deplorable suffering these one time normal people had been forced to suffer, many of whom were [once] our nation's ... finest, fittest and best men[;] ... [m]any of whom I knew would never feel the great blessing of robust health again. Anger that such sadistical brutality should have been so wantonly administered to such one time useful people. Hatred that any nation should have acquired through sheer lack of common decency and respect the free right to massacre, and torture, as their warped minds wished[.] ... [A]nd fear, that without the courage, tenacity and phenomenal tolerance and suffering that these heroic and gallant prisoners had portrayed, we could so easily have also been in their shoes.

Reflecting on her experiences, Mona Stanton wrote in a letter to Patricia Sewell:

Little did I know that while I was away on active service, New Zealand had come perilously close to an invasion by the Japanese. It was the Americans and Australians in the Coral Sea, and just a month later the fierce battle with very heavy casualties in the Battle of Midway, that stopped their advance further south in the Pacific, and brought relief from the threat of invasion. I do not think that many New Zealanders realize just how close it was.

Mona Stanton's memoir, Four Glorious Years, *was published by Pen Press Publishers. 39-41 North Road, Islington, London N7 9DP, England. The ISBN (for ordering) is 1 900796 05 8.*

Chapter Thirty-Three

Treating the Wounded in the Battle of the Bulge

Henry M. Hills, Jr., M.D.

Dr. Hills, along with nine other young army doctors and surgical technicians, was airdropped behind the perimeter defenses of the 101st Airborne Division at Bastogne, Belgium. The 101st was trapped inside the German offensive squeeze known as "The Bulge." With their medical teams cut off by the German advance, hundreds of wounded GIs lay untreated and dying in an old motor garage.

The following is a condensation of an interview with Dr. Hills (with comments from his wife, Willie) conducted by Dr. Michael O. Fidler on June 24, 1994, for the 50th anniversary of the events of December 1944.

Dr. Hills: I was at Massachusetts General Hospital when the war started [in 1941]. I was finishing my orthopedic training. Shortly thereafter I was supposed to go to Children's Hospital for another nine months, but the army decided I'd had enough children's, enough training altogether—they needed me in the army.

MOF: Were you drafted?

Dr. Hills: Well, no, I went ahead and signed up. And I went to Washington, D.C., to Walter Reed Army Hospital, and was there till I got assigned to the 12th Evac Hospital...

MOF: What other experiences in the army come to mind in the months prior to D-Day?

Dr. Hills: I was in England for 18 months. Our unit took care of the Eighth Air Force in all their bombing runs over France and Germany. And we worked like hell. We had a big clinic. The most notorious thing was the "3B fracture"—Beer, Blackout, and Bicycle—they all broke their radial heads.

Then, just before the invasion, we were put in Patton's army, the Third Army. The first directive we got was, "If you do not take the objective and are not killed or mortally wounded in the attempt, you will be court-martialed."

MOF: You mentioned casualties from the Eighth Air Force. What kinds of battlefield injuries did you take care of in England?

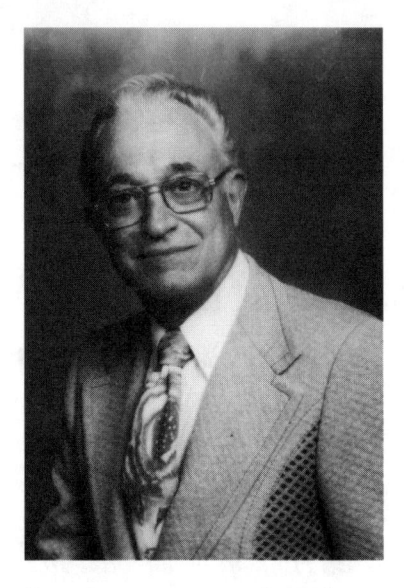

Dr. Henry M. Hills, Jr., today.
Courtesy of Dr. Henry M. Hills, Jr.

Dr. Hills: Well, all kinds of planes were shot down. Planes would come back with a lot of wounded. We took care of every kind of thing—gunshot wounds of the extremities.

MOF: Did you do strictly orthopedic surgery?

Dr. Hills: Oh, yes. There were two orthopedic surgeons in our unit—Fred Knocke, who was a friend of mine, and myself.

MOF: You would see all sorts of gunshot-inflicted open fractures and so forth?

Dr. Hills: Uh-huh. I remember that the B-26 was no good. They shot them completely to the ground. They went into low-level bombing, and they weren't made for that. [The Germans] would have guns set up in church steeples and hit them head-on, and destroyed the whole bunch. Didn't any of them come back.

The big bombing runs were, of course, to Ploeste and those places. Most of the Eighth Air Force was B-17s.

MOF: What were you doing on D-Day?

Dr. Hills: We were set up in a hospital on the English coast to receive patients from the D-Day invasion. We were up all night watching planes take off the night before—paratroopers and gliders and so forth. It went on for hours. We received patients from the D-Day landing and worked on them.

MOF: Were they different from things that you'd seen before in any way?

DR. HILLS: Pretty much the same. You couldn't do any open reduction work—but you could clean up the wound and leave it packed open.

MOF: Do you remember any particular patients from that day?

DR. HILLS: We took care of some of the Afrika Korps, and boy they were mean, tough bastards. They were scared to death, but they were mean.

MOF: Did you have an unusually long day of work on D-Day?

DR. HILLS: Well, the Third Army didn't go in until they had a real, good-sized beachhead. The Third Army was made up of two tank divisions for every infantry division, a heavy striking force. One infantry division would punch a hole, then the tanks would go up and down the line and tear the enemy to pieces. [The Germans] were scared to death of [General Patton], and they needed to be. We had a terrible striking force.

I thought of one thing [about D-Day]. One guy came back who had been on Omaha beach, and he had a buddy that was shot right beside him. And he went berserk. He found a rabbit running around there, and he got that rabbit and started carrying it around with him, and that was his "buddy." And then the rabbit was killed, and he really went to pot. He came into our unit wild as a coot—you couldn't hold him down or do anything with him. He got loose one time and ran around the fields there with no clothes on, trying to get somewhere, but he was completely out of his head. This was at the beachhead. But the funny thing was that when we got to Luxembourg, here came this guy, and he had two Silver Stars and a couple of Purple Hearts, and he said, "Once you go crazy and get over it, hell, nothing happens to you then!"

MOF: So we're on the beaches at Normandy now. Tell me about what happened to you next. What were some of your movements on the way to what became the Bulge?

DR. HILLS: We walked I don't know how many miles carrying a pack, but I know it was all night. It must have been 20 or 30 miles. We got to pitch a tent and lay down and rest a bit. I found a nice, soft spot and lay down to sleep—I came to learn in the morning that that was a covered-over latrine!

MOF: So you slept in a latrine in France!

Dr. Hills: They had German prisoners in wire enclosures along the way, and we had nurses marching along, and the prisoners would do a lot of yelling at the nurses.

MOF: You were carrying your own personal gear?

Dr. Hills: We had to carry all our stuff, our bedroll and so forth.

MOF: You were how old at the time?

Dr. Hills: Probably 24.

MOF: So when you got up out of that latrine, where did you head?

Dr. Hills: I can't remember specifically. We operated hospitals right along [with the movement of the front].

MOF: We've all seen the *M*A*S*H* movies and so forth. What was the routine at your field hospital? Did you typically operate for endless hours, for example?

Dr. Hills: Yes. We had a 12-hour shift [in surgery], but the other 12 hours you had to spend going over your records and charts and checking your patients, and so forth. So you probably got four or five hours' sleep, something like that. Then you'd come on your 12-hour shift, and they'd have them all packed up behind you waiting to be done. It would go on interminably.

MOF: Was much of the surgery fairly routine to you, or was it challenging?

Dr. Hills: Pretty much challenging. There were a lot of severe wounds such as hip wounds and so forth. And that's where I lost my cool. We were in Luxembourg, in a hospital building. I had a Luxembourger who was to help around my surgery unit, and he didn't know any English at all, and I didn't know his language. At that time I was working real hard, a lot of stressful things. I'd had 20 or 30 lined up when I came on duty—

MOF: Would that be typical, 20 or 30?

Dr. Hills: Yes. And I'd get them done and think, "Good, next time I come on there won't be so many." Well, next time there would be 20 or 30 or 40. So I'd get to the point where things would happen, like I was in a hip and a bleeder would get loose, and I'd utter a swear word or two, and I'd clamp the damn thing, and it would come loose, so I would clamp it and tie it again, and it would start to come loose. I'd utter some special words, and I finally got to where I was even throwing some instruments, getting kind of wild. And I made up my mind I wasn't going to say another word, wasn't going to do a thing, no matter what happened.

Well, I got into a hip again, and a gluteal vessel came loose, and I had a hell of a time with it, but I didn't say anything. But I picked up an instrument and I threw it down, and this Luxembourger says, "Gott dammit!"

MOF: So he picked up the language!

Dr. Hills: Yep!

MOF: I was going to ask you later whether you ever felt sort of inadequate, with the limitations in equipment and facilities and so forth.

Dr. Hills: I think we did a pretty good job really. When we were at Nancy we came under the long [German] siege guns. They shelled our hospital. We had a 750 pound shell buried twenty feet in the ground right below our unit, right at the corner of our hospital, of our orthopedic ward. It didn't go off, fortunately. They came in regular as time. Just as you'd go off to sleep—"WHEEEEEEE"—in would come another one. And then they would move the siege gun a little further down the line before anyone could hit it. It was on a railroad track.

MOF: Where were you when the Bulge became a focus of Allied concern?

Dr. Hills: I was at Nancy. They asked for volunteers. [Capt. Edward N.] Zinschlag and I volunteered. We volunteered to parachute in.

MOF: Which you had never done?

Dr. Hills: No. I had never been in a glider either, for that matter.

MOF: So, being a 24 year old, you just figured, "What the heck?"

Dr. Hills: No. I was so mad because we were back of the lines, and I was getting a bunch of crud, and it disgusted me so.

MOF: What would you mean by "crud"?

Dr. Hills: We were getting a bunch of crud sent in that were no-goods, soldiers who were trying to get out. And it made me so mad, and the way I felt about those people that were in [the Bulge] ... I thought, "Dammit, that's where I should be."

MOF: What was your unit at this point?

Dr. Hills: The 12th Evac Hospital, attached to the Third Army.

MOF: How many people were involved in an Evac hospital?

Dr. Hills: There were about six surgical teams. There were two orthopedic teams, a medical unit, and a neuropsychiatric unit. There was a neurosurgeon there, but not a full neurosurgery team. We had a couple of psychiatrists. We had a large medical unit with probably 20 internists. Patton wouldn't go to that. They were a bunch of gold bricks to him. The orthopedic teams each had a surgeon and two technicians. You had your ward, with nurses on your ward.

I did some special work while I was there. I don't know whether you know about "crush syndrome" that the English dealt with in the bombing raids?

MOF: No.

Dr. Hills: They lost a lot of people, limbs particularly, due to crushing injury. The arteries would go into spasm. We got a lot of those same problems when the Germans started using explosive-nosed bullets. They would penetrate with a small wound and then explode and just destroy the whole thigh. The major artery would be just like a little white cord. The British decided that you needed to cut the main artery, in that case, to let the collateral circulation take over. Well, I got into those and looked into what we could do to save those. I found that if you peeled off every bit of adventitia around that artery, it would expand again. I got a bunch of these, and my nurse got very capable [in recognizing them], and she would send a message up to me in surgery that we had another one.

I wrote a little article on it and sent it through channels. Then the 12th Evac was designated the "vascular injury center"! But the war ended before we started seeing any referrals.

With this technique, I never again had to cut the main artery. They all expanded with this local sympathectomy.

MOF: ...Were most of the wounds that you saw in the lower extremities?

Dr. Hills: No, arms and legs, both.

MOF: What about spinal injuries, did you see those?

Dr. Hills: I didn't see any spinal injuries. I suspect those were sent along to the general hospital without much done in the field, I suspect.

MOF: Did you see life-threatening wounds or only wounds that could be treated definitively for return to duty, or how was that divided?

Dr. Hills: We didn't see any minor wounds. Those could be handled by the general surgery teams. We only saw major injuries to the bones and joints and skeleton.

MOF: And your patients would typically be shipped back from the front after your care?

Dr. Hills: After we cleaned them up, got them into a spica cast or whatever. I even developed a thing for traction [for transport], but it didn't turn out because you just couldn't spend the time on it. I used a fish scale, and I would put a pin in the distal femur and a long leg cast with a projection at the lower end to attach the fish scale to, so you could adjust the tension to 25 pounds. But when you get two or three hundred patients in at one time, you don't have time to do those nice things.

MOF: What about all the cast work? That must have been a tremendous amount of physical work.

Dr. Hills: Oh, yes. And, of course, you had to do all the lifting yourself. You didn't have anybody to help you.

MOF: What was an operating table like in your hospital?

Dr. Hills: Most of the time we had fairly good tables, but sometimes it was just a cot on two saw horses. We did cast work on the same table. Some of the cast material was terrible; you couldn't use the damn stuff. Somebody was trying to make a lot of money on it. It was no good from the beginning.

MOF: What about wound management?

Dr. Hills: Clean it out good, pack it open, immobilize the fractures, medication. Close [the wound] later after they got back to the general hospital.

MOF: Did you do any kind of internal fixation?

Dr. Hills: We weren't allowed to. In fact, they insisted you couldn't put a cast on a fractured hand. Well, I just did it anyway—what a bunch of nonsense. They make rules for the least trained of anybody. I could take care of those hands and get some semblance of alignment and position so they had some hope of getting reasonable function.

I was sort of a renegade. In fact I had a sign—"Renegade Society"—that went with me wherever we went.

MOF: We've heard about the Kunscher nail for femur fractures being seen in returning POWs.

Dr. Hills: While I was in England, I did some temporary duty in Bristol, and some of those came back, the first they had seen. The story was the Germans were putting them in their troops and sending them back to the lines in two days.

The interesting thing is that if you can keep the injured guy close to the action and close to his buddies until he recovers, he will go back to the fight. But once he gets back to the general hospital, he's gone for good. Their attitude is, "Oh, what the hell. Let them do it." The same is true of workers compensation today. If you can keep the worker in touch with his workplace and fellow workers, he's more likely to go back to work.

MOF: Did you know any of the people trapped in the Bulge?

Dr. Hills: No. But I've had contacts with people who were there who have spoken to me about it back here since. I didn't know them while I was there because I was working all the time.

MOF: But you didn't hear about the Bulge situation and learn that someone you knew was out there in it?

Dr. Hills: Well, I had it happen to me. At the time I was in Nancy, when we volunteered to go, we had a fellow who was a commander of a tank corps, the Sixth Armored. And he was having too good a time. He was enjoying having the nurses in, having a drink in the evening at the officers' club and so forth—he didn't want to go back to work. He didn't want to go back in there. But, when I volunteered to go, he left the next morning. He said, "We'll get you out of there." And he did.

MOF: Do you remember who actually came around and asked for volunteers?

Dr. Hills: I don't know—some general I think, or possibly a full colonel in the Medical Corps. What the Germans had done was pinch out all the medical personnel from the 101st Airborne. They only had one medical officer for the whole unit. They had to get somebody in there. When we got there, they had been lying there in this garage for eight to ten days, dying like flies from gas gangrene.

MOF: How well did you know the other medical personnel you went in with?

Dr. Hills: Oh, the two sergeants and Dr. Zinschlag, I knew very well—we worked together. Now I didn't know the fellows from the other unit. They were from the Fourth Auxiliary Surgical Unit.

The anesthesiologist, Dr. Weslowski, could give spinal anesthesia and sodium pentothal. That's what we did work on. I even had one of the cooks give pentothal on the last case I did. Scared him to death.

MOF: When you volunteered, how much did you know about what you were getting into? Did they tell you much about conditions in the Bulge or about your chances?

Dr. Hills: They didn't say anything about the chances, they just said they needed help. They said there were about 800 casualties in a garage. My wife has never quite forgiven me.

MOF: I was about to ask you that. Did Willie have any idea at the time what you were getting into?

Dr. Hills: They were not supposed to have anything put in the papers about it. And we wrote letters and so forth in case we didn't come back. They were not supposed to put anything in the papers until we got back. But the next day they had it [in] the Chicago *Tribune* and Des Moines papers. Willie was in Iowa City at the time. She knew about it the next day. And [my son] Henry said, "Does that mean Daddy's coming home?"

MOF: So Willie couldn't forgive you?

Dr. Hills: Well, she didn't see how I could do it with a wife and small child at home. I just told her I felt that that's what I needed to do. The people saw it in the paper and came around and said, "Is this your husband that was in this?"

MOF (to Willie Hills): Henry says you never forgave him for going on this mission.

Willie: I never said any such thing.

MOF: What was going on with you at the time? What went through your mind?

Willie: Well, it was difficult. We had this child, two and a half, Henry had never even seen yet, and he was very smart and picked up on all the news around him. And he started jumping up and down and saying, "Oh, goody! Does this mean Daddy's coming home soon?" Which was about the worst statement he could make. It was hard to explain things to him.

MOF: Do you remember how you felt?

WILLIE: Well, I thought, it would be about the type of thing Henry would do. If I hadn't realized that, I'd probably be madder than heck. But I thought, "Sounds just like him."

MOF (to Dr. Hills): How much time did you have between volunteering and actually leaving?

DR. HILLS: Christmas Day. We wrote our letters and so forth.

MOF: Did you have a Christmas dinner or something special?

DR. HILLS: Nope. One of the nurses gave me a St. Anthony's necklace and wanted me to wear it, so I did. I gave it back to her when I got back. We had some Christmas presents to open, and then we put them aside and got our gear together to get ready to go.

MOF: Did anybody talk much about the way they felt?

DR. HILLS: Not really. It was cold, winter—snow all over.

MOF: Did you have any doubt that you would get in safely?

DR. HILLS: No. Never occurred to me. It was just something we had to do.

MOF: What did you know about glider operations at the time?

DR. HILLS: This was the first time medical personnel had ever been flown behind enemy lines. We knew of course that many gliders had wrecked on D-Day and that they wrecked pretty easily. We had two pilots in the glider, and they had their Tommy guns. They went into the [infantry] line as soon as they got the thing down.

MOF: When did you find out that you weren't going to have to parachute in?

DR. HILLS: At the airstrip. They decided at the last minute that they needed to send in a lot of supplies. So they loaded up the gliders with blood, plasma, instruments, and so forth.

MOF: But up to the last minute, you understood you were going to parachute in. You had never done that. How were you going to learn how to do it?

DR. HILLS: Well, I assumed somebody was going to tell us what to do. Of course, I'd never been in a glider either.

MOF: Do you remember how you felt as you were about to get yanked into the air in that glider?

Dr. Hills: Well, that's a funny feeling. You don't get yanked. You're sitting there on the ground, and along comes this C-47 and the rope gets picked up. It stretches out, and you just gently start moving and go up into the air, going faster and faster. But when they cut you loose, it's like hitting a brick wall.

MOF: How long were you in the air?

Dr. Hills: We had to go about a hundred miles. We were in the air I guess maybe an hour.

MOF: Did you carry a weapon?

Dr. Hills: No. The gliders had big red crosses on them. The Germans shot at them. They mostly missed, but put a few up through the tail. I understand some bullets came through the cabin, but I didn't personally see it. We came in for a nice, smooth landing. But we landed between the lines. There was a row of trees on each side and a nice field in the center. A GI with long whiskers came out and said, "What the hell are you doing out there? This is the outermost outpost of the 101st Airborne. Get the hell in here!"

About that time [rockets] started to take off. They sound like a covey of birds taking off. They were shooting over in the general area. So we got down in a shallow area for protection.

You can't build a foxhole in frozen ground with a helmet. You just can't do it! I tried!

Then they took us in two at a time, with supplies, in a jeep. We had to cover three miles of open road with sharp, hairpin turns. We got in, and the driver said, "Now look. We're going to go as fast as we can go, and we're going to go from the ditch on one side of the road to the one on the other side. We won't let up on the speed—if we do, the mortars will get us. [The Germans] have got it all zeroed in along the road." And we did. We got mortars coming in right behind us all the way "Whump. Whump. Whump." But as long as you kept up your speed you were alright. Nobody got hurt. We got to the garage, and it was a large area with a parachute for a door in front. As soon as you lifted up that parachute door to go in you could smell gas gangrene. Here were these creatures, lying on parachute cloths, no lights. There were some women from Bastogne there trying to help, giving them water and so forth. And [the men] were dying like flies. They'd been there for ten days with wounds that were now gas gangrene.

The only light was at the far side, where mechanics did repairs. There was a field stove there with coffee brewing. The light was not good light but some light. They had four tables set up—stretchers on saw horses. Once you used your instruments [the first time], they weren't sterile anymore. They had a great big vat filled with alcohol. After a case, we dumped all our instruments and gloves into the vat. We had no gowns or masks, of course. For the next case, you'd reach into the vat and put your gloves on wet, pick out the instruments you needed, and go to work.

One man in my group acted as triage officer. The bottom floor of the garage had 400 serious casualties. The top floor had 400 walking casualties. We didn't bother with them.

MOF: Do you remember any specific patients that you feel survived because of your efforts?

Dr. Hills: Oh, there were several, no question. The first night I was there the triage officer came to me and said there was a boy in terrible shape who was not going to survive until morning. We had lost all but six pints of our plasma [in the landing]. He said, "Let's give him a pint of blood and a couple of pints of plasma and get his leg off." So we took him in and did it. He was moribund—didn't need any anesthesia; he was out, he was dying. Fever of 105 degrees. The next morning one of the nurses came in and said he wanted to talk to me. And he thanked me. He made it.

During the course of doing this work, one of the [infantry] colonels got a little perturbed because I was taking limbs off. He came down to see what was going on and said, "I understand you're taking them off right and left here." I said, "Yep, those that need to come off." He said, "Well, I'm not quite sure they do." So I picked a limb up and handed it to him. He just about passed out. He never said another word.

MOF: Did you ever get a chance to assess the situation for the fighting men in the Bulge? Was it organized or chaotic?

Dr. Hills: Oh, they were organized. They were tough; they were tough boys. They only had nine rounds of artillery shells left when I went in. They couldn't get supplies in because of the weather.

MOF: Did they seem upbeat about getting out of the situation OK?

Dr. Hills: Well, they were glad to see us. I don't think they worried much about it. They needed supplies and ammunition. They broke through to them about 50 hours after I got there.

33. Treating the Wounded in the Battle of the Bulge

We got bombed where we were operating. It blew the doors in. It was common practice to listen for the planes coming over, droning. Then you'd hear the whistling of the bombs coming closer and closer. At a certain point you would dive under the table. Once Zinschlag and I dove under the table at the same instant, and we cracked heads, and neither one of us ended up under the table!

MOF: Was there any way to evacuate the worst patients, even to save a life?

DR. HILLS: No, not until the tanks broke through to us.

MOF: Did you have antibiotics?

DR. HILLS: We had sulfa, but no penicillin.

MOF: Did you see any cases of battle fatigue?

DR. HILLS: No. I wouldn't expect it in the 101st Airborne.

MOF: Did you ever see a soldier who shot himself in the foot intentionally?

DR. HILLS: Oh, I've got a story about that! They used to shoot the left little toe. Then they got the right little toe, then they got to the fourth toe. So it made a progression across.

Patton was making rounds on my ward. I had just gotten this guy in the night before who had been in a foxhole during an attack and had to shoot a guy entering his foxhole. In the process he accidentally shot himself in the ankle, a bad injury with destruction of the ankle joint. He was laying there in his long leg cast, and Patton comes along and says, "Son, what happened to you?" He replied, "I shot myself in the foot." Well, Patton blew up. He called him everything he could—I was embarrassed. This boy never said a word. Finally, when Patton was through scathing him, he said, "General, I've been in Africa, Sicily, Italy, France, and now Germany. If I was going to do this to get out of the service, I'd have done it a long time before." Patton went on down and saw two or three more, and then he came back and said, "Son, I'm sorry, I made a mistake."

MOF: So you worked without stopping at Bastogne?

DR. HILLS: We worked continuously for about 50 hours without a break until we were relieved at the breakthrough. My last case was a compound [fracture of the] forearm, a relatively minor case. The anesthesiologist was busy with another case, so I found this cook. I told him

I was going to start the anesthesia, and I would tell him when to push in on the syringe of pentothal a little more. He sat there sweating and did what I said. At the end he said, "Now I've done everything in the army."

MOF: What came next for you?

Dr. Hills: I went back to Nancy and went back to work. We stayed there until the war was over.

MOF: I take it you never had a need or opportunity to shoot at anybody?

Dr. Hills: I didn't have anything to shoot with.

Once, in Nancy, I had a weekend off. This medical officer from the field came by and wanted to see what we were doing there. One day he got hold of a jeep, and he said, "Let's go up to the front lines and see what's going on." So we went. We were stopped by a guard, and we asked where the front line was. He said, "This is it. That town over there, we haven't taken it yet." He offered to take us to the commanding officer. Well, this major was giving one of his captains hell, saying every time they were supposed to be leading a charge, there was something wrong with this captain's tank. "I'm beginning to think something's wrong with you," he said. "I've requested you be promoted to major to get you out of my outfit." Then he turned to me and said, "Doc, let's go into that town over there and see what's going on. I said "Fine," and he told me to take off my Red Cross arm band: "They like to shoot at those things." So we headed up the pavement, and he said to step where he stepped to avoid mines. The town was quiet. There was a disabled Tiger tank sitting there. It was an eerie feeling. We got to the center of town and found some Americans that had been shot in the head on a previous foray. The Germans had pulled out. Then some civilians came out and motioned for us to come down in a basement where they apparently had some patients. The major said, "That's fine, we've got a doc here." We went through the door and it was dark as pitch. You didn't know if you were getting into a trap or what. But they had several people who were hurt. When we came out, the sappers were there taking out mines. The major said, "It's alright. Doc and I have taken this place."

MOF: So there, you went through a dark doorway. Did you get to a point where you didn't think about things so much?

Dr. Hills: You're damn right I thought about it. That kind of got to me. You didn't know what was waiting for you down there. Really, it wasn't very smart.

MOF: Were you surprised at yourself for being able to step forward for this mission to the Bulge?

Dr. Hills: I don't think so. The fact that I was seeing crud from being back of the lines contributed to it. I thought, "Those worthless bastards. Somebody's got to do something to help those people [up front]."

MOF: You had no doubts about your preparedness?

Dr. Hills: In those days I had no doubts about anything. I could handle anything.

MOF: You hear over and over from World War II vets that "There was a job to do and we did it." Is that the way you feel, too?

Dr. Hills: That's it exactly. Somebody had to help those people in there, and better it be me.

MOF: Did your World War II experiences change you in any way?

Dr. Hills: Well, I wasn't as explosive as I used to be. I controlled my temper better. As long as it wasn't a damn motorcycle—that drove me crazy!

MOF: How about your approach to the difficulties of everyday life—did this experience make you handle them better?

Dr. Hills: I've never felt that I wasn't about to handle whatever comes along.

MOF: So who were the heroes of the Battle of the Bulge?

Dr. Hills: The 101st Airborne; they were the toughies. Of course, the Ninth Armored and some remnants of the 106th Infantry were in there, too.

MOF: You clearly admire the fighting GI.

Dr. Hills: Oh, they were something else. You don't win wars until you get down to the basics of being a beast. Until you get down to that level, you can't compete with somebody like a storm trooper. You have to be mean, ornery, with only one idea, to beat the hell out of the opponent. You have to get down to the animal instincts. If you don't have that, you're not going to win.

MOF: And you and your fellows were awarded the Silver Star for your contributions at Bastogne?

Dr. Hills: That's right.

MOF: Well, I think you earned it. Thank you.

Chapter Thirty-Four

Memories of Naval Medicine in World War II

NORTON L. FRANCIS, M.D.

Dr. Francis served in the navy from March 1942 to 1946 with ranks of lieutenant, junior grade, to lieutenant commander.

I was assigned to the United States Naval Hospital in March 1942. The chief purpose of the hospital was to care for the midshipmen. We did have some admissions for men who had been to sea and were sent to the hospital for care. We had to discontinue the use of telephones at night to the wards because, if the telephone rang, these individuals would jump out of bed and think they were at general quarters. We also found that the pharmacy did not have any sulfa drugs that had been on the market for seven years.

Midshipmen wanting to go in the submarine service were required to have surgery if they had deviation of the nasal septum. They were also required to have a psychiatric examination. After doing a week of these examinations our psychiatrist said the reason for this was that subconsciously the individual wished to get back in his mother's womb and be surrounded by all that fluid.

My next assignment in October 1943 was to Noumea, New Caledonia. It was at a receiving station. We would have ships come in from the States, and we would get from several hundred men to 3,000 men. We would send these individuals to various units that needed replacements. The only problem we had was that occasionally there would be groups who tried to disobey their orders. There was also a barracks for homosexuals. Usually when the number grew to 60 or 70, they would be returned to the States. Medical officers at the receiving station had to make rounds on them.

At Mobile Hospital #7 I was head of the ear, nose and throat (ENT) department. The purpose of the hospital was to care for local personnel of the base and receive patients from the hospital ships. A ship would arrive, and we would receive as many as 3,000 injured with Mobile Hospital #5. We had a system of triage to assess the injuries. Besides caring for the patients in my ward, I assisted the neurosurgeon in surgery. Then decisions were made to return the individual to duty or to send him back to the States.

I was transferred from there to Mobile Hospital #8. It was located on the small island of Beneka across a strait from Guadalcanal. The purpose of the hospital was to care for injuries and illnesses that occurred in personnel of the Third Marine Division located on a nearby island, where they were staging for their next invasion. We had just received penicillin for use. We found that if it was used on patients with fungus conditions, it flared the conditions up. This was particularly true in external otitis as the ear became very swollen and tender.

I found that unless one was connected to a marine division or a combat naval ship or a naval hospital ship, that most of the medicine was related to the care of incidental medical conditions associated with 18- to 28-year-old service personnel.

My next transfer was to the Great Lakes Naval Station where I was the ENT consultant. This was terminated, and I was transferred to Chicago Navy Pier to be one of five navy medical officers to set up the Model Naval Separation Center. Separation consisted of acquiring a short history of the patient to learn if there were any service-connected injuries or illness which might require pension evaluation; a physical examination and x-ray of the chest; and arrangements for their transfer home. When the model was accepted, then satellite separation centers were established. I was then assigned the officers' separation, as officer in charge.

I soon became eligible for discharge and was asked to join the regular navy. The last experiences I had indicated that I was headed for administration activities, and I preferred clinical medicine and was discharged.

Chapter Thirty-Five

More on the War
VARIOUS AUTHORS

Having received personal accounts and anecdotes that were too brief to give them a chapter, I have gathered them together and saved them for last. They represent the humorous as well as the poignant.

In 1943 a small field surgical unit of which I was 2 I.C. [second in command] (assistant surgeon and anesthetist), attached to the 24th New Zealand Field Ambulance, was stationed alongside U.S. marine forces on the island of Nissan (Green Island) just north of Bougainville and only a few miles from the Japanese base of Rabaul on New Guinea.

We had got to know U.S. troops quite well on Guadalcanal and Vela Lavella and invariably found them to be charming and generous hosts. After a particularly happy occasion in an American officer's mess on Nissan, we decided that we really must try and return their hospitality. But we lacked even the most basic of resources. We had chilli con carne and Spam and K rations designed for the Aleutian Islands rather than the tropics and New Zealand beer—good in itself but not up to the standard of the luxuries offered us by our friends.

So we did some research.

One thing we *did* have was a large container of absolute alcohol—for surgical purposes. It was decided that this should be sacrificed in the interest of international relations. After some study we came up with the idea of suspending cut limes by cotton thread over the alcohol so that the juice would drip slowly into it and give it a subtle flavor. The result was good but rather acidic. So next we added pure glycerol, a fine sweetening agent. The final ingredient was designed to give a distinctive and unforgettable color. For this we used Castellani's Carbol Fuchsin, a beautiful deep red,

35. More on the War

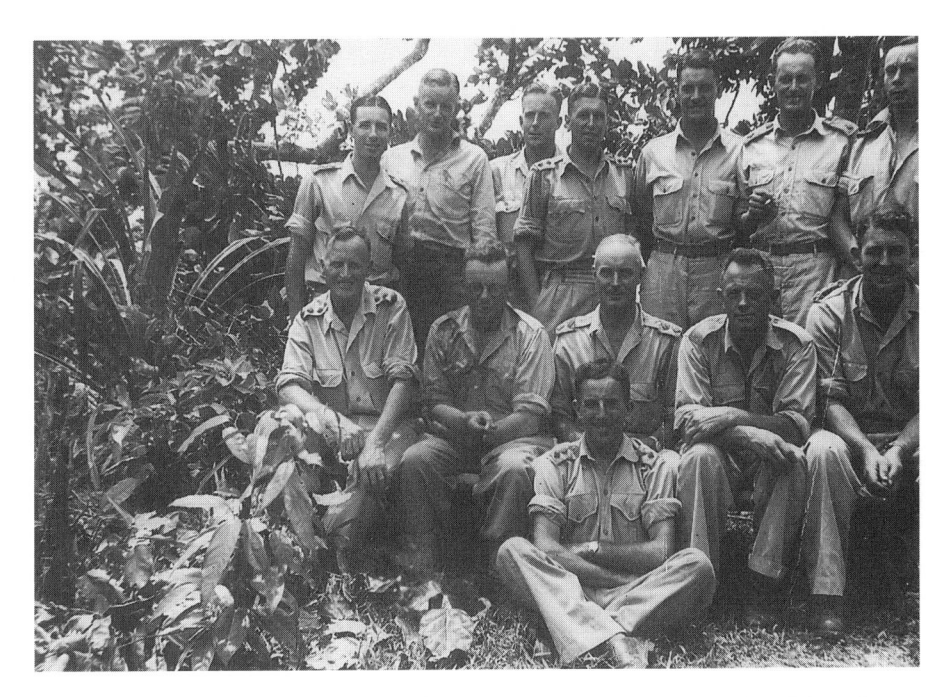

Officers' Mess, 22nd Field Ambulance and 1st Field Surgical Unit, Guadalcanal. *Standing:* Capt. Walter Ruthven Lang, Capt. Derek Ryder, Lt. Alex Fraser, Lt. Jack Betteridge, Lt. Ray Saunders, "Smithy," Capt. Tom Clouston. *Seated:* "Solomon Sam" otherwise Padre Francis, Major "Ossie" Bennett, Lt. Col. "Bill" Shirer, Major Percy Brunette, Major "Rod" Ferguson. *Seated on ground:* "Lou" (surname unknown). *Courtesy of Dr. Walter Ruthven Lang.*

normally applied as a cure for ringworm affecting the feet and groin but, thankfully, in the amounts used, harmless when swallowed. Finally, the vehicles to hold our concoction. These were self-suggesting—bottles from Abbotts Blood Transfusion sets.

The night of the party remains memorable to this day. We and our American friends reached the height of happiness. No one remembered what he had eaten. And next day there were no hangovers—thanks to absolute alcohol.

Walter Ruthven Lang, M.D.
Pacific Theater (New Caledonia and Solomon Islands)
New Zealand

At one stage during World War II, I was attached to a medical unit to set up and service an electrical generator to supply power to the field hospital. While with the unit they were sent forward along with divisional troops. We had attached to our unit two United States members as observers for the landing and hopefully occupation of Nissan, Green Island.

As it happened the first casualty was unfortunately one of our American guests who was rather a little shot up, and a call went out for a blood donor. I volunteered. After the required amount of blood had been taken, the orderly said he had been told to give me a brandy, and evidently it was his first time called to perform such a function as he asked me how much. I had never given blood previously, nor for that matter had I even tasted brandy, so told him I just had no idea. He said, "Well, you have donated a pint of blood so I guess I had best replace it with a pint of brandy."

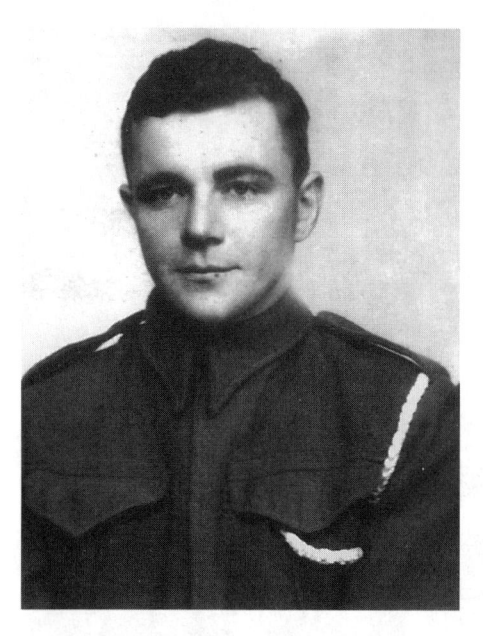

Basil J. Crompton. *Courtesy of Basil J. Crompton.*

One sip was more than enough, so I took the mug still full back to the lines and shared it with my mates—may I add, well diluted. I have been a regular donor ever since, but have never found anyone quite so generous. In fact, in latter years the opinion appears to be that a cup of tea or coffee is better for you.

I have at times wondered just how the American casualty got on, as he was transferred back to a base hospital and I never heard just what happened to him. I must admit that at times I have wondered if he is still, shall I say, running around with a mixture of Kiwi blood.

Basil J. Crompton
New Zealand

Your enquiry to the NZ Returned Services REVIEW has brought back vivid memories of the exceptional heroism of the young Americans who served with the American Field Service as ambulance drivers during the desert battles in North Africa in the early 1940s.

35. More on the War

This dedicated group of young men who volunteered as noncombatants driving American ambulances attached to our Medical Corps, through their sterling effort, earned the very highest regard for their selfless devotion to saving our injured comrades.

As a dispatch rider with an infantry battalion moving about the open battlefields of the desert, I witnessed many individual rescue sorties carried out under enemy fire.

There is one memorable occasion in June 1942 when General Rommel began his advance on Egypt. The New Zealand Division was recalled from garrison duty in Syria and made a hasty return to the Western Desert. At a place called Minqar Qaim, about 25 miles south of Mersa Matruh, a small port West of Alexandria, we were ordered to prepare defensive positions. The following date, the 27th of June, in the early afternoon, large clouds of dust on the horizon indicated the arrival of German tanks and vehicles. We were soon under enemy artillery fire, and during the later part of the afternoon while making my way to our brigade H.Q., I observed a small group of engineers laying a protective minefield in front of our infantry positions. Clearly visible to the enemy, they soon came under heavy fire and suffered casualties. From seemingly nowhere an American Field Service ambulance appeared, heading directly into the danger area. Some of the casualties were obviously beyond help, but the others were quickly loaded aboard and rushed to the nearest aid post. That driver's cool assessment of the situation and apparently fearless devotion to the wounded made an unforgettable impression on me and no doubt on those he saved.

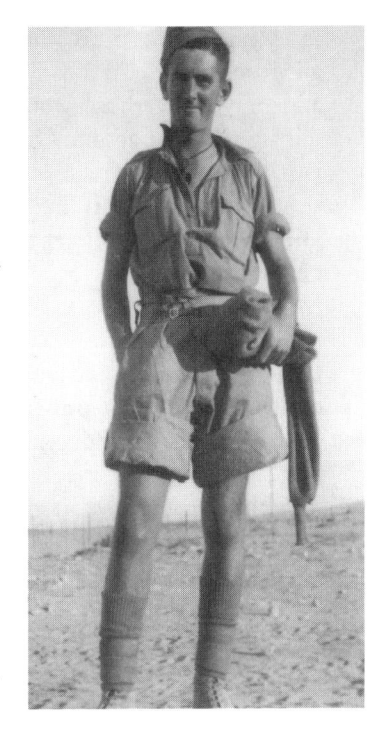

Noel F. Wootton, Western Desert (Sahara). *Courtesy of Noel F. Wootton.*

Sadly, I can find no recognition of these valiant men in the official histories of the units in which I served, but hopefully there is a fitting tribute to them published in the NZ forces medical histories.

Noel F. Wootton
New Zealand

Experiences during my two years of service have left memories pleasant from a comradeship point of view, whereas others recall the courage and bravery of those wounded soldiers who came through our theater during times of action. One particular incident, even after 50 odd years, is still vivid in my memory.

Rimini, on the Italian East Coast, 1943. Our operating theater [operating room] tent was set up to receive casualties. Behind us, an English heavy battery was attracting attention from the German 88, bursting shrapnel in the area. Our activities were concentrated on assisting the surgeon, Graham Cowie, attending to a wounded soldier. A piercing whistle and then an explosion left myself and a fellow orderly lying prostrate on the ground—self-preservation! I happened to look up and see our surgeon with his body draped over the hapless soldier—unselfishness at its best. No comment was made. We regained our composure, and in a very humble way, I carried on my duties. This incident has left a lasting impression.

George H. Hedges, Private
4th Field Ambulance
Operating theater orderly
Italian Campaign
1943–45

My incident was for me very dramatic and unique, in that it was the only bit of surgery that I performed in 4½ years of service overseas as a medical officer of Second NZ Expeditionary Force, mostly in the field.

By 1st December '41 (as Pearl Harbor was being attacked) [sic], the 21st NZ Infantry, along with the Fourth and Sixth brigades, having advanced into Libya and opened a corridor to relieve Tobruk, were under counterattack by the Afrika Korps. Our line was broken by tanks, and troops fell back from the high ground hotly pursued.

With my medical truck I was on the flat of the Trigh Capuzzo along with the

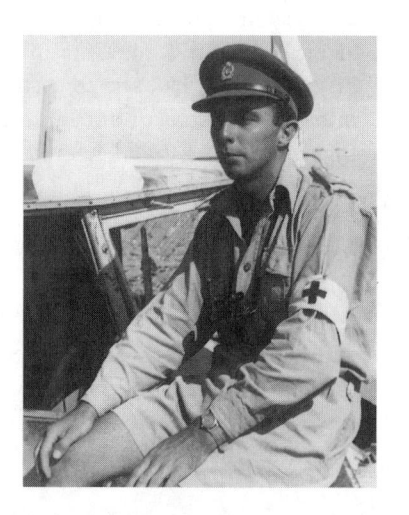

Dr. G.H. Levien, Alamein Line, Egypt, August 1942. *Courtesy of Dr. G.H. Levien.*

transport vehicles, with two ambulances and several open trucks loaded with wounded. Having no orders, I took off with my small flotilla southeast to the open desert. Shells and antitank shot followed us, and a mile or two along, we stopped to assess the wounded. One man was in extreme agony. A piece of shrapnel, the size of a walnut, had entered his hand and lodged just beneath the skin on the other side of the web between thumb and finger, so pressing on nerves and tendons. Our convoy being under sporadic fire, urgent action was indicated, and there was no time for a local anaesthetic to act. I took a scalpel, made an incision over the lump, and, with a long and strong pair of bullet forceps (recently acquired from a burnt-out German truck), hauled out the piece of metal. The poor man almost fainted, I was none too happy, but the excessive pain had gone. A field dressing was applied, morphine injected, and off we flew until out of range.

It did not cross my mind to keep the souvenir of my first and only surgery!

G.H. Levien, Major, ret. R.N.Z.A.M.C.
New Zealand

The following account is compiled from articles in the New Zealand Returned Services Association Journal, *August 1997; the newspaper,* The Dominion, *Wellington, New Zealand, July 7, 1996; and a letter from Grace Mitchel.*

Romance bloomed for many men and women who served during the war. The courtship of Grace Sopp, a nurse with the Second New Zealand General Hospital, and Colin Mitchel of the Australian Headquarters Signals, was so heart-warming that it brought military personnel of three nations together. Theirs was the first wedding to take place between members of the Allied Occupation Forces in Japan.

Grace had arrived in Japan direct from active duty in Italy. Colin had come from active service in New Guinea and was recovering from pneumonia. Colin remarked that she had seen beyond the mere "handsome New Zealanders" she had previously met. They were international news when they were married in a New Zealand hospital in Kiwa, Japan, on July 20, 1946.

The ceremony and reception were provided by the hospital staff. Transport for the Australian guests was arranged by Mr. Mitchel's CO, while the Americans (General R. Eichelberger's headquarters) paid for a second wedding supper and a honeymoon trip to Nara, near Kyoto. Their

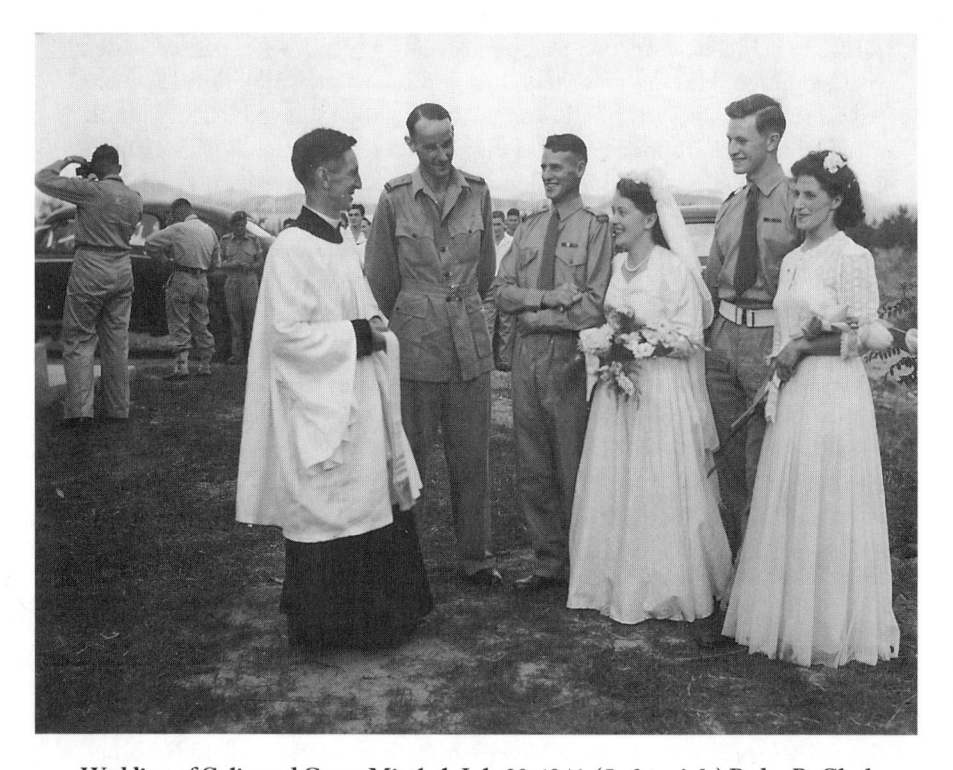

Wedding of Colin and Grace Mitchel, July 20, 1946. (*Left to right*) Padre R. Clarke, Capt. Mike Gilmore (NZ), Colin Mitchel, Grace Sopp (Mitchel), the best man, Sgt. Frank Raywood, and bridesmaid, Nurse Murial Williams. *Courtesy of Colin and Grace Mitchel.*

supper included a magnificent wedding cake and floor show and dance at the Nara Hotel. The wedding was covered by *The Stars and Stripes* and other nations' press.

When interviewed for their 50th wedding anniversary, Colin stated that the secret to living happily together "is letting Mum have the say; she always wins."

Grace and Colin Mitchel
New Zealand

Now age 93, I am an Englishman living in New Zealand since 1960. I served right through World War II in the Royal Artillery, British army, joining the Territorial Army in April 1939, age 33, being embodied in the Regular Army on mobilization in August. We were one of the first

35. More on the War

regiments in France in September and were on the Belgian border until the terrible retreat to Dunkirk in May and June 1940. I rose from gunner to captain. (Just in case you don't know it, in the British army the lowest rank of gunner is exactly equal to private. And private has no gradations.)

I had three medical examinations in the army. The first was on mobilization when the medical officer asked: "Are you fit?" I replied: "Yes, sir." He said with a smile: "You look fit. Next, please."

The second was in India in 1942 when almost exactly the same words were used.

The third was very thorough and on demobilization. The army did not want any claims against it.

In the Middle East in 1943 I broke two ribs, and the M.O. gave me morphine. At no other time in my life have I known such happiness. If someone had told me I was to be shot at dawn I would have smiled and said "OK." The M.O. returned, and said he was sorry. He did not notice it was a new bottle and double strength.

At dinner that evening the colonel remarked: "I hear David has been having a pissup with the doctor."

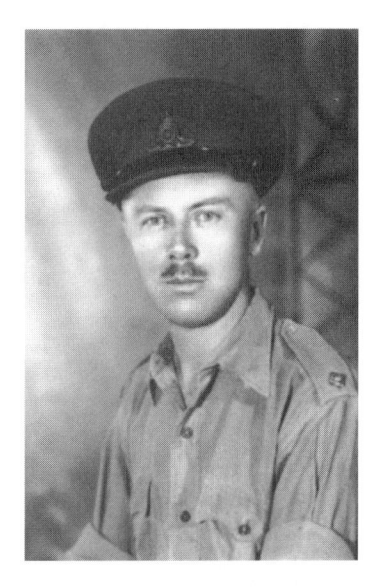

David More after recovering from malaria and jaundice, India 1942. *Courtesy of David More.*

David More
New Zealand

The following account of the experiences of Otto Wood Dickey was contributed by Dickey's son, who notes, "My dad never talked too much about what happened over there. He was a modest and quiet person." Otto Dickey served in the CBI Theater with the 14th Army Air Force, 19th Liaison Squadron.

Otto Dickey talked about being on several of the old AVG Flying Tiger bases seeing the P-40s and P-51s. There was an incident where a P-40 crash-landed and ground crew and medics (including him) ran out. The aircraft was on fire. The emergency crews put out the fire, and he jumped up on the wing, unbuckled the pilot's straps and tried to pull him out.

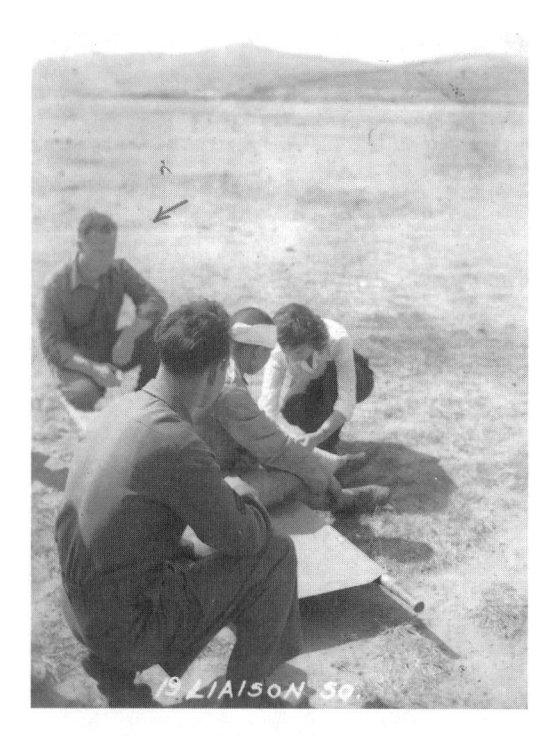

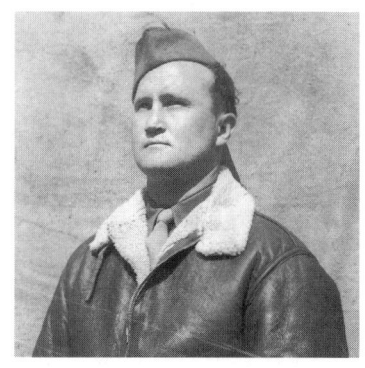

Left: Otto Wood Dickey (facing camera) kneeling at foot of litter of injured mechanic. *Above:* Otto Wood Dickey. *Below:* Otto Wood Dickey (at foot of litter) helping load injured mechanic onto waiting plane. *All photographs courtesy of Otto Wood Dickey, Jr.*

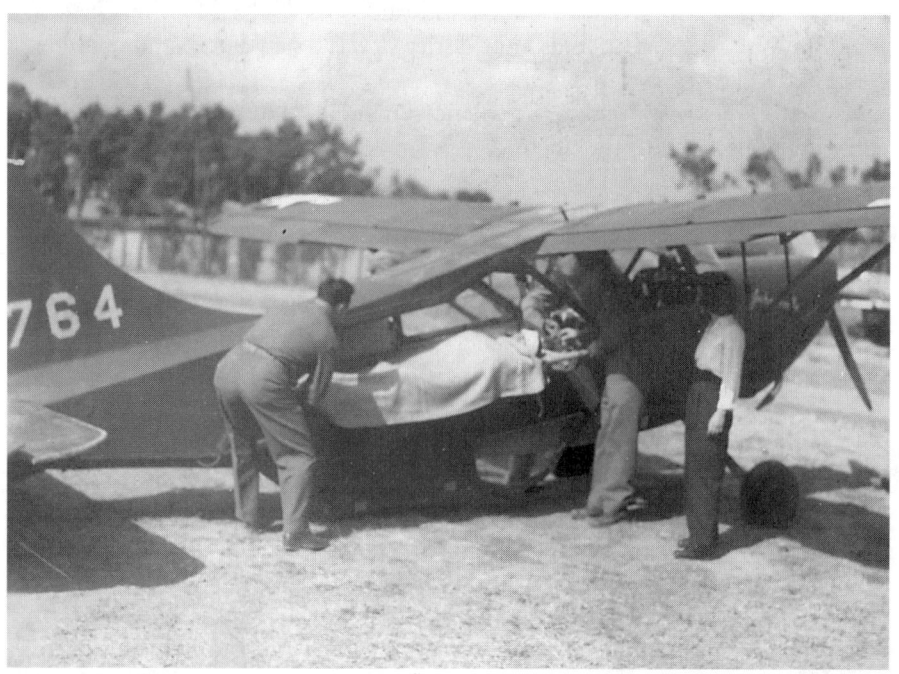

The pilot was burned so badly that everything came off in Otto's hands. The pilot died. Otto remarked, "You'll never forget the smell of burning human flesh."

Once a crew chief, while marshaling an airplane out of the revetments, slipped and stumbled. Because the airplane was a "tail dragger," the pilot couldn't see over the nose and lost sight of the crew chief. Then he hit him with the propeller, instantly killing him.

A Japanese aircraft was shot down over the base and the pilot parachuted out. Some GIs along with Otto ran out to capture the pilot and bring him back to base a couple of miles away. When they got there the Chinese villagers had hung the guy up by his arms and legs, stripped him of his uniform, and had started skinning him alive. They were about half-finished when the GIs arrived (including Otto). They ended up shooting the pilot to put him out of his misery.

On a happier note, Otto and several other GIs adopted a young Chinese boy. He was in several photos with Otto and others. His nickname was Buttercup (his Chinese name sounded similar to buttercup, so that's what he became). There are conflicting reports as to the boy's outcome.

Otto W. Dickey, Jr.

Axel Lagergren was a medic with the 169th Infantry Regiment, 43rd Division, which saw action in New Guinea and Luzon, Philippines. A Meritorious Service Unit Plaque notes that as casualties among the medical personnel increased in the Philippines, the medical detachment became understaffed. The aid men became mentally and physically exhausted, but they continued their often hazardous and indispensable care of the wounded.

Axel Lagergren was awarded the Combat Medical Badge and the Bronze Star Medal.

The following account was contributed by his wife.

My husband and I were married November 16, 1940. He was almost 24. I was 19. Our first child, a daughter, was born December 23, 1942. My husband was inducted May 24, 1943, at Camp Blanding, Florida, and entered active service May 31, 1943. He was 26 years old. Then he went to Fort McClellan in Alabama. After basic training he came home for about a week. From Pensacola, he went to California for overseas duty. We didn't see him again until November 1945. Our daughter was almost three years old.

He sailed from San Francisco to New Caledonia. There he was

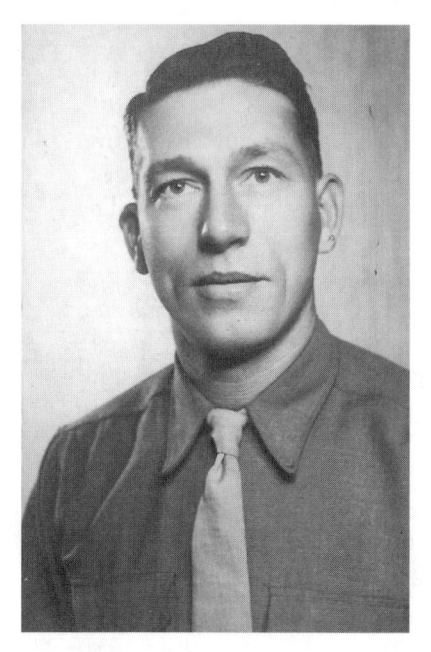

Axel E. Lagergren. *Courtesy of Dorothy M. Lagergren.*

assigned to the 43rd Division. He left New Caledonia for New Zealand. There he joined the 43rd and was assigned to Company A–169th Infantry as an aid man.

In July 1944 he went into combat in New Guinea. In November 1944 he was detached from Company A to the aid station as clerk.

On December 26, 1944, he left New Guinea for Lingayen Gulf, Luzon, Philippines. There he made the beachhead on Luzon. From January 1945 until September 1945 he was on Luzon. From there he went to Japan with the occupation forces. In October 1945 he had enough points to return to the States.

He and a younger brother got together in the Philippines. His brother was on Leyte in the air corps. He told me of a time when my husband was an aid man. He took some bottles of plasma to the foxhole. After climbing in, he reached up for the plasma to find the bottles had been shattered by sniper fire.

Another incident I recall was after an engagement with the Japanese, he was taking information from the dog tags on the men who had been killed. The chaplain was saying words over the deceased men as the unit was moving out.

He didn't talk much about what he went through. He was fortunate to escape any injury while in combat.

He kept a book with all the photographs I sent to him. He saw our daughter as she grew from a baby into a little girl.

Dorothy Lagergren

Afterword

I have been asked why I wrote this book. Was my father a doctor? Was I a military brat? The answer to both of these questions is "no."

The desire to write this book has developed over many years. I have a great curiosity about things "medical," having once thought I was destined for a career in medicine until I realized, while in my teens, that I didn't have the dedication and tenacity it took to accomplish that goal.

My interest in World War II came quite naturally as the daughter of an Army Air Corps, Ninth Air Force, aircraft mechanic working on B-26 Marauders in the European Theater of War. My uncles served in the Pacific, European, and Mediterranean theaters of war. A family friend, Julia Sadler, whose account appears here, was a recent graduate of nursing school when she volunteered.

I have always felt that the medical personnel in the war received little recognition. The sick and wounded never forgot the men and women who cared for them, sometimes under circumstances so adverse that they are inconceivable to those of us who have never experienced combat conditions.

When I began my quest for accounts I was compiling my father's personal history and searching for the men who served with him in England, France, Belgium, and Holland. As I began placing messages on various Internet websites, I became aware that many stories remained to be told. I encouraged family members of veterans to tape or write down those accounts that veterans were willing to share, whether I received them or not. We must not let these recollections be lost to future generations.

Some veterans have stated that they thought no one was interested in what they might have to tell. Perhaps that was so in years past, through no fault of their own. More people are becoming aware of just how much was sacrificed by those who fought the war, so that we might have the freedom we enjoy and so often take for granted. As we their children are now in our middle years and moving rapidly toward our senior years, we have gained insight into what our parents faced over half a century ago. I wonder if we would have dealt with such challenging times as nobly and unselfishly as they did.

To all who served: you are my heroes.
Patricia W. Sewell

The Eisenhower Center has entered into a three-year project focusing on U.S. personnel in the Pacific Theater, but accounts from personnel in all theaters of war are gladly welcomed. They encourage anyone who has a story to tell to write to them and request "oral history guidelines."

Eisenhower Center
923 Magazine Street
New Orleans, LA 70130, USA

Index

Airborne Division, 101st 245, 257, 259
The Army Nurse Corps: A Commemoration of World War II Service (Bellafaire) 147, 148, 149
Army Specialized Training Reserve Program(ASTRP) 79
Artificial pneumothoraces 19
Aviation Medical Examiners (AMEs) 67

B-17s 246
B-26s 246
Balkan Nurses vii,147
Ball, Des 122, 128; at Forli church bombing 133; at Po River 136; Battle for the Senio 134; Battle of the Gaiana River 136; burying the dead 131–132; first contact with Yougoslav army 137; helping civilians 126–127; Italian-Scottish family 129–130; Italian train ride 137; partisans with German soldier 131
Barnes, George S. 1, 67
Battle of St. Lo 97
Battle of the Bulge 25, 52, 60, 94, 119, 245, 249, 252–258
Battle of the Gaiana River 136
Battle of the Rhine River 60
Bellafaire, Judith 147–149
Biak Island 74–75
Bing, Richard J. 81; assigned to report on progress of German medicine 82–84; at Edgewood Arsenal 82; basic training in chemical warfare 82; demonstration of cardiac catheter 83; research on DDT 82
Blondeau, Maurice: Tuberculosis specialist 19
Bolger, Ray 93
Boyington, Greg "Pappy" 226
Breeding, Mary A. 24; Battle of the Bulge 25; 174th General Hospital, U.S. 24; the Little General 26; treating German wounded 26
Bren carriers 136
Brokaw, Tom 114
Brooks Army Hospital at Fort Sam Houston 45
Buzz bombs 50

C-47 145, 148, 181, 182, 184
C-54, aircraft 147
C-130s (Flying Boxcars) 52
Camp Adair 3, 6
Camp Blanding 77, 271
Camp Butner 70, 102, 110
Camp Claiborne 22
Camp Dix 56
Camp Ellis 60
Camp Grant 60
Camp Hood 46–48
Camp Livingston 71
Camp McCoy 111
Camp Miles Standish 3, 41
Camp Old Gold 40
Camp Pendleton 140
Camp Pickett 111
Camp Polk 70

276

Index

Camp Robinson 94
Camp Shanks 214
Camp Shelby 69, 77, 110
Camp Shoemaker 224
Camp White 3
Canary (wireless/radio) 161
Carlisle Barracks 67, 87, 101–102
Cassino 126, 129
Castillo, Al 105 106, 110
Castillo, Luis 57, 58, 59
CBI (China, Burma, India) 47, 48, 53, 181, 269
Cholera 184
Churchill tanks 136
Churchill, Winston 115, 215
Coblenz 204
Combat Infantry Badge 77, 91, 110
Combat Medical Badge 77, 85, 91
Conti, Rose 22
Conti, Vincent Stephen 21; Typhus Commission Medal 21, 22
Corregidor 85, 88, 90, 92
Crocodiles and Wasps (Churchill tanks and Bren Carriers) 136
Crompton, Basil J. 263–264

DDT(dichloro diphenyl trichloroethane) insecticide 82, 88
Dickey, Otto Wood 269–271
Dickey, Otto W., Jr. 271
DiIaconi, Daniel E. 117, 118, 119; Atlantic crossing home 121; attacked by drunken, American soldier 117; Battle of the Bulge 119–120; champagne 121; Coblenz, Officer's Club 120; mascot, white goose 119–120; shot at by sniper at Rhine 117; Welsh family 120
Doss, Desmond T. 63; as medic with Seventy-seventh Infantry Division 112; at Maeda Escarpment 63; awarded Congressional Medal of Honor 114; conscientious objector 111; Miracle Day 63, 65; Seventh Day Adventist 63; Signal corps report 65; wounded 65, 66
Doss, Frances 66

Early ambulation 50, 53
El Alamein 123, 150, 151

Ellis, Frank R. 10; *Nordwind* offensive 10, 11

Fairest, Shirley Ann 122
Feltham, Richard John 150, 153; as POW at Bari, 152, 153, 156; as POW at Benghazi, 152; at Castel San Pietro 154; at Einheit III 168, 171; at Fort XIII 161, 164, 165, 166, 167; at Mersa Matruh 152; at Oflag 9A/Z 157; at "Russian hager"/"Copernicusharger" 169; at Thorn, Stalag XXA, Fort Fifteen 158, 163; "canary" (wireless/radio) 157, 170; capture by Germans 151; conditions at Einheit III 168; execution of wounded German officer 176; Fort XV, Gestapo search at 161–162; freedom/rescue by Russian troops 173; medical officer, Twentieth Battalion, NZ 150; POW, insists on privileges of rank 154; reaction to capture 174; realization of freedom 174; taken ill 152, 167–168; taking shelter in cookhouse cellars 171; tempers short 155, 168; treatment of Russian POWs at Einheit III 169
Fessler, Diane Burke vii, 147, 148
Fidler, Michael O., Dr. 245
Field Ambulance, The Italian Campaign, Recollections of an Ambulance Driver (Shirley Ann Fairest) 122
Flying Boxcars *see* C-130s
Flying Fortresses 155
Fookes, Glen A.: at box factory 97; at Fort Custer, Camp Robinson 94; cow in tree 97; dealing with black market 98; drinking cider 97; Fort Knox 96; in Atlanta 95; in South Hampton, England 96; in Toledo 95; medic training 94; medical depot at Carrington 96; Mojave Desert depot 95; St. Lo, destruction of 97; seeing casualties from Battle of the Bulge 99
Forsyth, Grady 60; homecoming of 62; in Philippines 61; 1303 Engineers, Third Army, U.S. bridge over Rhine, 60–61
Fort Benjamin Harrison 4
Fort Benning 60, 67

Fort Bragg 79, 214
Fort Custer 94
Fort Devons 214
Fort Dix 144
Fort Hamilton 44
Fort Jackson 95, 144
Fort Knox 27, 96
Fort Leonard Wood 3, 6, 79
Fort McClellan 271
Fort McPherson 144
Fort Meade 111
Fort Miles Standish 103
Fort Moultrie 69
Fort Ord 77
Fort Rucker: basic training and segregation at 144
Fort Sam Houston 45, 77
Fort Sill 45–46
Four Glorious Years (Stanton, Mona) vii, 244
Francis, Norton L., M.D. 260
Freyberg: effect of prolonged artillery bombardment 135

Gaiana River 136
Gelborn, Martha: war correspondent in Belgium, wife of Ernest Hemingway 40
Geneva Convention 34, 91
God Is My Co-Pilot (Scott) 184
Goolsbee, Daniel 139; Acting Chief Master-at-Arms at Civilian hospital (Guam) 142; administering castor oil to children 142; amphibious training at Tan Farine Race Track 140; as diagnostician 142; as instructor at Treasure Island Naval Hospital 140; as navy corpsman 139; as Pharmacist Mate Second Class 140; as Qualified Assistant in Operating Room Technique 139; at Camp Pendleton 140; at General Dispensary (Treasure Island) 140; Baragada, Japanese straggler at 141; boot camp in San Diego 139; Christmas on Guam 142; delivering babies 142; discovering a suicide 142; Hawaii, Marshall Islands, and Guam 140; homemade camera and X-ray film 142; military experience, knowledge gained from 142; milk, filtering and pasteurizing of 141; promoted to Pharmacist Mate First Class 142; treating wounded returned to United States 140;

Habegger, Les viii, 3, 5, 7; confronted with German infiltrator 8; hometown 4, 5; in combat, first time 6; lost youth 5
Hedges, George H. 266
Hemingway, Ernest 33, 34, 38, 40
Higgins boats 29
Hills, Henry M, Jr., M.D. 245; Battle of the Bulge 252–258; D-Day patients 246–247; Eighth Air Force casualties 246; Evac Hospital, 12th 245, 250
Hills, Willie 245, 253–254
Holleman, Agnes Smith 100, 101, 104
Holleman, Jeremiah Henry vii, 100; assigned to 89th Infantry Division, U.S. 102; assigned to 314th Combat Engineers Battalion, U.S. 102; at Camp Butner 102, 110; at Camp Shelby 110; at Carlisle Barracks 101–102; at Ohrdurf concentration camp 107–108; construction of Rhine pontoon bridge 107; crossing the Atlantic 104; in Paris, R&R (Rest and Relaxation) 107; in the combat zone 104; relationship with the French couple 109; Russian Army encounter 108; sightseeing in Rouen 109; volunteered for Pacific duty 109; wedding of 101
Hovis, Logan W. 85; aid station under sniper fire 87–88; at Japanese surrender on Negros 92; Bronze Star Citation 86–87; care of injured and wounded (Corregidor) 87; Corregidor assault 85–86; evacuating casualties, tending brigadier general 89; identifying bodies at morgue 87; letters to parents during Negros Campaign 89–93; living conditions during Negros Campaign 90; medical laboratory acquired 91–92; parachute jump 86; reaction to injured medics 90; transfer from Third Battalion, assigned as Regimental Surgeon 91; treating trooper with

phosphorus burns 88; under attack at Monkey Point 88
Hurtgen Forest, Battle of "The Place of Death" 35–39, 51
The Hump (Himalayas) 181, 182

King, Alan: at Elsterhorst, Stalag IVA 19; at Hohenstein-Ernstahl, Charity Home 19; at Konigswartha 19; at Lamsdorf Stalag VIIIB 17, 19; at Turkish Barracks 17; Battle of Bardia 16; Battle of Tobruk 16; Brallos Pass, *Last Post* 16; evacuation to Crete, Neon Korion capture 16; Greek Campaign 16; in Dresden 19; in United States of America 20; liberation of 20; medical officer near Maleme 17; return to Australia 20; solitary confinement 17; treatment of tuberculosis 19
Kippenberger, Brigadier 129
Kirchner, Gregory S. 111; at Camp Picket 111; Fort Meade 111; furlough in London 115; medical training in United States, use of 111–112; mine field incident 112–114; ski training 111, 113; V-E Day celebration 115
Kirtley, James Marion 27, 31, 37; Ansbach needle factory 73; appendectomy performed aboard ship 28; at Camp Old Gold 40; at St. Martin de Varreville 30, 31; at Siegfried Line 35; bath unit with showers 35; Battle of Hurtgen Forest 35, 36, 37, 38, 39; "Beanie," Jeep 29, 30, 31, 32, 33, 34; Cat "Robert" 39, 40; Cherbourg 32; Christmas in Belgium 40; crossing Atlantic 27–28; Field Marshall Montgomery, visit by 28; in Belgium 34; in Paris 32–33; Pearl Harbor announcement 27, 38, 40; Portsmouth 29; treats Ernest Hemingway 33, 34, 38, 40; Utah Beach 29, 30
Kirtley Kronicles, the Life and Times of James Marion Kirtley, M.D. (Kirtley) 27; *see also* Kirtley, James Marion
Kirtley, Lee (Leolia) Black 27
Kornblum, Caroline E. Holts 104
Kornblum, Stanley A. 44, 49; almost AWOL 52; army physical 44–45; at Camp Hood 46–48; at Fort Sill 45–46; at Orly Field 53; "black market" in France 102; courtship of 46; crossing North Atlantic 48–49, 56; experiences at Camp Hood 46–48; father's visit 47; hernia repair 53–54; in London, "buzz bombs" 50; in Orly Field "house-of-ill repute" 55; in Paris with wife 54; Kornblum, Caroline 56; 189th General Hospital, U.S. 51; playing chess 54; poker game in France 55; R&R 55, 56; shot at by DP guard 100; transferred to 189th General Hospital, U.S. 54; treating German POW 47, 48; visit by wife 53

Lagergren, Axel 271–272
Lagergren, Dorothy 272
Lang, Walter Ruthven, M.D. 262–263
Lekisch [Lokeisch], Kurt 13, 15
Levien, G.H., Major, ret., R.N.Z.A.M.C. 266–267

Maeda Escarpment 63
Malinta Hill 88
Malinta tunnel 87–88
Maness, Ava 149
Mangerich, Agnes Jensen 148
Marshall, George C. 103
M*A*S*H 13, 25, 42, 248
Maunganui, H.M.N.Z.H.S. 187
McArthur, Douglas 110
McKenna, Thomas J. 181, 185; at Luichow airstrip 184; China, Burma, India Theater (CBI) 181; Flight Surgeon, Fourth Combat Cargo Squadron, First Combat Cargo Group, U.S. 181; landing in Likiang 182; Lister Bags, contamination of 185; Lister Bags, preventing contamination of 186; purifying drinking water 185; visit with missionary 183
Mckenzie, Lois Watson 148
Mindoro 85, 88
Mitchel, Colin 267–268
Mitchel, Grace Sopp 267–268
Monkey Point 88
Montgomery, Bernard Law 28
More, David 268–269
Moses, Helen 238
Mursa Matruh 150, 152

Index

Navy-Army Medical Research Unit (NAMRU) on Guam 141
The Neapolitan Typhus Epidemic (Conti) 44
Ninth Evac Hospital, U.S. Reserve hospital (Roosevelt Hospital), enlisted personnel, Brooklyn 42
No Time for Fear, Voices of American Military Nurses in World War II (Fessler) vii, 147
Nordwind 10–11

O'Connell, Arthur V.: Silver Star, Combat Medical Badge 77, 78
101st Airborne Division 245, 257, 259
Osowski, Stanley 29, 30, 31, 32, 33, 34

Pearl Harbor 27, 44, 70
Phillipsbourg 4, 6, 11
Plymouth 29
Port Said 123
Portsmouth 29

Red Cross 55, 142, 153, 168, 169, 210, 214, 239; ditty bags for patients 142; insignia 258; insignia not worn in Pacific Theater 91
Robson, Grace 187, 197, 198; service in V.A.D. (Voluntary Aid Detachment) 188, 210
Robson, Herbert Matthew 187, 188; arrival in Scotland 192; bodies of German gun crew 190; German sailors 189; H.N.Z.H.S. *Maunganui*, service of 187–210; leave in Great Britain 193; winter guard duty aboard *Maunganui* 192
Roosevelt, Franklin D. 70; death of 40, 75, 89, 108, 200

Sadler, Julia Parrish 143, 145, 273; army Nurse Corps, enlists in 144; at Ft. Dix 144; emergency appendectomy 144; Hattiesburg army hospital 144; in Hawaii and Saipan 144; in Seoul 144; in Yokohama 144; intimidation by army officer 146; Korean hospital tour 146; life in Taejon 145; nurses' quarters burned 145; sent to Pacific Theater 144; survives typhoon 144; Taejon Mayor's residence, banquet at 145; Taejon, plane crash in 145; 377th Station Hospital, U.S., Taejon 145; training at Ft. Jackson 144
Sandberg, Amy 94
Sangro River 124, 214
Schistosomiasis japonicum 75
Schwartz, Sol 13, 14; observing medical care of wounded 13
Scott, Robert L. 184
Seftel, Daniel: basic training in field artillery at Fort Bragg 79; enlisted in army 79; Fort Leonard Wood, 1292 Combat Engineer Battalion, U.S., medic 79; in ASTRP 79; Philippines, invasion of Japan, youngest among medical personnel 80; with occupation troops in Japan 80
Segregation: in military 144
Setchell, Jenny Feltham 150
Seventieth Infantry Division, U.S. 3, 11
SHAEF 50
Siegfried Line 35
Silver Star 77, 78, 259
Sopp, Grace 267–268
Stanton, Mona vii, 239, 241
Stars and Stripes 51
Strain, Shelleu M. 41; army induction 41; basic training 41; Case Western Reserve University Medical School 41; faltboating 43; in ETO 41; Liverpool 41; Nineth Evac Hospital, U.S. 42; Rheims 42
Suez 123, 124, 189, 191
Suicide Cliff (on Saipan) 144

Task Force Herren 3, 11
Threlkeld, Lee 213, 215; Fort Bragg 214; lieutenant, fighter pilot injured 216
Tobruk 152
Topside, Corregidor 86, 87–88
Treasure Island Naval Hospital 139
Tropical syphilis (Yaws): Guam civilians 142
Truman, Harry S 75, 131; as president 73, 202
Tuberculosis 171
Typhus: epidemic form, body louse transmission (periculus corporis),

symptoms 21, 22; special delousing station 17; Typhus Commission 21; Typhus Commission Medal 21, 22

An Unbroken Chain, Memoirs by Jeremiah Henry Holleman (Holleman) 100
Utah Beach 24, 29, 30

V.A.D. (Voluntary Aid Detachment) 1, 187, 210, 211, 240
Von Rundstedt 40, 52

Walker, Forrest 218, 219, 231; arrival of nurses 235; boot camp, San Diego Naval Training Station 218; Christmas Eve, 1944 235; dispensary duty 224; Espiritu Santo 226; food poisoning 227–228; Hospital Corps School 220; Moses, Helen 238; Physical Therapy Training 222, 223; Roger or Stater external fixation or splinting 234; Russell Islands, Banika 228; tendon stretchers 223; Tulagi 236; USO 233

Warshauer, Samuel E. 69; accidental discharge of .45 automatic pistol 74; bridge game 74; bridge player 72; Camp Livingston, 171st Station Hospital 71; Chief of the Medical Service 72; completes medical exam 73; in Auckland 71; in Melbourne 71; in New Guinea 72; marriage 71; on Biak Island 74–75; on troop train home 76; taking oral part of medical exam 76; *War Medicine*, paper published in 73

Warshauer, Miriam Miller 71
Wootton, Noel F. 264–265